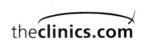

MEDICAL CLINICS
OF NORTH AMERICA

Hospital Medicine

GUEST EDITORS
Scott A. Flanders, MD
Vikas I. Parekh, MD
Lakshmi Halasyamani, MD

March 2008 • Volume 92 • Number 2

SAUNDERS

An Imprint of Elsevier, Inc.
PHILADELPHIA LONDON TORONTO MONTREAL SYDNEY TOKYO

W.B. SAUNDERS COMPANY
A Division of Elsevier Inc.

1600 John F. Kennedy Boulevard • Suite 1800 • Philadelphia, Pennsylvania 19103-2899

http://www.theclinics.com

MEDICAL CLINICS OF NORTH AMERICA	**Volume 92, Number 2**
March 2008	**ISSN 0025-7125**
Editor: Rachel Glover	**ISBN-13: 978-1-4160-4987-6**
	ISBN-10: 1-4160-4987-8

The ideas and opinions expressed in *Medical Clinics of North America* do not necessarily reflect those of the Publisher. The Publisher does not assume any responsibility for any injury and/or damage to persons or property arising out of or related to any use of the material contained in this periodical. The reader is advised to check the appropriate medical literature and the product information currently provided by the manufacturer of each drug to be administered to verify the dosage, the method and duration of administration, or contraindications. It is the responsibility of the treating physician or other health care professional, relying on independent experience and knowledge of the patient, to determine drug dosages and the best treatment for the patient. Mention of any product in this issue should not be construed as endorsement by the contributors, editors, or the Publisher of the product or manufacturers' claims.

Medical Clinics of North America (ISSN 0025-7125) is published bimonthly by W.B. Saunders, 360 Park Avenue South, New York, NY 10010-1710. Business and editorial offices: 1600 John F. Kennedy Boulevard, Suite 1800, Philadelphia, PA 19103-2899. Accounting and circulation offices: 6277 Sea Harbor Drive, Orlando, FL 32887-4800. Periodicals postage paid at New York, NY, and additional mailing offices. Subscription prices are USD 173 per year for US individuals, USD 306 per year for US institutions, USD 89 per year for US students, USD 220 per year for Canadian individuals, USD 389 per year for Canadian institutions, USD 131 per year for Canadian students, USD 250 per year for international individuals, USD 389 per year for international institutions and USD 131 per year for international students. To receive student/resident rate, orders must be accompanied by name of affiliated institution, date of term, and the *signature* of program/residency coordinator on institution letterhead. Orders will be billed at individual rate until proof of status is received. Foreign air speed delivery is included in all *Clinics* subscription prices. All prices are subject to change without notice. POSTMASTER: Send address changes to *Medical Clinics of North America*, Elsevier Periodicals Customer Service, 6277 Sea Harbor Drive, Orlando, FL 32887-4800. **Customer Service: 1-800-654-2452 (US). From outside the United States, call: 1-407-563-6020. Fax: 1-407-363-9661. E-mail: JournalsCustomerService-usa@elsevier.com.**

Reprints. For copies of 100 or more, of articles in this publication, please contact the Commercial Reprints Department, Elsevier Inc., 360 Park Avenue South, New York, New York 10010-1710. Tel.: (+1) (212) 633-3813; Fax: (+1) (212) 462-1935; E-mail: reprints@elsevier.com.

Medical Clinics of North America is also published in Spanish by McGraw-Hill Interamericana Editores S. A., P.O. Box 5-237, 06500 Mexico, D.F., Mexico.

Medical Clinics of North America is covered in *Index Medicus, Current Contents, ASCA, Excerpta Medica, Science Citation Index*, and *ISI/BIOMED*.

Printed in the United States of America.

GOAL STATEMENT

The goal of *Medical Clinics of North America* is to keep practicing physicians up to date with current clinical practice by providing timely articles reviewing the state of the art in patient care.

ACCREDITATION

The *Medical Clinics of North America* is planned and implemented in accordance with the Essential Areas and Policies of the Accreditation Council for Continuing Medical Education (ACCME) through the joint sponsorship of the University of Virginia School of Medicine and Elsevier. The University of Virginia School of Medicine is accredited by the ACCME to provide continuing medical education for physicians.

The University of Virginia School of Medicine designates this educational activity for a maximum of 90 *AMA PRA Category 1 Credits™*. Physicians should only claim credit commensurate with the extent of their participation in the activity.

The American Medical Association has determined that physicians not licensed in the US who participate in this CME activity are eligible for *AMA PRA Category 1 Credits™*.

Credit can be earned by reading the text material, taking the CME examination online at http://www.theclinics.com/home/cme, and completing the evaluation. After taking the test, you will be required to review any and all incorrect answers. Following completion of the test and evaluation, your credit will be awarded and you may print your certificate.

FACULTY DISCLOSURE/CONFLICT OF INTEREST

The University of Virginia School of Medicine, as an ACCME accredited provider, endorses and strives to comply with the Accreditation Council for Continuing Medical Education (ACCME) Standards of Commercial Support, Commonwealth of Virginia statutes, University of Virginia policies and procedures, and associated federal and private regulations and guidelines on the need for disclosure and monitoring of proprietary and financial interests that may affect the scientific integrity and balance of content delivered in continuing medical education activities under our auspices.

The University of Virginia School of Medicine requires that all CME activities accredited through this institution be developed independently and be scientifically rigorous, balanced and objective in the presentation/discussion of its content, theories and practices.

All authors/editors participating in an accredited CME activity are expected to disclose to the readers relevant financial relationships with commercial entities occurring within the past 12 months (such as grants or research support, employee, consultant, stock holder, member of speakers bureau, etc.). The University of Virginia School of Medicine will employ appropriate mechanisms to resolve potential conflicts of interest to maintain the standards of fair and balanced education to the reader. Questions about specific strategies can be directed to the Office of Continuing Medical Education, University of Virginia School of Medicine, Charlottesville, Virginia.

The authors/editors listed below have identified no professional or financial affiliations for themselves or their spouse/partner:
Vineet M. Arora, MD, MA; Jeanne M. Farnan, MD; Kristin M. Flammer, MD; Scott A. Flanders, MD (Guest Editor); Leanne B. Gasink, MD, MSCE; Rachel Glover (Acquisitions Editor); Paul J. Grant, MD; Lakshmi Halasyamani, MD (Guest Editor); Margaret Isaac, MD; William J. Janssen, MD; Daniel R. Kaul, MD; Derek J. Linderman, MD; Tracy Minichiello, MD; Nelson Nicolasora, MD; Steven Z. Pantilat, MD; Vikas I. Parekh, MD (Guest Editor); Paula M. Podrazik, MD; Sumant R. Ranji, MD; Kaveh G. Shojania, MD; and Chad T. Whelan, MD.

The authors/editors listed below identified the following professional or financial affiliations for themselves or their spouse/partner:
Thomas W. Donner, MD is on the Speaker's Bureau for Merck, Pfizer, Amylin, Novartis, and Aventis.
Patrick F. Fogarty, MD received travel reimbursement for travel to Investigator's meeting from GlaxoSmithKline.
Ebbing Lautenbach, MD, MPH, MSCE is a consultant for Ortho-McNeil and Bristol Myers Squibb and has received research support from Merck.
Robert M. Wachter, MD is on the Advisory Committee/Board of ABIM, Google, Intellidot, and Hoana Medical.
Joseph Ming Wah Li, MD is on the Speaker's Bureau for Ortho-McNeil.
David H. Wesorick, MD received a one-time honorarium from GlaxoSmithKline and Adolor Co.

Disclosure of Discussion of non-FDA approved uses for pharmaceutical products and/or medical devices:
The University of Virginia School of Medicine, as an ACCME provider, requires that all faculty presenters identify and disclose any "off label" uses for pharmaceutical and medical device products. The University of Virginia School of Medicine recommends that each physician fully review all the available data on new products or procedures prior to instituting them with patients.

TO ENROLL

To enroll in the Medical Clinics of North America Continuing Medical Education program, call customer service at 1-800-654-2452 or visit us online at http://www.theclinics.com/home/cme. The CME program is available to subscribers for an additional fee of USD 205.

FORTHCOMING ISSUES

RECENT ISSUES

GUEST EDITORS

SCOTT A. FLANDERS, MD, Associate Professor, Hospitalist Program, Department of Internal Medicine, University of Michigan Health System, Ann Arbor, MI

VIKAS I. PAREKH, MD, Assistant Professor, Hospitalist Program, Department of Internal Medicine, University of Michigan Health System, Ann Arbor, MI

LAKSHMI HALASYAMANI, MD, Associate Chair , Department of Medicine, St. Joseph Mercy Hospital, Ypsilanti, MI

CONTRIBUTORS

VINEET M. ARORA, MD, MA, Assistant Professor of Medicine, Department of Medicine, University of Chicago, Chicago, Illinois

THOMAS W. DONNER, MD, Associate Professor of Medicine, Division of Endocrinology, Diabetes and Nutrition; Director, Joslin Diabetes Center Affiliate, University of Maryland School of Medicine, Baltimore, Maryland

JEANNE M. FARNAN, MD, Instructor, Department of Medicine, University of Chicago, Chicago, Illinois

KRISTIN M. FLAMMER, MD, Clinical Fellow, Division of Endocrinology, Diabetes and Nutrition, University of Maryland School of Medicine, Baltimore, Maryland

PATRICK F. FOGARTY, MD, Assistant Clinical Professor of Medicine, Division of Hematology/Oncology, Department of Medicine; Director, Comprehensive Hemostasis and Antithrombotic Service, University of California, San Francisco, California

LEANNE B. GASINK, MD, MSCE, Instructor of Medicine; Associate Hospital Epidemiologist, Department of Medicine, University of Pennsylvania, Hospital of the University of Pennsylvania, Philadelphia, Pennsylvania

PAUL J. GRANT, MD, Clinical Instructor, University of Michigan Medical School, Division of General Medicine, Department of Internal Medicine, Ann Arbor, Michigan

MARGARET ISAAC, MD, Clinical Instructor, University of Washington School of Medicine, Harborview Medical Center, Seattle, Washington

WILLIAM J. JANSSEN, MD, Assistant Professor, Department of Medicine, National Jewish Medical and Research Center; Division of Pulmonary Sciences and Critical Care Medicine, University of Colorado Health Science Center, Denver, Colorado

DANIEL R. KAUL, MD, Assistant Professor of Medicine; Director, Transplant Infectious Disease Service, Division of Infectious Disease, University of Michigan Medical Center, Ann Arbor, Michigan

EBBING LAUTENBACH, MD, MPH, MSCE, Assistant Professor of Medicine and Epidemiology, Associate Hospital Epidemiologist; Senior Scholar, Center for Clinical Epidemiology and Biostatistics, University of Pennsylvania School of Medicine, Philadelphia, Pennsylvania

JOSEPH MING WAH LI, MD, Assistant Professor in Medicine, Harvard Medical School; Director, Hospital Medicine Program, Beth Israel Deaconess Medical Center, Boston, Massachusetts

DEREK J. LINDERMAN, MD, Instructor, Division of Pulmonary Sciences and Critical Care Medicine, University of Colorado Health Science Center, Denver, Colorado

TRACY MINICHIELLO, MD, Associate Clinical Professor of Medicine, Division of Hospital Medicine, Department of Medicine; Director, Anticoagulation Clinic, University of California, San Francisco, California

NELSON NICOLASORA, MD, Fellow, Division of Infectious Disease, University of Michigan Medical School, Ann Arbor, Michigan

STEVEN Z. PANTILAT, MD, Professor of Clinical Medicine, Alan M. Kates and John M. Burnard Endowed Chair in Palliative Care; Director, Palliative Care Program, Department of Medicine, UCSF Medical Center, University of California, San Francisco, San Francisco, California

PAULA M. PODRAZIK, MD, Associate Professor of Medicine, Section of Geriatrics, Department of Medicine, University of Chicago, Chicago, Illinois

SUMANT R. RANJI, MD, Assistant Clinical Professor of Medicine, Division of Hospital Medicine, Department of Medicine, University of California, San Francisco, San Francisco, California

KAVEH G. SHOJANIA, MD, Associate Professor of Medicine, University of Ottawa; Scientist, Clinical Epidemiology Program, Ottawa Health Research Institute, Ottawa, Ontario, Canada

ROBERT M. WACHTER, MD, Professor; Associate Chairman; Chief, Division of Hospital Medicine, Department of Medicine, University of California, San Francisco; Chief, Medical Service, UCSF Medical Center, San Francisco, California

DAVID H. WESORICK, MD, Clinical Assistant Professor, University of Michigan Medical School, Division of General Medicine, Department of Internal Medicine, Ann Arbor, Michigan

CHAD T. WHELAN, MD, Associate Professor of Medicine, Section of General Internal Medicine, Department of Medicine, University of Chicago, Chicago, Illinois

CONTENTS

In the mid 1990s, a new model for hospital care began to take hold in the United States, in which a separate physician, who I dubbed a "hospitalist," assumed the responsibility for managing the inpatient stay in place of the primary care physician. A 2006 American Hospital Association survey indicated that there are more than 20,000 hospitalists in the United States, making this the fastest growing medical specialty in American medical history. In this article, I briefly trace the reasons for the field's remarkable growth, describe some of hospital medicine's key issues and concerns, and speculate about the future shape of the field.

Hospitalists play an important role in improving patient safety through clinical expertise and leadership in hospital quality improvement activities. The evidence base in patient safety remains incomplete, despite an increasing body of published research in recent years. Thus, physicians must consider other factors in addition to the strength of evidence supporting a practice when deciding which patient safety interventions to implement. These factors include the prevalence of the safety problem targeted, the potential for unintended consequences of the intervention, the costs and complexity of implementing the intervention, and the potential of the intervention to generate momentum for further safety initiatives. In this article, the authors define a framework for evaluating patient safety interventions and discuss specific interventions hospitalists should consider.

wishes unheeded by physicians. Hospitalists can improve end-of-life care in hospitals dramatically. Hospitalists must relieve symptoms, such as pain, dyspnea, nausea, vomiting, delirium, and depression; communicate clearly; and provide support to patients and families. Hospitalists can increase the number and the timeliness of hospice referrals, allowing more patients to die at home. Finally, physicians must attend to their own sense of grief and loss to avoid burnout and to continue to reap the rewards end-of-life care provides.

Effective management of acute pain should be a primary goal of each health care provider. Acute pain is a complex medical problem with multiple possible etiologies. This article describes the pathophysiology of pain, discusses the ways to assess pain, and reviews the principles of acute pain management, including the use of both pharmacologic and nonpharmacologic measures to treat pain.

A significant portion of hospital care involves elderly patients who have frequent and severe disease presentations, higher risk of iatrogenic injury during hospitalization, and greater baseline vulnerability. These risks frequently result in longer and more frequent hospitalizations. The frailty and complication rates of the elderly population underscore the importance of hospital-based programs of education and screening for cognitive and functional impairments to determine risk and needed additional care and services during hospitalization and at discharge. In addition, physicians are needed to take the lead in instituting programs of prevention and improving the systems of care. It is such a multi-tiered approach, with interventions in the areas of education, screening, prevention, and systems of care improvements, that is needed to improve the clinical care and outcomes of the hospitalized elderly patient.

Hyperglycemia is an increasingly common and often complex condition to manage in the inpatient setting. Numerous clinical trials have demonstrated associations between uncontrolled diabetes and poor clinical outcomes in a number of inpatient settings. Insulin remains the treatment of choice for the majority of hyperglycemic hospitalized patients and should be prescribed in a physiologic manner, employing basal and bolus insulin.

Intravenous insulin should be used liberally in the ICU setting where randomized studies have demonstrated improved outcomes. Recommendations for insulin use in the inpatient setting are provided.

THE MEDICAL
CLINICS
OF NORTH AMERICA

ELSEVIER
SAUNDERS

Med Clin N Am 92 (2008) xi–xii

Preface

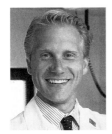 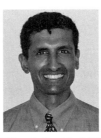 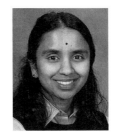

Scott A. Flanders, MD   Vikas I. Parekh, MD   Lakshmi Halasyamani, MD

Guest Editors

Over the past decade, the field of hospital medicine has experienced meteoric growth and is now the predominant model of inpatient care in many hospitals across the United States. This growth has been fostered by a variety of organizational, financial, and clinical factors. One critical factor is the increasing complexity of hospitalized medical patients and the necessity of accountability for quality and efficiency of care delivery. Similar to the site-based specialties of emergency medicine and critical care, hospital medicine has emerged as a focus of practice, which over the years has defined its own set of core knowledge and core competencies. Hospitalist physicians have become leaders and scholars in a variety of domains in the inpatient setting, including patient safety, perioperative medicine, and palliative care, in addition to their traditional focus on the comprehensive medical care of hospitalized patients.

This issue of *Medical Clinics of North America* is the second dedicated to the field of hospital medicine. In the six years since the last issue, there has been rapid growth in both the number of practitioners, which now exceeds 20,000, as well as in the scope of knowledge that is required to effectively practice hospital-based medicine. This issue begins with an update on the current state of the field of hospital medicine followed by articles on core areas of hospitalist expertise, including patient safety, prevention of nosocomial infection, transitions in care, perioperative medicine, and palliative care. This issue also covers core clinical topics in the management of hospitalized patients, including pain management, geriatric care, diabetic management, life-threatening infectious diseases, and thromboembolic disease.

doi:10.1016/j.mcna.2008.01.007   *medical.theclinics.com*

It concludes with a review of critical care management topics essential to non-critical care specialists. The subject matter was chosen, not so much to cover the entire body of knowledge required of hospitalists, which would be impossible in one issue, but rather to represent those areas that we feel are at the core of clinical practice and scholarship in the specialty of hospital medicine in 2008. We hope it will be valuable to hospitalists and non-hospitalists alike.

Scott A. Flanders, MD
Department of Internal Medicine
University of Michigan Health System
3119 Taubman Center
1500 E. Medical Center Drive
Ann Arbor, MI 48109, USA

E-mail address: flanders@umich.edu

Vikas I. Parekh, MD
Department of Internal Medicine
University of Michigan Health System
3119 Taubman Center
1500 E. Medical Center Drive
Ann Arbor, MI 48109, USA

E-mail address: viparekh@umich.edu

Lakshmi Halasyamani, MD
Department of Medicine
St. Joseph Mercy Hospital
5301 McAuley Drive
Ypsilanti, MI 48197, USA

E-mail address: halasyal@trinity-health.org

THE MEDICAL
CLINICS
OF NORTH AMERICA

Med Clin N Am 92 (2008) 265–273

The State of Hospital Medicine in 2008

Robert M. Wachter, MD

*Division of Hospital Medicine, Department of Medicine, University of California,
San Francisco, Room M-994, 505 Parnassus Avenue, San Francisco,
CA 94143-0120, USA*

In the mid 1990s, a new model for hospital care began to take hold in the United States, in which a separate physician, who I dubbed a "hospitalist" [1], assumed the responsibility for managing the inpatient stay in place of the primary care physician. This separation of the inpatient and outpatient physician was new in the United States (although it was quite familiar in most other medical systems around the world), and concerns about it led to considerable controversy. A parallel controversy erupted in academia, where the emergence of the hospitalist model often meant the replacement of the traditional one-month-per-year ward attending (often a subspecialist or basic science researcher) with a dedicated inpatient teaching attending whose primary professional focus was inpatient care.

Despite these controversies, the field has enjoyed explosive growth. A 2006 American Hospital Association survey indicated that there are more than 20,000 hospitalists in the United States, making this the fastest growing medical specialty in American medical history (Fig. 1) [2]. The field, already about the same size as emergency medicine and cardiology and far larger than established internal medical specialties such as infectious disease and endocrinology, continues to grow by 10% to 20% each year, and the growth shows no signs of abating. The field has grown larger than predicted in earlier estimates [3], and its ultimate size may be in the 30,000 to 50,000 range, making it the largest specialty (other than primary care) of internal medicine.

In this article, I briefly trace the reasons for the field's remarkable growth, describe some of hospital medicine's key issues and concerns, and speculate about the future shape of the field.

E-mail address: bobw@medicine.ucsf.edu

doi:10.1016/j.mcna.2007.10.008   *medical.theclinics.com*

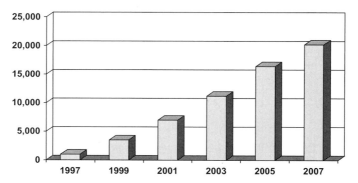

Fig. 1. The growth of hospitalists in the United States during the field's first decade. (*Data from* the Society of Hospital Medicine and the American Hospital Association.)

Drivers of early growth

To understand the early growth of the hospitalist field, one needs to understand the United States payment system for hospital care. Beginning in 1983, Medicare, the primary payer for inpatient care, switched to a system of diagnosis-related groups in which hospitals received fixed payments for given diseases (eg, exacerbation of heart failure, pneumonia with complications). Even though physician reimbursement continued to largely be on a fee-for-service, per-day basis, the fact that hospital reimbursement was now fixed based on discharge diagnosis created a powerful incentive for hospitals to support strategies that could safely shorten lengths of stay (LOSs) and decrease hospital costs.

Until the mid-1990s, these efforts mostly took the form of care pathways and practice guidelines, both of which had relatively little effect on physicians' practice patterns. Even the hiring of nonphysician case managers, whose charge was to look for excessive resource use and prolonged hospitalizations, often had little impact. Why? In most health systems, the inpatient physician was also the patient's outpatient physician, spending only a short period of time in the hospital each day before running back to an office full of patients. In community settings, this physician was an independent entrepreneur whose financial incentives were not to shorten LOS but were, if anything, to increase it (because the physician payment was per diem, and late days in a hospitalization are usually less labor intensive than early days—he or she had no "alignment of incentives" with the hospital operating under the diagnosis-related groups system). Many older physicians developed their practice styles in an era in which 2-week LOSs for pneumonia or myocardial infarction were commonplace, and many saw little reason to change tactics. The result was that many of the methods hospitals used to try to change physician practice patterns in the hospital were surprisingly unsuccessful, and many hospitals continued to experience prolonged LOSs and excessive hospital expenditures that added little to patients' quality of care or outcomes.

In the early 1990s, some large health systems—particularly those with employed physicians who did have aligned incentives with their hospitals—began reconsidering the dominant model of having the same physician serve as inpatient and outpatient attending. As they analyzed the nature of hospital care, they realized that inpatients were increasingly few (per physician) and increasingly sick, that physicians were busier than ever in their offices, and that the old system was unlikely to lead to efficient hospital care [4]. Extending the notion that "practice makes perfect" and the theoretically attractive notion that on-site availability by a dedicated inpatient physician would likely lead to improved quality and throughput, a few forward-thinking organizations began to reorganize their hospital care, dichotomizing the inpatient and outpatient work between two physicians. Recognizing the potential harm from such a split, strong organizations immediately began focusing on ensuring a smooth "handoff" to prevent any "voltage drops" at the inpatient–outpatient interface [5]. The hospitalist model was born.

Data soon began to emerge supporting the hypothesis that hospitalists could improve the "value" of care (ie, quality divided by cost) largely by decreasing the denominator significantly (an average of 15% reduction in hospital LOS and costs). A 2002 review found that virtually all the published literature to that point supported this premise [6], and a recent study of hospitalist versus nonhospitalist care involving 75,000 patients at 45 hospitals found similar LOS and cost advantages [7]. Despite these impressive efficiency advantages, no study has shown a decrease in quality associated with hospitalist care, and a few studies have indicated that hospitalist care might improve quality in the form of decreased risk-adjusted mortality rates or fewer readmissions [8–10]. Moreover, several studies of hospitalist programs in academic settings demonstrated markedly improved teaching evaluations when hospitalists became the ward attendings for students and residents [11–13].

More recent drivers of hospitalist growth

The early motivation for hospitalist programs was largely economic, and the return-on-investment that hospital leaders anticipated was a key driving force for the field's growth. This return-on-investment was vitally important because a new field of largely nonprocedural and often coordinative inpatient care would not have emerged based on professional fee reimbursements alone. Instead, thousands of hospitals were willing to supplement hospitalists' professional fee billings with additional support, monies that they regarded as an investment that was more than paid back through the economic advantages (to hospitals) of shorter LOSs and lower hospital costs [14].

In late 1999, the Institute of Medicine published *To Err is Human*, which placed the issue of medical mistakes (particularly in hospitals) squarely on the public's radar screen [15]. Two years later, the Institute of Medicine followed up with another report, *Crossing the Quality Chasm*, highlighting the poor quality and marked variations of care in the United States [16]. Because the stakes are the highest there and the data are more readily available, the public, media, and Congress turned to hospitals as the place to begin to address these shocking quality and safety gaps. Hospitals quickly realized that they needed an army of physicians—preferably ones who were open to new models of care, were innovative, were computer savvy, practiced evidence-based medicine, spent time in many areas of the hospital (wards, intensive care unit, emergency department, surgical floors), enjoyed systems thinking and teamwork, and had financial and professional interests aligned with those of the hospital. Because hospitalists fit this bill to a "t," even hospitals that had hesitated getting into the hospitalist business began to reconsider that decision: Having a strong hospitalist program now seemed like not just an economic advantage but potentially a quality and safety imperative. For hospitalists, being known as the doctors whose main task was to save hospitals money was professionally unsatisfying; being branded as a field that, while contributing to positive financial outcomes, was also focused on improving quality and safety was much more rewarding. The field's growth and stability were assured.

Other forces catalyzed even more expansion. In pediatric settings, many of the same issues were at play (although achieving a critical mass of pediatric hospitalists was harder in small, all-purpose hospitals), leading to a rapidly growing hospitalist workforce, particularly in large childrens' hospitals [17]. Many primary care physicians who resisted the hospitalist model at first began to embrace it, particularly if well-organized systems with high-quality hospitalists had emerged in their region [18]. Finally, in teaching hospitals, the duty hour restrictions enacted by the Accreditation Council for Graduate Medical Education in 2003 created a massive amount of work that could no longer be done by residents [19]. Although a variety of solutions have been tried to fill this breach, in many systems hospitalists became the favored ones, resulting in the hiring of large numbers of hospitalists to staff newly "uncovered" (by residents) services. In my program at UCSF, for example, we have grown from 15 hospitalists in 2004 to 38 hospitalists in 2007 largely because of the development of nonteaching, hospitalist–based services on general internal medicine, oncology, cardiology, and even neurosurgery.

The latter service may be the harbinger of the largest catalyst for growth in the second decade of the hospitalist field. Early hospitalists generally practiced inpatient internal medicine, caring for typical medical problems (eg, heart failure, sepsis, and stroke) and performing medical consultations on nonmedical services (eg, surgery, psychiatry, and ob-gyn). But if hospitals were now to be judged—and perhaps even paid—based on the quality of care divided by the cost (ie, value), how should a busy neurosurgery or orthopedics surgery service be organized? Just as one of the catalysts for hospitalist growth in internal medicine was the fact that general internists were so busy in their office that their hospital patients often languished (or were being "managed" by an uncoordinated horde of subspecialists), the same is true for many surgical patients who have medical comorbidities. With the surgeon in the operating room throughout the day, and in an environment where the quality of the medical care (eg, venous thromboembolism and antibiotic prophylaxis, pain management, and vaccinations and other preventive care) is being publicly measured and reported, it seems likely that more systems will embrace hospitalist–surgical comanagement, particularly for older surgical inpatients who have chronic diseases. Although early evidence regarding the value of improvements from this strategy is limited [20,21], it is growing rapidly across the United States.

Key issues and concerns

Although the explosive growth of the hospitalist field has validated the premise of the model and has been a source of strength and pride, it has also created problems. Recruiting has become a constant concern for many hospitalist programs, and there are hints that the quality of people entering the field is being compromised by the relentless demand for physicians [22]. Hospitalists worry about being placed in positions in which they are managing problems (particularly management of complex surgical patients) beyond their expertise. Particularly in programs that are understaffed or rapidly expanding their clinical roles (comanagement, night coverage, ICU coverage, etc.), there are concerns about burnout, though early studies are relatively reassuring in this regard [23]. In fact, a 2005 study by the Press Ganey organization found that the job satisfaction of hospitalists was second highest among physician specialties, trailing only radiation oncology [24]. This survey preceded the most recent growth spurt.

Similar concerns have emerged in teaching hospitals, where hospitalist programs have rapidly expanded to fill the gap created by implementation of residency duty hour restrictions. Many academic hospitalist programs are struggling to carve out an academic identity for themselves, which generally entails research productivity and teaching excellence, in an environment in which their primary role is to replace clinical tasks formerly performed by residents. Although some programs are managing this tension successfully, it is likely to be an ongoing challenge for virtually every academic hospitalist program [25].

Despite these challenges, the field has managed to achieve a tremendous amount in a very short time. Consider that in a decade, the field has achieved the following milestones:

- Unprecedented growth
- About a dozen fellowship programs, and growing [26]

- Tremendous name recognition (a Google search on "hospitalist" produces approximately 700,000 entries, and a Pubmed search yields approximately 700 articles)
- Two textbooks (*Hospital Medicine* and *Comprehensive Hospital Medicine*) [27,28]
- A thriving professional society (Society of Hospital Medicine), with more than 7000 members
- A well-respected journal (*Journal of Hospital Medicine*)
- A published list of core competencies [29]

Together, these accomplishments paint a picture of a field that is a bona fide specialty. In the early years of the hospitalist movement, its leaders were reluctant to seek a special designation or certification, fearing that such a certification would have led some managed care organizations to block primary care physicians from providing hospital care for their patients. That would have led to a major backlash, one that hospitalist leaders wanted to avoid.

Today, however, the field has matured to the point that the Society of Hospital Medicine is seeking specialty recognition from the relevant specialty boards. At this writing, the American Board of Internal Medicine (the certifying organization for internists) has tentatively approved such a designation through a "Recognition of Focused Practice" achieved through the Maintenance of Certification process [30]. It seems likely that hospitalists will undergo additional training (a focus during their internal medicine or pediatrics residency or additional fellowship training); at that point, the field will probably pursue a more traditional subspecialty designation. In the short term, the challenge will be to find a way to credibly recognize the competencies that bona fide hospitalists accrue through their practice in the absence of specific additional training. And the old concerns, particularly about primary care physicians being prohibited from providing hospital care for their patients if they lack a hospitalist certification, endure.

Summary

In its first decade, the hospitalist field has become the fastest growing specialty in American history. As a "site-defined generalist specialty," it has filled a niche similar to (but far larger than) the ones filled a generation earlier by the then-new fields of Emergency Medicine and Critical Care Medicine. The pattern is now unmistakable: When a site of care becomes sufficiently complex, a new specialist with generalist skills and sensibilities (someone comfortable with interdisciplinary collaboration, using consultants, and caring for a wide array of disorders and patient populations) emerges to manage patients in that location. Such site-defined specialists tend to take on the dual responsibility of caring for two "patients": the sick individual and the "sick" site of care itself, the latter through systems improvement work.

Table 1
Hospitalist leadership roles now and in the future

Domains	Presently	In the future
Medical student leadership	Clerkship director	Dean for students
Residency leadership	Associate residency director	Residency director or Dean for Graduate Medical Education
Physician leadership	Assistant director for Quality and Patient Safety	Chief Medical Officer
Information technology leadership	Assistant director for implementation of electronic health record	Chief Information Officer or Chief Medical Information Officer

For individual hospitalists, this systems improvement work has provided an opportunity to improve patient care outside their direct clinical content. Even relatively junior hospitalists often emerge with key roles in their institutions: directing quality, helping with implementing complex information technology systems, or leading medical student or residency educational programs. It seems likely that such individuals, as they mature (presently, the average age of hospitalists in the United States is 37 and of group leaders is 41 [31]), will assume even greater responsibilities in their hospitals, medical schools, and national organizations (Table 1).

With that as background, the fact that hospitalists entered the scene just as the United States health care system became focused on improving quality, safety, and efficiency was an extraordinary bit of serendipity, particularly because most hospitalists receive support from their hospitals and thus have uniquely aligned incentives with their organizations. These conditions have meant that hospitalists have quickly become indispensable to their patients, their hospitals, and to the health care system as a whole. There are no indications that the situation is likely to change in the foreseeable future.

References

[1] Wachter RM, Goldman L. The emerging role of "hospitalists" in the American health care system. N Engl J Med 1996;335:514–7.
[2] Society of Hospital Medicine. Hospital medicine specialty shows 20 percent growth. Available at: http://www.hospitalmedicine.org/AM/Template.cfm?Section=Press_Releases&;Template=/CM/ContentDisplay.cfm&ContentID=12507. Accessed December 12, 2007.
[3] Lurie JD, Miller DP, Lindenauer PK, et al. The potential size of the hospitalist workforce in the United States. Am J Med 1999;106:441–5.
[4] Wachter RM. An introduction to the hospitalist model. Ann Intern Med 1999;130:338–42.
[5] Vidyarthi AR, Arora V, Schnipper JL, et al. Managing discontinuity in academic medical centers: strategies for a safe and effective resident sign-out. J Hosp Med 2006;1:257–66.
[6] Wachter RM, Goldman L. The hospitalist movement 5 years later. JAMA 2002;282:487–94.

[7] Lindenauer PK, Rothberg MB, Pekow PS, et al. Outcomes of patients treated by hospitalists, general internists, and family physicians. Abstract, presented at the Society of Hospital Medicine annual meeting. Dallas, May, 2007.

[8] Auerbach AD, Wachter RM, Katz P, et al. Implementation of a voluntary hospitalist service at a community teaching hospital: improved clinical efficiency and patient outcomes. Ann Intern Med 2002;137:859–65.

[9] Meltzer D, Manning WG, Morrison J, et al. Effects of physician experience on costs and outcomes on an academic general medicine service: results of a trial of hospitalists. Ann Intern Med 2002;137:866–74.

[10] Diamond HS, Goldberg E, Janosky JE. The effect of full-time faculty hospitalists on the efficiency of care at a community teaching hospital. Ann Intern Med 1998;129:197–203.

[11] Hauer KE, Auerbach AD, McCulloch CM, et al. Effects of hospitalist attendings on trainee satisfaction with teaching and with internal medicine rotations. Arch Intern Med 2004;164: 1866–71.

[12] Kripalani S, Pope AC, Rask K, et al. Hospitalists as teachers: how do they compare to subspecialty and general medicine faculty? J Gen Intern Med 2004;19:8–15.

[13] Hunter AJ, Desai SS, Harrison RA, et al. Medical student evaluation of the quality of hospitalist and nonhospitalist teaching faculty on inpatient medicine rotations. Acad Med 2004; 79:78–82.

[14] Wachter RM. Hospitalists in the United States: mission accomplished or work-in-progress. N Engl J Med 2004;350:1935–6.

[15] Kohn L, Corrigan J, Donaldson M, editors. To err is human: building a safer health system. Washington, DC: Committee on Quality of Health Care in America, Institute of Medicine: National Academy Press; 2000.

[16] Crossing the quality chasm: a new health system for the 21st century. Washington, DC: Committee on Quality of Health Care in America, Institute of Medicine: National Academy Press; 2001.

[17] Bellet PS, Wachter RM. The hospitalist movement and its implications for the care of hospitalized children. Pediatrics 1999;103:473–7.

[18] Auerbach AD, Aronson MD, Davis RB, et al. How physicians perceive hospitalist services after implementation: anticipation vs. reality. Arch Intern Med 2003;163:2330–6.

[19] Philibert I, Friedmann P, Williams WT. ACGME work group on resident duty hours. accreditation council for graduate medical education: new requirements for resident duty hours. JAMA 2002;288:1112–4.

[20] Huddleston JM, Long KH, Naessens JM, et al. Medical and surgical comanagement after elective hip and knee arthroplasty: a randomized controlled trial. Ann Intern Med 2004; 141:28–38.

[21] Roy A, Heckman MG, Roy V. Associations between the hospitalist model of care and quality-of-care-related outcomes in patients undergoing hip fracture surgery. Mayo Clin Proc 2006;81:28–31.

[22] Auerbach AD, Chlouber R, Singler J, et al. Trends in internal medicine advertisements: an analysis of advertisements published between 1996 and 2004. J Gen Intern Med 2006;21: 1079–85.

[23] Hoff TH, Whitcomb WF, Williams K, et al. Characteristics and work experiences of hospitalists in the United States. Arch Intern Med 2001;161:851–8.

[24] Clark-Cox K. Physician satisfaction and communication. National findings and best practices. Available at: http://www.pressganey.com/files/clark_cox_acpe_apr06.pdf. Accessed December 12, 2007.

[25] Sehgal NL, Wachter RM. The expanding role of hospitalists in the United States. Swiss Med Wkly 2006;136:591–6.

[26] Ranji SR, Rosenman DJ, Amin AN, et al. Hospital medicine fellowships: works in progress. Am J Med 2006;119:72, e1–7.

[27] Wachter RM, Hollander H, Goldman L, editors. Hospital medicine. 2nd edition. Philadel-phia: Lippincott, Williams & Wilkins; 2005.

[28] Williams MV, Flanders SA, Whitcomb W, et al. Comprehensive hospital medicine. Philadel-phia: Elsevier; 2007.

[29] [No authors listed]. The core competencies in hospital medicine: a framework for curriculum development by the Society of Hospital Medicine. J Hosp Med 2006;1(Suppl 1):2–95.

[30] Wachter RM. What will board certification be–and mean –for hospitalists. J Hosp Med 2007;2:102–4.

[31] Society of Hospital Medicine. 2005–2006 SHM Survey. Available at: http://www.hospitalmedicine.org/Content/NavigationMenu/PracticeResources/Survey/SHM_Survey.htm. Accessed December 12, 2007.

ELSEVIER
SAUNDERS

THE MEDICAL
CLINICS
OF NORTH AMERICA

Med Clin N Am 92 (2008) 275–293

Implementing Patient Safety Interventions in Your Hospital: What to Try and What to Avoid

Sumant R. Ranji, MD[a],*, Kaveh G. Shojania, MD[b,c]

[a]Division of Hospital Medicine, Department of Medicine, University of California,
San Francisco, 533 Parnassus Avenue, Box 0131, San Francisco, CA 94143, USA
[b]University of Ottawa, Ottawa, ON, Canada
[c]Ottawa Health Research Institute, 1053 Carling Avenue, Room C403, Box 683,
Ottawa, ON K1Y 4E9, Canada

In the response to the Institute of Medicine report, *To Err is Human* [1], and the widespread interest in patient safety that it generated, the US Agency for Healthcare Research and Quality (AHRQ) was asked to study and improve the safety of the health care system. One of the initial projects funded by the AHRQ under this initiative was a comprehensive review of the literature that summarized the evidence supporting more than 75 specific patient care interventions [2,3].

Interventions that received the highest ratings for strength of evidence and potential impact tended to be clinical (eg, venous thromboembolism prophylaxis, perioperative beta-blockers, and measures to reduce nosocomial infections). Some leaders in the patient safety field criticized the emphasis on such clinical interventions over more explicitly safety-oriented interventions such as computerized provider order entry (CPOE) [4]. However, the advantages of this more evidence-oriented approach to improving patient safety, focusing on specific interventions that reduce complications of care, has gained greater acceptance [5]. In fact, the Institute for Healthcare Improvement's well-publicized "100,000 Lives" campaign [6] was based on the principle of leveraging widespread implementation of evidence-based interventions, rather than more general approaches to improving patient safety.

Despite the growing acceptance of using evidence to inform decisions about what to implement, the evidence base in patient safety remains young and has not yet stabilized. Increased publication of patient safety research in

* Corresponding author.
E-mail address: sumantr@medicine.ucsf.edu (S.R. Ranji).

recent years [7] has resulted in serious questions about several interventions that had high ratings in the 2001 AHRQ report. For instance, perioperative beta-blockers received the second-highest rating in the AHRQ report on the basis of five randomized trials that, although relatively small, all demonstrated consistent and substantial benefits [8,9]. However, 5 years later, more than 20 randomized controlled trials had been published, and meta-analysis of their results revealed questionable benefit and definite harm [10]. Similarly, N-acetylcysteine had shown a dramatic 90% reduction in contrast nephropathy in a single randomized controlled trial [11] and received a fairly high evidence rating [3]. However, numerous subsequent studies have shown inconsistent results [12,13]. In addition to contradictory evidence about benefit, new studies can reveal potentially unrecognized problems (analogous to side effects of clinical therapies), such as new opportunities for error from complex interventions such as CPOE and bar coding [14,15].

Evidence may change, but the need to respond to patient safety problems nonetheless remains. In this article, the authors outline a framework for choosing candidate patient safety interventions and discuss specific patient safety practices hospitalists should consider implementing at their hospitals.

Definitions and target audience

The authors define a patient safety intervention as any practice that reduces the probability of adverse events resulting from exposure to the health care system [3,16]. The use of the phrase "exposure to the health care system" makes it clear that adverse events can result not just from active treatments and procedures but also from simply being hospitalized, as with nosocomial infections. Although this definition makes no reference to the concept of "error," errors clearly play a causal role in the development of many adverse events. In this broader view of patient safety, errors take on the role of an intermediate clinical outcome. Just as we target blood pressure control to reduce myocardial infarction and stroke, targeting errors plays a role in preventing many adverse events.

Hospitalists have a natural role to play in improving patient safety, given their broad clinical expertise and frequent leadership roles in hospital quality improvement activities [16,17]. Hospitalists may work with administration to spearhead organizational change; however, in this article, the authors focus on interventions that hospitalists could decide to implement without the need for major institutional investment.

Choosing patient safety interventions to implement

Quality improvement efforts often focus on disseminating firmly established processes of care (eg, aspirin and beta-blockers for patients who have acute myocardial infarction). However, patient safety has yet to find its "aspirin and beta-blocker" because few, if any, interventions have such robust supporting evidence. Thus, considerations other than just evidence must play a role in the decision to implement specific patient safety interventions. These factors include the prevalence and severity of the safety problem targeted by the intervention, the strength of the evidence supporting the intervention, the potential for undesirable side effects of the intervention, the costs and complexity of efforts to implement the intervention, and the potential of the intervention to generate momentum for further safety initiatives (Box 1).

Box 1. Framework for selecting candidate safety interventions to implement

Scope of the problem
The scope combines the prevalence and severity of the safety problem; common problems with modest impact would score highly, as might less common but serious problems (eg, incorrect patient wrist bands).

Effectiveness
The effectiveness is the strength of evidence in support (eg, their validity) combined with the magnitude of effect (how well the intervention seems to work).

Need for vigilance
Does implementation of the practice require monitoring for unintended consequences (eg, problems due to increased handoffs after reducing work hours or new errors created by a CPOE system)?

Implementation issues
Cost and complexity should be considered; some interventions are costly but not complex (eg, hiring more nurses or pharmacists), whereas others are both, and thus at high risk for implementation failure (eg, any major change in how care is organized across disciplines, or implementation of a bar-coding system).

Momentum or synergy with other interventions
Of the various interventions one could implement at a given institution, some will have the potential to create momentum for additional initiatives or will relate to existing interests of clinical, administrative, or research leaders in the institution.

Data from Shojania KG, Duncan BW, McDonald KM, et al. Making health care safer: a critical analysis of patient safety practices. AHRQ Publication No. 01-E058; July 2001. Available at: http://www.ahrq.gov/clinic/ptsafety. Accessed December 1, 2007.

The existing literature often provides data on the first two factors (the scope of the problem and the effectiveness of a candidate solution), but less often on implementation issues and unintended consequences. However, the literature in this arena is growing. Examples involving unintended consequences from CPOE and bar coding have already been mentioned [14,15]. Examples also exist for less technical interventions. For instance, although patient isolation for infection control may help reduce transmission of nosocomial infections, it also increases the risk of adverse events, perhaps because isolated patients receive less careful attention from physicians and nurses [18]. Even apparently simple interventions, such as elevating the head of the bed to prevent ventilator-associated pneumonia, can prove surprisingly difficult to implement [19].

When data on implementation issues are not available, hospitalists should consider the following factors: the need for involving personnel from different disciplines, new education and training, impacts on workflow, and changes in organizational culture. Interventions requiring fundamental changes in any of these areas are less likely to succeed [20,21]. The easiest interventions to implement are those that fit well with what clinicians already do (ie, prescribing drugs [eg, to prevent venous thromboembolism] and using medical devices [eg, ultrasound guidance for central line insertion]). More substantive changes are easier to accomplish if they involve only one group of providers (eg, a new patient sign-out system for physicians), or involve adding more staff to perform ongoing activities (eg, hiring more nurses or pharmacists). That said, sometimes more complex interventions can lead to far greater rewards. The suggested framework (see Box 1) will help physicians evaluate this tradeoff between the resources required to implement a given patient safety intervention and the magnitude of the expected benefits. The authors recommend a "balanced diet" of patient safety interventions that hospitalists should consider implementing, consisting of some "low-hanging fruit" (practices that are easy to implement and supported by a strong evidence base), some momentum-generating projects (practices with a smaller evidence base, but that are likely to positively affect the institution's culture of safety), and some system-wide interventions where hospitalist involvement will be beneficial.

Important patient safety practices for hospitalists: "low-hanging fruit"

The following practices should be considered for implementation by all hospitalists, because they address common patient safety problems, are supported by strong evidence, are relatively easy to implement, and have low potential for harm (Box 2). In general, the authors considered practices to have a strong evidence base if a systematic review reported clear benefit, or the only randomized trials to have evaluated the intervention demonstrated effectiveness.

Box 2. "Low-hanging fruit"

Practices with a relatively strong evidence base (or strong face validity) that target broad problems, are easy to implement, and have low potential for harm
Ultrasound-guided central venous catheter insertion
Prevention of catheter-related bloodstream infection
Automatic stop orders to reduce urinary catheterization
"Read-backs" for critical communications

Interventions targeting patient safety at the time of hospital discharge (lower-quality supporting evidence, but high impact)
Postdischarge telephone calls to patients
Structured discharge summaries
Structured handoff communications

Ultrasound-guided central venous catheter insertion

More than 5 million patients in the United States receive central venous catheters every year, and in some series, up to 19% of these patients experience a mechanical complication (ie, arterial puncture, hematoma, or pneumothorax) [22,23]. A 2005 meta-analysis of seven studies comparing ultrasound guidance to the standard landmark method showed a significantly reduced overall failure rate of central venous catheter insertion attempts [24], particularly for internal jugular venous catheterization, and a reduction in mechanical complications. Ultrasound equipment and training of operators costs $10,000 to $15,000, although one analysis suggested this expense would be offset by complications averted [3]. Use of ultrasound guidance has not been associated with harm, although the concern exists that operators trained only in catheter placement using ultrasound guidance may be unable to use the traditional landmark method when ultrasound equipment is unavailable. This concern can be addressed by periodically permitting clinicians to perform catheterization without the use of ultrasound guidance to maintain skills with the landmark method.

Prevention of central venous catheter–related bloodstream infection

Approximately 80,000 patients in the United States experience catheter-related bloodstream infections (CRBSI) yearly, most of which occur in ICU patients [25–27]. The Centers for Disease Control and Prevention recommends several proven strategies to prevent CRBSI [25], which center around improving sterility at the catheter insertion site:

- Appropriate hand hygiene before insertion and during catheter maintenance

- Maximal sterile barrier precautions (use of a mask, cap, sterile gown, and gloves when inserting a catheter)
- Use of chlorhexidine (instead of povidone-iodine) for skin antisepsis
- Avoidance of femoral vein catheterization, except in emergencies
- Prompt removal of unnecessary catheters

The effectiveness of these simple, easy-to-implement strategies was demonstrated in the Keystone ICU project [28], in which 103 ICUs demonstrated significant reductions in CRBSI incidence over an 18-month follow-up period. The Institute for Healthcare Improvement also included prevention of CRBSI in its "100,000 Lives" campaign [6] through its central line "bundle," which includes the above interventions. Implementation of strategies to reduce CRBSI will go toward satisfying the Joint Commission for Accreditation of Healthcare Organizations' (JCAHO)'s National Patient Safety Goal 7 ("Reduce the risk of healthcare-associated infections") [29].

Prevention of catheter-associated urinary tract infections

Nearly all hospital-acquired urinary tract infections (UTIs) are associated with indwelling urinary catheter use [30–32]. Although urinary catheters are usually inserted for appropriate reasons, they often remain in place without clear indications for continued use, perhaps because physicians frequently overlook their presence. Unnecessary catheter use predisposes to bacterial colonization and eventual symptomatic UTI [33]; thus, effective catheter-associated UTI prevention strategies target duration of catheterization. A systematic review [34] found that automatic stop orders, in which urinary catheters were removed after 48 to 72 hours, unless a physician specifically countermanded the order, were effective at reducing duration of catheterization and asymptomatic bacteriuria, although the effect on symptomatic UTI rates was less clear. This intervention resulted in minimal harm to patients (a low rate of catheter reinsertion) and was easy to implement. Moreover, physicians also tend to overlook the extent to which urinary catheters bother patients [30]. Even if the magnitude of the impact on clinical UTI rates remains unclear, the impact on patient satisfaction is probably substantial.

"Read-backs" for laboratory results and other high-priority communications

The Joint Commission's 2007 National Patient Safety Goal 2 requires hospitals to "improve the effectiveness of communication among caregivers" [29], and specifically includes communication of critical laboratory test results as part of this goal. Similarly, failure to accurately identify patients being called for procedures or to confirm verbal orders correctly has resulted in several high-profile errors [35]. "Read-back" protocols (asking the recipient to repeat the information just communicated) are an easy-to-implement intervention that has the potential to prevent such communication errors [36,37]. Although fewer studies address this issue than the other "low-hanging fruit," the strategy should have minimal cost and low potential for harm, and thus is appropriate for widespread implementation. One proof of concept study [36] showed that, among 822 outgoing calls from clinical laboratories for the purpose of communicating critical laboratory results, the process of "read back" revealed errors in 3.5% of cases.

Interventions highly relevant to hospitalist practice: improving safety around transitions in care

The period immediately following hospital discharge may be dangerous for patients. Two studies contacted patients within 3 weeks of their discharge from the medical service at academic teaching hospitals and found that approximately 20% experienced adverse events (defined as new symptoms, unanticipated visits to a health care provider, or death) [38,39], most commonly adverse drug events or health care–associated infections. In 3% to 6% of cases, serious injury or death was attributable to a preventable adverse event. Overall, one half of the adverse events could have been prevented (or at least ameliorated) by the inpatient physicians. Patient harm may also result from failure to follow up appropriately on tests performed during hospitalization. In one study, 41% of patients discharged from the medical service at an academic medical center had test results pending at the time of discharge, but the patient's outpatient physician was unaware of the pending results 60% of the time [40]. Hospitalists are well positioned to address these problems at the inpatient–outpatient interface, and interventions to improve patient follow-up and communication between clinicians (especially inpatient and outpatient physicians) could significantly improve patient safety [41]. Practices in this group generally have lower-quality supporting evidence than the "low-hanging fruit" and may require more resources to implement, but are relevant to virtually all patients cared for by hospitalists and have little or no potential for harm.

Postdischarge follow-up phone calls

Given the prevalence of complications soon after discharge, early telephone contact with recently discharged patients could identify at-risk patients in need of immediate assistance or close follow-up. Although a recent Cochrane Collaboration systematic review did not find that such interventions were effective overall [42], most studies included in the review did not evaluate patients discharged from general medical wards and contacted patients up to several weeks after discharge, which may have led to the null result. Two studies more relevant to hospitalists [43,44] used nonphysician providers (pharmacists in one study and nurses in the other) to contact patients within 1 week of discharge. As in other studies, a considerable proportion of patients had developed new symptoms or concerns requiring contacting the inpatient physicians or other assistance (15% and 44% in the two studies); patient satisfaction was improved in both studies, and telephone follow-up by pharmacists resulted in a significantly reduced risk of emergency department visits after discharge [43]. Although follow-up phone calls should benefit patients, additional costs will be incurred, and dedicated resources will be required for adequate implementation. If resources are limited, physicians may consider targeting high-risk patients (eg, elderly patients, patients prescribed multiple new medications, or patients who have pending test results).

Structured discharge summaries

Similarly, structured communication between inpatient and outpatient physicians can help avert adverse outcomes due to postdischarge adverse events. The traditional dictated discharge summary is of limited value for patient safety purposes because it generally does not reach the outpatient physician before the patient follows up, and does not necessarily contain the information outpatient physicians need to ensure continuity of care [41,45]. A structured discharge summary should contain a complete medication list and information on new diagnoses, changes in medications since admission, pending investigations, and recommended investigations for nonacute problems identified during hospitalization. Ideally, this basic information should be transmitted directly to the outpatient physician at the time of discharge. Less important elements of the discharge summary, as identified in a survey of outpatient physicians [46], include inpatient laboratory data and radiology reports.

Structured sign-out systems

Discontinuity among providers has become an inevitable reality of medical practice [47], and managing this discontinuity is particularly relevant for hospitalists in both academic and community settings. Prior research has demonstrated that patients are at an increased risk of preventable adverse events while they are cared for by a covering physician [48]. Structured sign-outs should include accurate administrative information, specific tasks, and contingency planning. "Closing the loop" by accurately relaying events that occurred during cross coverage is equally important [49]. Trials of standardized sign-out systems, largely performed in residency programs [50,51], have successfully reduced the incidence of adverse events and have also improved physician efficiency and perception of continuity of care.

Implementing mechanisms for targeting patient safety during care transitions addresses three of the JCAHO National Patient Safety Goals: "Improve the effectiveness of communication among caregivers" (goal 2), "Improve the safety of using medications" (goal 3), and "Accurately and completely reconcile medications across the continuum of care" (goal 8).

Medication reconciliation

To comply with goal 8 (and the "100,000 Lives" campaign), many hospitals are investing resources in ensuring patients' medications are not stopped or changed inappropriately. This process of "medication reconciliation" [52] is undoubtedly important because, as multiple studies demonstrate, medications are changed without a clear indication at admission [53], at transitions during hospitalization (ie, when a patient is discharged from the ICU [54,55]), and at discharge [56]. However, many caveats remain regarding medication reconciliation. No study has yet documented an improvement in patient outcomes through reconciling medications, and the best method of accomplishing reconciliation remains unclear. Basic questions, such as when reconciling medications is most important (at admission, during in-hospital transitions, or at discharge), which patients will benefit the most (all patients versus patients who have complex medication regimens), and who should carry out the process (nurses, pharmacists, or physicians), remain unanswered. Given the complexities of hospital workflow, the answers will likely vary from hospital to hospital. Medication reconciliation will likely benefit some patients (eg, patients on many medications or on high-risk medications), but, as with many problems in the new field of patient safety, more data are needed on the scope of the problem and the types of patients most likely to be affected. Although many hospitalists likely will be involved in medication reconciliation activities, the authors believe that postdischarge follow-up calls, structured discharge summaries, and structured sign-out systems will provide more immediate benefits to patients, with fewer implementation difficulties.

Momentum-generating projects

Some practices have weak evidence, but substantial face validity and a low risk of harm, and offer the potential to establish collaborative relationships across disciplines that may generate momentum for future patient safety projects. These include

- Rapid response teams
- Executive walk rounds
- Teamwork training

Hospitalists might consider implementing some of these momentum-generating interventions to establish patient safety as a priority at their institution, improve morale among frontline providers, and generate support from senior administrators for future activities.

Rapid response teams

Because of their inclusion in the Institute for Healthcare Improvement's "100,000 Lives" campaign, rapid response teams (RRTs) have become one of the most widely implemented patient safety interventions in American hospitals, with nearly 3,000 hospitals committing to the implementation of an RRT. The concept behind RRTs is intuitively appealing: at the first sign of clinical deterioration, a team of providers is immediately summoned to the bedside to initiate treatment, ideally preventing further deterioration and adverse clinical outcomes such as ICU transfer or cardiac arrest. Although many uncontrolled studies claim great improvement in patient outcomes [57–61], careful analysis of these studies demonstrates serious problems in outcome measurement and reporting of co-interventions, calling their results into question [62–64]. The only controlled trial of RRTs (the cluster-randomized MERIT trial performed in Australia [65]) failed to show any benefit of the RRT on any clinical outcome. In fact, the control group hospitals (which received an educational intervention on caring for critically ill patients) experienced the same reduction in inpatient mortality and cardiac arrest rates as the intervention group hospitals (which received the educational intervention and started an RRT) [62]. The lack of benefit seen in this well-designed trial has been attributed by some to inadequate implementation in the intervention arm [66], but, in fact, implementation (as measured by calls per 100 patients) was greater than reported in all but one previous trial [62].

Given the plausibility of the idea underlying RRTs, some form of the intervention probably does improve patient outcomes, further highlighting the importance of the specifics of implementation. Although the optimal format for implementing RRTs remains unclear, compelling reasons nonetheless exist for hospitalists to proceed with this intervention (or maintain an RRT that has already been implemented). Anecdotal and some empiric evidence [67,68] indicates that they are extremely popular among nursing staff. Moreover, those staffing RRTs are well positioned to notice recurring problems that jeopardize patient safety [69]. A 2005 survey showed that one third of hospitalists have the primary responsibility for the RRT [70]. Hospitalists may consequently find that RRTs reveal important safety problems to target, and that the enthusiasm they generate among nurses and other staff provides the organizational support required to solve these problems.

Thus, although hospitalists should not consider establishing an RRT a top priority, RRT implementation may be used as a vehicle to promote interprofessional collaboration, identify patient safety issues that are important to bedside providers, and lay the foundation for future projects. Major barriers to implementing an RRT are the need for dedicated time and resources, the extensive implementation process needed to introduce this new system of care and ensure appropriate usage, and the need to monitor patient outcomes carefully to document RRT effectiveness. Unfortunately, despite the widespread implementation of RRTs, few reports are available to guide hospitalists in these matters [69].

Executive walk rounds

In addition to addressing specific patient safety issues, hospitalists should strive to create a "culture of safety" [37,71,72] at their hospitals. Key elements of safety culture include establishing a blame-free environment, creating an environment conducive to collaboration across disciplines and hierarchies, and committing leadership and resources to patient safety initiatives. Executive walk rounds, in which senior hospital leadership conduct informal visits to different areas of the hospital along with physicians and nurse leaders, have been associated with significant improvements in perceptions of the culture of safety [73,74]. For executive walk rounds to be successful, leaders should encourage nonjudgmental discussion of factors that led to adverse events or near misses, and should provide concrete and timely follow-up when issues are raised. In surveys, hospital executives frequently identify low physician participation as a barrier to inpatient quality improvement activities [75]. Hospitalists are uniquely positioned not only to lead quality improvement and patient safety projects but to liaise with senior management to identify and address safety concerns.

Teamwork training

Crew resource management (CRM), a concept initially studied in aviation, encompasses various training strategies designed to promote teamwork among groups of providers by teaching communication skills, de-emphasizing hierarchies, and promoting collaborative approaches to solutions. Medical applications of CRM have been conducted in the operating room and emergency department [76–78], with some success at improving participants' attitudes and behaviors. However, the bulk of the evidence (including a recent cluster-randomized trial of CRM conducted in obstetrics and gynecology units [79]) has not demonstrated improvement in patient outcomes [78]. Formal CRM training has not yet been evaluated in medicine or pediatrics units, but may have a role in resuscitation and ICU care, responsibilities that fall to many hospitalists. Given the positive effects on teamwork attitudes and behaviors, CRM potentially can be an important component of improving the safety culture. Hospitalists should thus consider participating in CRM activities to generate momentum for widespread patient safety activities, with the caveat that CRM's effect on patient outcomes remains unknown.

Interventions that are commonly used but lack demonstrated benefits

All hospitals are required to maintain an incident reporting system so that frontline providers may report patient safety and quality problems in an anonymous fashion. Although these systems are ubiquitous, thus far they have not proved useful in addressing specific patient safety issues [80]. Given the voluntary nature of incident reporting systems, the data gathered from them are subject to reporting bias [81] and do not represent a comprehensive picture of patient safety within an institution. Furthermore, reports often reach management too late to address a specific incident, causing providers to lose faith in the system and fail to file reports. Physicians, in particular, rarely file incident reports [82], in part because of a widespread perception that issues are not addressed. Thus, the authors do not believe that hospitalists should focus on incident reporting as a priority tool to improve patient safety.

One major goal of incident reporting systems is to identify serious adverse events that should be investigated further. Root cause analysis (RCA) is a widely recommended tool for investigating such incidents [83]. An RCA is performed retrospectively, by forming a multidisciplinary team to investigate possible contributing factors to an adverse event in each of several predefined causal categories (eg, personnel, training, equipment, and scheduling). The goal of an RCA is to identify latent errors (errors caused by system flaws) in addition to active errors (errors at the point of human interface with the system).

The Joint Commission mandates performance of an RCA when so-called "sentinel events" occur, but their value as a routine tool is limited. One of the authors (KGS) has had the chance to participate in a number of RCAs (or observe their results) at institutions that had investigated incidents that typically involved numerous errors [35] and substantial harm (including death) to patients [84–86]. Instead of identifying systematic problems and developing appropriate solutions, many institutions focused on only the most superficial of contributing causes and instituted changes that were unlikely to reduce the likelihood of subsequent events similar to the index cases. In hindsight, this experience should not have come as a surprise. System problems contributing to errors include issues such as staffing ratios and work schedules better designed to meet resource constraints than targets for safe operation; poor communication within and across disciplines; inadequate or poorly designed information technology support; and fragmentation of care, to name just a few. Identifying such problems is easy but solving them is difficult.

RCAs can have an effect on improving safety through identifying active errors and simply raising awareness of both latent and active errors. Because hospitalists will likely be asked to participate in RCAs, they should be aware that in most cases, the RCA itself is only the diagnostic arm of addressing a safety problem. The therapeutic arm often will require intensive, concerted efforts by multiple personnel from across various departments and disciplines within an institution. Such efforts should be made when warranted, but simply performing a series of RCAs has the potential to lead to frustration if problems are identified but not addressed. Perhaps after succeeding with a few "low-hanging fruit" and one of the above momentum-generating projects, a hospital might be in a position to tackle successfully some of the system problems that come to light in a well-conducted RCA.

System-level interventions benefiting from hospitalist involvement

Recommended interventions to improve safety include the clinical interventions discussed above and interventions that promise to fundamentally alter day-to-day practice for hospitalists. Chief among those are

Computerized physician order entry (CPOE)
Electronic medical records (EMR)

The authors strongly recommend that hospitalists become involved in the implementation of such systems, rather than view themselves as mere end users, to ensure optimal implementation and integration into provider work flow.

Computerized provider order entry

CPOE has been widely recommended as a means of reducing medication errors, yet in practice, few institutions have successfully implemented CPOE and achieved the touted benefits [87]. CPOE systems are difficult to implement because careful attention must be paid to integrating CPOE into clinician workflow; conflict between the system designers and physicians was in part responsible for one high-profile implementation failure [88]. In another case, CPOE implementation may have contributed to increased mortality in pediatric ICU patients [89]. This increase was attributed to failure to integrate CPOE properly into provider workflow, taking clinicians away from the bedside and resulting in an inability to obtain medications when urgently needed. Implementation issues and cost likely explain the slow uptake of CPOE systems in American hospitals [90–92].

Nevertheless, although CPOE implementation is time consuming, it can be performed well; when the same CPOE system associated with increased mortality was subsequently implemented in another pediatric ICU, careful attention to implementation factors (in consultation with the institution that originally implemented the system) resulted in no adverse consequences for patients [93]. CPOE provides many opportunities to improve safety; institutions with longstanding CPOE systems have seen reductions in medication errors [87]. Moreover, CPOE can be used as a tool to promote adherence to recommended care and provide decision support for physicians [94]. Because increased computerization in the hospital environment is inevitable, hospitalists will be well served to play an active role in CPOE implementation at their institution. Lack of physician input has been consistently identified as a factor in failed CPOE implementation [91,92], but by involving themselves early in the process, hospitalists can help customize CPOE systems to maximize their usefulness while minimizing interference with workflow.

Electronic medical records

Similarly, although many American hospitals already have an EMR, full implementation has still not been achieved [95] and many hospitals are substantially updating existing systems. EMRs can improve a provider's efficiency [96] but, as with CPOE, poorly designed systems can interfere with provider workflow. Unintended consequences of EMR systems, such as the perpetuation of incorrect information by cutting and pasting [97,98], have also been documented. Hospitalists are particularly reliant on EMRs to obtain and transmit clinical information at the time of care transitions; thus, when the opportunity to help implement an EMR system presents itself, hospitalists should avail themselves of the opportunity. Hospitalists will also be well positioned to monitor for potential adverse consequences of CPOE and EMR, and early collaboration with the system developers will help address these problems if they arise.

Summary

The "balanced diet"

When considering a patient safety project, hospitalists should think about not only the scope of the problem and projected effectiveness of the intervention but also the ease of implementing the intervention, its cost, and its potential for harm. Based on these factors, the authors have reviewed several candidate patient safety practices that hospitalists should consider implementing. The spectrum of patient safety problems varies from hospital to hospital, as do the resources available to tackle quality improvement in general. Thus, hospitalists should carefully prioritize the patient safety initiatives they undertake, to avoid spending limited resources on projects that are difficult to implement or less likely to succeed.

The authors thus recommend that hospitalists choose a "balanced diet" of patient safety projects, starting with high-impact interventions that are easy to implement, along with interventions that will promote interprofessional collaboration and lay the groundwork for future projects. Thus, initial projects, such as preventing CRBSI and instituting structured discharge communications, combined with a momentum-generating project such as executive walk rounds, should provide immediate clinical benefits and improve the culture of safety and climate for future interventions. They also strongly believe that hospitalists should be involved in hospital-wide interventions that will affect their day-to-day practice, such as implementation of CPOE.

The authors prioritized interventions that target common patient safety problems, according to a framework that also takes into account the strength of evidence supporting the intervention, the ease and cost of implementation, the potential for unintended consequences, and the potential for the intervention to promote other patient safety projects. They did not specifically recommend several interventions that, although commonly used, provide fewer benefits for patients in relation to the effort required to implement and perform them. These include medication reconciliation, incident reporting, and RCA. Although each of these interventions may be beneficial in specific patients or groups of patients, the authors believe that, in the setting of limited time and resources, hospitalists should prioritize their involvement in other interventions.

Hospitalists should be aware that the field of patient safety is changing rapidly, and interventions that were highly recommended as recently as a few years ago are now considered to be of questionable benefit. Several print and Web-based resources are available for those interested in staying current in the field. The AHRQ's Web sites WebM&M (webmm.ahrq.gov) and Patient Safety Net (psnet.ahrq.gov) are respectively a case-based journal and an annotated library dedicated to patient safety resources and education. The Veterans Affairs National Patient Safety Center Web site (www.patientsafety.gov) also includes practical patient safety resources and educational material, including detailed information on performing RCA. Organizations dedicated to patient safety, such as the Institute for Healthcare Improvement and the National Patient Safety Foundation, also carry out programs centered on patient safety education, leadership, and inpatient quality improvement.

References

[1] Corrigan JM, Donaldson MS, Kohn LT, et al, for the Committee on Quality of Health Care in America. To err is human: building a safer health system. Washington, DC: National Academy Press; 2000.

[2] Shojania KG, Duncan BW, McDonald KM, et al. Safe but sound: patient safety meets evidence-based medicine. JAMA 2002;288(4):508–13.

[3] Shojania KG, Duncan BW, McDonald KM, et al. Making health care safer: a critical analysis of patient safety practices. Evid Rep Technol Assess (Summ) 2001;43:1–668, i–x.

[4] Leape LL, Berwick DM, Bates DW. What practices will most improve safety? Evidence-based medicine meets patient safety. JAMA 2002;288(4):501–7.

[5] Brennan TA, Gawande A, Thomas E, et al. Accidental deaths, saved lives, and improved quality. N Engl J Med 2005;353(13):1405–9.

[6] Berwick DM, Calkins DR, McCannon CJ, et al. The 100,000 lives campaign: setting a goal and a deadline for improving health care quality. JAMA 2006;295(3):324–7.

[7] Stelfox HT, Palmisani S, Scurlock C, et al. The "To Err is Human" report and the patient safety literature. Qual Saf Health Care 2006;15(3):174–8.

[8] Auerbach AD, Goldman L. Beta-blockers and reduction of cardiac events in noncardiac surgery: clinical applications. JAMA 2002;287(11):1445–7.

[9] Auerbach AD, Goldman L. Beta-blockers and reduction of cardiac events in noncardiac surgery: scientific review. JAMA 2002;287(11):1435–44.

[10] Devereaux PJ, Beattie WS, Choi PT, et al. How strong is the evidence for the use of perioperative beta blockers in non-cardiac surgery? Systematic review and meta-analysis of randomised controlled trials. BMJ 2005;331(7512):313–21.

[11] Tepel M, van der Giet M, Schwarzfeld C, et al. Prevention of radiographic-contrast-agent-induced reductions in renal function by acetylcysteine. N Engl J Med 2000;343(3):180–4.

[12] Bagshaw SM, McAlister FA, Manns BJ, et al. Acetylcysteine in the prevention of contrast-induced nephropathy: a case study of the pitfalls in the evolution of evidence. Arch Intern Med 2006;166(2):161–6.

[13] Nallamothu BK, Shojania KG, Saint S, et al. Is acetylcysteine effective in preventing contrast-related nephropathy? A meta-analysis. Am J Med 2004;117(12):938–47.

[14] Koppel R, Metlay JP, Cohen A, et al. Role of computerized physician order entry systems in facilitating medication errors. JAMA 2005;293(10):1197–203.

[15] Patterson ES, Cook RI, Render ML. Improving patient safety by identifying side effects from introducing bar coding in medication administration. J Am Med Inform Assoc 2002; 9(5):540–53.

[16] Shojania KG, Wald H, Gross R. Understanding medical error and improving patient safety in the inpatient setting. Med Clin North Am 2002;86(4):847–67.

[17] Wachter RM, Goldman L. The hospitalist movement 5 years later. JAMA 2002;287(4): 487–94.

[18] Stelfox HT, Bates DW, Redelmeier DA. Safety of patients isolated for infection control. JAMA 2003;290(14):1899–905.

[19] van Nieuwenhoven CA, Vandenbroucke-Grauls C, van Tiel FH, et al. Feasibility and effects of the semirecumbent position to prevent ventilator-associated pneumonia: a randomized study. Crit Care Med 2006;34(2):396–402.

[20] Grimshaw JM, Shirran L, Thomas R, et al. Changing provider behavior: an overview of systematic reviews of interventions. Med Care 2001;39(8 Suppl 2):II2–45.

[21] Shojania KG, Grimshaw JM. Still no magic bullets: pursuing more rigorous research in quality improvement. Am J Med 2004;116(11):778–80.

[22] Mansfield PF, Hohn DC, Fornage BD, et al. Complications and failures of subclavian-vein catheterization. N Engl J Med 1994;331(26):1735–8.

[23] McGee DC, Gould MK. Preventing complications of central venous catheterization. N Engl J Med 2003;348(12):1123–33.

[24] Hind D, Calvert N, McWilliams R, et al. Ultrasonic locating devices for central venous cannulation: meta-analysis. BMJ 2003;327(7411):361–7.

[25] O'Grady NP, Alexander M, Dellinger EP, et al. Guidelines for the prevention of intravascular catheter-related infections. Am J Infect Control 2002;30(8):476–89.

[26] O'Grady NP. Applying the science to the prevention of catheter-related infections. J Crit Care 2002;17(2):114–21.

[27] Saint S, Savel RH, Matthay MA. Enhancing the safety of critically ill patients by reducing urinary and central venous catheter-related infections. Am J Respir Crit Care Med 2002; 165(11):1475–9.

[28] Pronovost P, Needham D, Berenholtz S, et al. An intervention to decrease catheter-related bloodstream infections in the ICU. N Engl J Med 2006;355(26):2725–32.

[29] Joint Commission 2007 National Patient Safety Goals for Hospitals. Available at: http://www.jointcommission.org/PatientSafety/NationalPatientSafetyGoals/07_hap_cah_npsgs.htm. Accessed May 11, 2007.

[30] Saint S, Lipsky BA, Goold SD. Indwelling urinary catheters: a one-point restraint? Ann Intern Med 2002;137(2):125–7.

[31] Tambyah PA. Catheter-associated urinary tract infections: diagnosis and prophylaxis. Int J Antimicrob Agents 2004;24(Suppl 1):S44–8.

[32] Tambyah PA, Maki DG. Catheter-associated urinary tract infection is rarely symptomatic: a prospective study of 1,497 catheterized patients. Arch Intern Med 2000;160(5): 678–82.

[33] Saint S, Wiese J, Amory JK, et al. Are physicians aware of which of their patients have indwelling urinary catheters? Am J Med 2000;109(6):476–80.

[34] Ranji S, Shetty K, Posley K, et al. Healthcare-associated infections. vol. 5. In: Shojania KG, McDonald KM, Wachter RM, editors. Closing the quality gap: a critical analysis of quality improvement strategies. Technical review 9 (prepared by the Stanford University-UCSF Evidence-based Practice Center under Contract No. 290-02-0017). AHRQ Publication No 04(06)-0051-4. Rockville (MD): Agency for Healthcare Research and Quality; 2007.

[35] Chassin MR, Becher EC. The wrong patient. Ann Intern Med 2002;136(11):826–33.

[36] Barenfanger J, Sautter RL, Lang DL, et al. Improving patient safety by repeating (read-back) telephone reports of critical information. Am J Clin Pathol 2004;121(6):801–3.

[37] Patterson ES. Communication strategies from high-reliability organizations: translation is hard work. Ann Surg 2007;245(2):170–2.

[38] Forster AJ, Clark HD, Menard A, et al. Adverse events among medical patients after discharge from hospital. CMAJ 2004;170(3):345–9.

[39] Forster AJ, Murff HJ, Peterson JF, et al. The incidence and severity of adverse events affecting patients after discharge from the hospital. Ann Intern Med 2003;138(3):161–7.

[40] Roy CL, Poon EG, Karson AS, et al. Patient safety concerns arising from test results that return after hospital discharge. Ann Intern Med 2005;143(2):121–8.

[41] Kripalani S, LeFevre F, Phillips CO, et al. Deficits in communication and information transfer between hospital-based and primary care physicians: implications for patient safety and continuity of care. JAMA 2007;297(8):831–41.

[42] Mistiaen P, Poot E. Telephone follow-up, initiated by a hospital-based health professional, for postdischarge problems in patients discharged from hospital to home. Cochrane Database Syst Rev 2006;4:CD004510. DOI: 10.1002/14651858:CD004510.pub3.

[43] Dudas V, Bookwalter T, Kerr KM, et al. The impact of follow-up telephone calls to patients after hospitalization. Am J Med 2001;111(9B):26S–30S.

[44] Epstein K, Juarez E, Loya K, et al. Frequency of new or worsening symptoms in the post-hospitalization period. J Hosp Med 2007;2(2):58–68.

[45] van Walraven C, Seth R, Austin PC, et al. Effect of discharge summary availability during post-discharge visits on hospital readmission. J Gen Intern Med 2002;17(3):186–92.

[46] O'Leary KJ, Liebovitz DM, Feinglass J, et al. Outpatient physicians' satisfaction with discharge summaries and perceived need for an electronic discharge summary. J Hosp Med 2006;1(5):317–420.

[47] Patterson ES, Roth EM, Woods DD, et al. Handoff strategies in settings with high consequences for failure: lessons for health care operations. Int J Qual Health Care 2004;16(2):125–32.

[48] Petersen LA, Brennan TA, O'Neil AC, et al. Does housestaff discontinuity of care increase the risk for preventable adverse events? Ann Intern Med 1994;121(11):866–72.

[49] Vidyarthi AR, Arora V, Schnipper JL, et al. Managing discontinuity in academic medical centers: strategies for a safe and effective resident sign-out. J Hosp Med 2006;1(4):257–66.

[50] Petersen LA, Orav EJ, Teich JM, et al. Using a computerized sign-out program to improve continuity of inpatient care and prevent adverse events. Jt Comm J Qual Improv 1998;24(2):77–87.

[51] Van Eaton EG, Horvath KD, Lober WB, et al. A randomized, controlled trial evaluating the impact of a computerized rounding and sign-out system on continuity of care and resident work hours. J Am Coll Surg 2005;200(4):538–45.

[52] Pronovost P, Weast B, Schwarz M, et al. Medication reconciliation: a practical tool to reduce the risk of medication errors. J Crit Care 2003;18(4):201–5.

[53] Midlov P, Bergkvist A, Bondesson A, et al. Medication errors when transferring elderly patients between primary health care and hospital care. Pharm World Sci 2005;27(2):116–20.

[54] Bell CM, Bajcar J, Bierman AS, et al. Potentially unintended discontinuation of long-term medication use after elective surgical procedures. Arch Intern Med 2006;166(22):2525–31.

[55] Bell CM, Rahimi-Darabad P, Orner AI. Discontinuity of chronic medications in patients discharged from the intensive care unit. J Gen Intern Med 2006;21(9):937–41.

[56] Rodehaver C, Fearing D. Medication reconciliation in acute care: ensuring an accurate drug regimen on admission and discharge. Jt Comm J Qual Patient Saf 2005;31(7):406–13.

[57] Bellomo R, Goldsmith D, Uchino S, et al. Prospective controlled trial of effect of medical emergency team on postoperative morbidity and mortality rates. Crit Care Med 2004;32(4):916–21.

[58] Bellomo R, Goldsmith D, Uchino S, et al. A prospective before-and-after trial of a medical emergency team. Med J Aust 2003;179(6):283–7.

[59] Buist MD, Moore GE, Bernard SA, et al. Effects of a medical emergency team on reduction of incidence of and mortality from unexpected cardiac arrests in hospital: preliminary study. BMJ 2002;324(7334):387–90.

[60] DeVita MA, Braithwaite RS, Mahidhara R, et al. Use of medical emergency team responses to reduce hospital cardiopulmonary arrests. Qual Saf Health Care 2004;13(4):251–4.

[61] Tibballs J, Kinney S. A prospective before-and-after trial of a medical emergency team. Med J Aust 2004;180(6):308–10.

[62] Ranji SR, Auerbach AD, Olson CJ, et al. The effect of rapid response systems on clinical outcomes: a systematic review and meta-analysis. J Hosp Med, in press.

[63] Winters BD, Pham J, Pronovost PJ. Rapid response teams–walk, don't run. JAMA 2006; 296(13):1645–7.

[64] Winters BD, Pham JC, Hunt EA, et al. Rapid response systems: a systematic review. Crit Care Med 2007;35(5):1238–43.

[65] Hillman K, Chen J, Cretikos M, et al. Introduction of the medical emergency team (MET) system: a cluster-randomised controlled trial. Lancet 2005;365(9477):2091–7.

[66] The "MERIT" Trial of Medical Emergency Teams in Australia: an analysis of findings and implications for the 100,000 Lives Campaign. Institute for healthcare improvement, 2006. Available at: http://www.ihi.org/NR/rdonlyres/F3401FEF-2179-4403-8F67-B9255C57E207/0/LancetAnalysis81505.pdf. Accessed May 11, 2007.

[67] Galhotra S, Scholle CC, Dew MA, et al. Medical emergency teams: a strategy for improving patient care and nursing work environments. J Adv Nurs 2006;55(2):180–7.

[68] Jones D, Baldwin I, McIntyre T, et al. Nurses' attitudes to a medical emergency team service in a teaching hospital. Qual Saf Health Care 2006;15(6):427–32.

[69] King E, Horvath R, Shulkin D. Establishing a rapid response team (RRT) in an academic hospital: one year's experience. J Hosp Med 2006;1(5):296–305.

[70] The Society of Hospital Medicine 2005–2006 Survey: the authoritative source on the state of the hospitalist movement. Available at: www.hospitalmedicine.org. Accessed May 11, 2006.

[71] Weick K, Sutcliffe K. Managing the unexpected: assuring high performance in an age of complexity. San Francisco (CA): Jossey-Bass; 2001. ISBN: 0787956279.

[72] Grabowski M, Roberts K. Risk mitigation in large scale systems: lessons from high reliability organizations. Calif Manage Rev 1997;39:152–62.

[73] Thomas EJ, Sexton JB, Neilands TB, et al. The effect of executive walk rounds on nurse safety climate attitudes: a randomized trial of clinical units [ISRCTN85147255] [corrected]. BMC Health Serv Res 2005;5(1):28.

[74] Frankel A, Grillo SP, Baker EG, et al. Patient safety leadership walkrounds at partners healthcare: learning from implementation. Jt Comm J Qual Patient Saf 2005;31(8):423–37.

[75] Levey S, Vaughn T, Koepke M, et al. Hospital leadership and quality improvement: rhetoric versus reality. Journal of Patient Safety 2007;3:9–15.

[76] Shapiro MJ, Morey JC, Small SD, et al. Simulation based teamwork training for emergency department staff: does it improve clinical team performance when added to an existing didactic teamwork curriculum? Qual Saf Health Care 2004;13(6):417–21.

[77] Morey JC, Simon R, Jay GD, et al. Error reduction and performance improvement in the emergency department through formal teamwork training: evaluation results of the MedTeams project. Health Serv Res 2002;37(6):1553–81.

[78] Salas E, Wilson KA, Burke CS, et al. Does crew resource management training work? An update, an extension, and some critical needs. Hum Factors 2006;48(2):392–412.

[79] Nielsen PE, Goldman MB, Mann S, et al. Effects of teamwork training on adverse outcomes and process of care in labor and delivery: a randomized controlled trial. Obstet Gynecol 2007;109(1):48–55.

[80] Cullen DJ, Bates DW, Small SD, et al. The incident reporting system does not detect adverse drug events: a problem for quality improvement. Jt Comm J Qual Improv 1995;21(10):541–8.

[81] Ashcroft DM, Cooke J. Retrospective analysis of medication incidents reported using an on-line reporting system. Pharm World Sci 2006;28(6):359–65.

[82] Schectman JM, Plews-Ogan ML. Physician perception of hospital safety and barriers to incident reporting. Jt Comm J Qual Patient Saf 2006;32(6):337–43.

[83] Wald H, Shojania K. Root cause analysis. In: Shojania KG, Duncan BW, McDonald KM, et al, editors. Making health care safer: a critical analysis of patient safety practices. Rockville (MD): Agency for Healthcare Research and Quality: Evidence Report/Technology Assessment No. 43 from the Agency for Healthcare Research and Quality: AHRQ Publication No. 01–E058; 2001. p. 51–6.

[84] Gandhi TK. Fumbled handoffs: one dropped ball after another. Ann Intern Med 2005; 142(5):352–8.

[85] Bates DW. Unexpected hypoglycemia in a critically ill patient. Ann Intern Med 2002;137(2): 110–6.

[86] Wachter RM, Shojania KG, Markowitz AJ, et al. Quality grand rounds: the case for patient safety. Ann Intern Med 2006;145(8):629–30.

[87] Kaushal R, Shojania KG, Bates DW. Effects of computerized physician order entry and clinical decision support systems on medication safety: a systematic review. Arch Intern Med 2003;163(12):1409–16.

[88] Connolly C. Cedars-Sinai doctors cling to pen and paper: transition to electronic medical records proves difficult. Washington Post. March 21, 2005:A01.

[89] Han YY, Carcillo JA, Venkataraman ST, et al. Unexpected increased mortality after implementation of a commercially sold computerized physician order entry system. Pediatrics 2005;116(6):1506–12.

[90] Poon EG, Blumenthal D, Jaggi T, et al. Overcoming barriers to adopting and implementing computerized physician order entry systems in U.S. hospitals. Health Aff (Millwood) 2004; 23(4):184–90.

[91] Poon EG. Universal acceptance of computerized physician order entry: what would it take? J Hosp Med 2006;1(4):209–11.

[92] Lindenauer PK, Ling D, Pekow PS, et al. Physician characteristics, attitudes, and use of computerized order entry. J Hosp Med 2006;1(4):221–30.

[93] Del Beccaro MA, Jeffries HE, Eisenberg MA, et al. Computerized provider order entry implementation: no association with increased mortality rates in an intensive care unit. Pediatrics 2006;118(1):290–5.

[94] Kuperman GJ, Bobb A, Payne TH, et al. Medication-related clinical decision support in computerized provider order entry systems: a review. J Am Med Inform Assoc 2007;14(1): 29–40.

[95] Longo DR, Hewett JE, Ge B, et al. The long road to patient safety: a status report on patient safety systems. JAMA 2005;294(22):2858–65.

[96] Poissant L, Pereira J, Tamblyn R, et al. The impact of electronic health records on time efficiency of physicians and nurses: a systematic review. J Am Med Inform Assoc 2005; 12(5):505–16.

[97] Hirschtick RE. A piece of my mind. Copy-and-paste. JAMA 2006;295(20):2335–6.

[98] Thielke S, Hammond K, Helbig S. Copying and pasting of examinations within the electronic medical record. Int J Med Inform 2007;76(Suppl 1):122–8.

ELSEVIER
SAUNDERS

Med Clin N Am 92 (2008) 295–313

THE MEDICAL
CLINICS
OF NORTH AMERICA

Prevention and Treatment of Health Care–Acquired Infections

Leanne B. Gasink, MD, MSCE[a,b,*], Ebbing Lautenbach, MD, MPH, MSCE[a,b]

[a]*Department of Medicine, University of Pennsylvania, Hospital of the University of Pennsylvania, Penn Tower Ground Floor, Suite 101, 3400 Spruce Street, Philadelphia, PA 19104, USA*
[b]*Center for Clinical Epidemiology and Biostatistics, University of Pennsylvania School of Medicine, 825 Blockley Hall, 423 Guardian Drive, Philadelphia, PA 19104-6021, USA*

Infections are the most common adverse events encountered in health care affecting approximately 2 million people, resulting in 90,000 deaths, and costing in excess of $4.5 billion each year in the United States [1]. Unfortunately, the risk of acquiring a health care–associated infection (HAI) is rising. An estimated 5% to 10% of patients admitted to acute care hospitals will become infected [2].

More than 80% of HAIs are caused by four types of infections: urinary tract infections, surgical site infections, bloodstream infections, and pneumonia [3]. Among identified pathogens in intensive care units (ICUs), 70% are resistant to at least one antibiotic [4]. This chapter aims to provide current data relating to the prevention of HAIs among patients admitted to an acute care hospital. As such, we will focus on hand hygiene, multidrug resistance, and *Clostridium difficile*, as well as the prevention of bloodstream infections, pneumonias, and urinary tract infections.

Hand hygiene

Hand hygiene (ie, hand washing with soap and water or the use of alcohol-based hand rubs), is paramount to the prevention of HAIs. Transmission of health care–associated pathogens has long been demonstrated to occur via the contaminated hands of health care providers [5]. Studies have also shown a temporal relationship between improved hand hygiene practices and

* Corresponding author. Department of Medicine, University of Pennsylvania, Hospital of the University of Pennsylvania, Penn Tower Ground Floor, Suite 101, 3400 Spruce Street, Philadelphia, PA 19104.
E-mail address: leanne.gasink@uphs.upenn.edu (L.B. Gasink).

decreased infection rates [6]. The "Guidelines for Hand Hygiene in Health Care Settings," published by the Health Care Infection Control Practices Advisory Committee (HICPAC), provides a comprehensive review of available data regarding hand washing and hand antisepsis, makes detailed recommendations for selection of hand hygiene agents, and describes appropriate indications and techniques [6]. In brief, hands should be decontaminated with soap and water or alcohol-based hand rubs before and after all contact with patients, when moving from a contaminated body site to a clean body site during patient care, and after contact with inanimate objects in the vicinity of patients. Soap and water, rather than alcohol-based hand gels, should be used when hands are visibly soiled, before eating, after using the restroom, and when exposed to *Bacillus anthracis* because antiseptics have poor activity against spores. Similarly, soap and water is preferred over alcohol hand rubs after exposure to *C difficile,* especially during outbreaks.

Although hand hygiene is considered one of the most important measures to decrease spread of pathogens in the health care setting, adherence to recommended hand hygiene procedures is typically low [7]. In more than 30 observational studies between 1980 and 2000 the rates of appropriate hand hygiene were reported to range from 5% to 81%, with an average rate of 40% [6]. Reported barriers to hand hygiene adherence include skin irritation due to hand hygiene products, inaccessibility of hand hygiene supplies, insufficient time available to perform hand hygiene, prioritization of patient care needs over hand hygiene, inadequate knowledge regarding the importance of hand hygiene, and lack of institutional support and/or prioritization of hand hygiene [8].

Alcohol-based hand rubs may improve hand hygiene adherence. Use of alcohol hand rubs requires less time to perform and results in less skin irritation and dryness [9,10]. Alcohol hand rub dispensers can be strategically placed and available at many more locations than hand-washing sinks. In addition, studies have shown that alcohol solutions reduce hand bacterial counts to a greater degree and are more effective compared with washing hands with soap and water [6]. Nonetheless, achieving sustained improvements in hand hygiene compliance is difficult. Success requires multimodal, multidisciplinary promotional campaigns that include administrative support, education, motivational materials, and ongoing monitoring of compliance with feedback to health care workers [6,11]. Guidance for the implementation of effective hand hygiene campaigns is available [6,11] and materials useful in the practical implementation of such programs are available at the Centers for Disease Control and Prevention (CDC) Web site (www.cdc.gov/handhygiene) and the Institute for Healthcare Improvement Web site (www.ihi.org).

Prevention of health care–acquired blood stream infections

Health care–acquired bloodstream infections (BSIs) are important causes of morbidity and mortality in the health care setting [3]. Since the 1980s, the incidence of health care–associated BSIs has been rising steadily, and the majority of these are related to the use of intravascular devices, especially central venous catheters (CVCs) [12,13]. Approximately 250,000 to 500,000 hospital-acquired BSIs occur in the United States annually [14–19]. BSIs are associated with a high case-fatality rate, exceeding 25% in many reports. In addition, they cause a significant economic burden with a marginal cost estimate of $25,000 per episode [16].

Pathogens most often reflect patient skin flora or pathogens transferred via the contaminated hands of health care workers. Microorganisms migrate to the bloodstream intraluminally though the end of the catheter or extraluminally, at the exit site [2]. Coagulase-negative staphylococci, *Staphylococcus aureus,* and *Enterococcus* are most commonly identified followed by gram-negative rods and *Candida* species. Catheter-related BSIs are BSIs that clearly originate from a catheter as defined by standard criteria [20]. In contrast, catheter-associated BSIs include BSIs that occur in patients with CVCs when other sites of infection have been excluded.

Given the importance of BSIs, much attention has been focused on their prevention. Most available data focus on strategies to decrease catheter-related BSIs. Although few randomized trials exist, evidence-based guidelines have been developed by the CDC and HICPAC and several standard practices have been widely accepted [20]. Full barrier precautions, which include sterile gloves, sterile gown, mask, cap, and large sterile sheet drape, have been shown to decrease the incidence of catheter-related BSI compared with sterile gloves and small drapes alone [21]. Chlorhexidine gluconate was found to be superior to povidone-iodine, in a meta-analysis and should be used preferentially for skin antisepsis [22]. The femoral CVC insertion site should be avoided, as it is clearly associated with higher rates of infection [20,23]. Many experts also advocate use of the subclavian rather than internal jugular insertion site as prospective, observational data have suggested higher infection risk in the latter [16,24]. Because the risk of infection is associated with length of CVC usage, catheters should be promptly removed when no longer needed [20]. Routine replacement of CVCs has not been shown to affect infection rates [25]. Finally, adherence to proper hand hygiene is strongly recommended [20]. HICPAC guidelines also provide specific recommendations regarding catheter site dressing regimens and replacement of administration sets [20].

A wide variety of alternative approaches to the prevention of BSIs have been investigated. Success in BSI reduction has been found with antibiotic-impregnated and antiseptic-impregnated (eg, chlorhexidine/silver-sulfadiazine) catheters in several randomized trials [26,27]. The use of instillation, or locking of anti-infective solutions into CVC lumens, and the placement of a chlorhexidine-impregnated sponge at the catheter exit have also been investigated as promising techniques [28,29]. However, conflicting data, questionable cost-effectiveness, and the potential for adverse events (eg, anaphylaxis, emergence of drug resistance) has limited the widespread use of these novel devices. Current guidelines state that antibiotic/antiseptic-impregnated catheters should be used if the rate of infection is high despite adherence to other strategies [20].

Despite strong evidence, adherence with recommendations for the prevention of catheter-related BSIs appears to be low. For example, only 28% of US internists reported greater than 90% compliance in using maximum barrier precautions during insertion of CVCs [30]. Adherence to evidence-based practices seems to depend heavily on skilled and motivated health care workers. Specialized "intravenous teams" have been shown to be effective in reducing catheter-related BSIs [20,31]. Well-organized programs that focus on the promotion of evidence-based practice, monitoring, feedback, and a team-oriented approach to prevention have been successful in decreasing BSIs and sustaining low rates [24,32,33]. Specific techniques implemented in these published reports can be used to model similar programs in other institutions. Updated consensus guidelines for the prevention of intravascular catheter-related infections are expected in 2008.

Prevention of health care–acquired pneumonia

Health care–acquired pneumonia (HAP) includes pneumonias that develop in ventilated and nonventilated patients 48 hours after admission. The overwhelming majority of available data pertain to ventilator-associated pneumonias (defined as pneumonia occurring within 48 to 72 hours of intubation) in critically ill patients in ICUs [34]. Because of the paucity of information regarding HAP occurring outside of an ICU, available data must be extrapolated to other settings and interpreted cautiously.

HAP causes significant morbidity and mortality. It is the second most common hospital-acquired infection occurring at an estimated rate of 5 to 10 cases per 1000 hospitalizations [35,36]. HAP is 20 times more likely to occur in ventilated patients compared with nonventilated patients and can affect up to a third of patients requiring mechanical ventilation [37]. Reported attributable mortality rates range from 33% to 50% and overall case-fatality rates may be as high as 70% [34]. In addition, HAP is associated with longer lengths of stay and an excess cost of up to $40,000 per incident [38].

HAP primarily results from microbial invasion of the normally sterile lower respiratory tract due to micro aspiration of oral secretions. Infected biofilms on endotracheal tubes also play an important role in pathogenesis [39]. The role of the stomach as a potential reservoir for oropharyngeal pathogen colonization is controversial, but gastric secretions may play a role, especially in certain conditions (eg, high gastric pH) [34,35,37]. Similarly, whether the sinuses act as a clinically important reservoir for HAP pathogens is debatable [34]. Patient factors (such as immunosuppression) and treatment-related factors (such as intubation and enteral feeding) are also important contributors to the development of HAP. Etiologic agents include a wide variety of bacterial pathogens. Infection may be polymicro-bial; however, anaerobes are infrequently implicated [40,41]. Fungal and viral pathogens are not significant causes of HAP, although they may be found in immunocompromised patients with HAP and during outbreaks (eg, nosocomial influenza), respectively [42,43].

HAP prevention strategies focus on the reduction of risk factors for oropharyngeal and gastric colonization and the subsequent aspiration of pathogens, especially among intubated patients [37]. Given the 20-fold higher incidence of HAP among ventilated patients, intubation and mechan-ical intubation should be avoided whenever possible. Noninvasive positive pressure ventilation has been effective at preventing mechanical ventilation and is associated with lower rates of health care infections and HAP [44]. Protocols to facilitate weaning may reduce the duration of mechanical ven-tilation and possibly decrease rates of HAP [45]. Notably, re-intubation is associated with an increased risk of HAP and should be avoided [46]. Among patients who require intubation, special attention should be given to the endotracheal tube and the ventilator circuit. Endotracheal and oro-gastric, rather than nasotracheal and nasogastric tubes are preferred because they reduce the incidence of sinusitis, although a link between sinusitis and HAP has not been clearly established [47]. Ventilator circuit management strategies have also received attention as a potential focus for treatment strategies. Although HAP may be related to colonization of the ventilator circuit, several prospective studies have found that the frequency of circuit changes does not affect the incidence of HAP [48,49]. Heat-moisture exchangers have been used to eliminate condensate accumulation; however, several randomized trials have reported conflicting results and further trials are needed before recommendations regarding the use of this expensive intervention can be made [35,49]. Drainage of subglottic secretions to min-imize aspiration has been shown in some, but not all studies, to decrease the incidence of HAP [49,50]. Although these specialized endotracheal tubes are expensive, at least one study concluded that they are cost effective [51]. A recent meta-analysis concluded that subglottic secretion drainage is most effective at preventing early-onset HAP among patients expected to receive more than 72 hours of mechanical ventilation [52].

Several other strategies aimed at minimizing aspiration have been inves-tigated. Semi-recumbent positioning (elevation of the head of the bed at least 45 degrees) has been shown to decrease reflux and aspiration events and reduce the incidence of HAP; therefore, it should be used in all patients who can tolerate head elevation [35,53,54]. Oscillating beds appear to have no benefit in the general population of medical patients and are associated with a high cost and potential for complications (eg, disconnected catheters, pressure sores) [49]. Recommendations in other patients, such as surgical and neurosurgical patients requiring prolonged mechanical ventilation and immobilization, remain unresolved [34,35,49]. Enteral feeding has been shown to increase the risk of HAP, but because of the risk of complications associated with administration of nutrition through CVCs, enteral nutrition is still preferred over parenteral nutrition based on the overall risk/benefit ratio [34,55]. Studies evaluating postpyloric feeding, intermittent enteral feeding, and the use of motility agents have shown no benefit [37].

Finally, there has been substantial interest in decreasing pathogen colonization of the oropharynx and stomach. Much data have been published regarding selective digestive decontamination (SDD) with topical and/or intravenous antibiotics. Seven meta-analyses of more than 40 randomized trials showed a decreased risk of HAP with SDD [49]; however, the methodological quality of many of these studies has been questioned and the benefits of SDD may be overstated [56]. Because of serious concerns regarding the long-term effects on antimicrobial resistance patterns, SDD is not recommended [49]. In contrast, an emphasis on oral care may be beneficial. A meta-analysis of seven randomized trials of topical application of an antiseptic, chlorhexidine, to oral mucosa concluded that chlorhexidine is beneficial, especially in cardiac surgery patients [57]. In a large, multicenter randomized trial of elderly persons in nursing homes, good oral care was shown to result in lower rates of pneumonia [58]. Finally, medications used to prevent stress ulcers in critically ill patients may allow for greater colonization of the upper gastrointestinal tract by increasing gastric pH, thus conferring a greater risk of HAP. Several meta-analyses found a lower rate of HAP and lower overall mortality among ventilated patients on sulcralfate compared with H2 antagonists, but other meta-analyses found no significant differences [49]. Given the questionable efficacy of sulfacrate in preventing gastrointestinal bleeding compared with H2 antagonists, clinicians should carefully consider the risks and benefits when choosing stress ulcer prophylactic therapies [59]. Of note, acidification of enteral feeds has been shown to have no benefit in decreasing HAP [60].

Guidelines for HAP prevention and a comprehensive review of available data behind these guidelines have been published by HICPAC, as well as the American Thoracic Society in collaboration with the Infectious Diseases Society of America (IDSA) [34,35]. In addition, a recent evidence-based systemic review provides a comprehensive review and synthesis of strategies for prevention of ventilator-associated pneumonia [49].

Prevention of health care–acquired urinary tract infections

Urinary tract infections (UTIs) are the most common hospital infections, accounting for between 30% and 40% of all nosocomial infections [61–64]. Most UTIs in the health care setting result from catheterization of the urinary tract. The most recent report of the CDC's National Nosocomial Infection Surveillance (NNIS) System revealed a median rate of catheter-associated UTI (ie, number of urinary catheter-associated UTIs per 1000 urinary catheter days) of 3.9 (10th to 90th percentile = 1.3 to 7.9) [3]. This rate ranged from 3.0 in cardiothoracic ICUs to 6.7 in neurosurgical

ICUs. A recent study that investigated device-associated infections in 55 ICUs of 46 hospitals in eight countries noted a median rate of 8.9 catheter-associated UTIs per 1000 urinary catheter days (10th to 90th percentile = 1.7 to 12.8) [65].

Although UTI is typically characterized by dysuria, urinary urgency, bacteriuria, and pyuria [66], these findings may be attenuated or absent in the elderly or in immunocompromised patients, and difficult to evaluate in patients with indwelling catheters. The most common causes of nosocomial UTI are *Escherichia coli, Enterococcus, Pseudomonas aeruginosa, Klebsiella pneumoniae*, and *Candida* species [62,67].

Nosocomial UTI results in secondary bacteremia in up to 4% of patients [68–71]. Furthermore, the urinary tract is the second most common source of nosocomial bloodstream infection; approximately 15% of nosocomial bloodstream infections are secondary to antecedent UTI [68–71]. Nosocomial UTI has been associated with a case-fatality rate between 13% and 30% [68–70]. Increased morbidity and mortality independent of the infection's progression to sepsis has been noted in patients with nosocomial UTI [72,73].

Urinary catheterization is a common practice; approximately 15% to 25% of hospital patients have a urinary catheter at some time during their hospital stay, with rates of use varying by unit type within the hospital [74]. The risk of contracting a catheter-associated UTI increases with the duration of catheterization [75]. Furthermore, females, the elderly, and persons with severe underlying illness are also at increased risk of health care–acquired UTI [76–78].

The overall risk of bacteriuria in hospitalized patients with indwelling catheters is about 25% [79]. Bacteria gain access to the catheterized bladder by either of two routes. They may migrate from the collection bag or the catheter drainage tube junction, or ascend extraluminally within the periurethral space [77]. Bacteria can adhere to and grow on the inner surface of the catheter, leading to a biofilm that also includes urinary proteins and salts. Bacteria embedded in this biofilm are less susceptible to antibiotics [80,81].

Asymptomatic bacteriuria (ie, bacteria identified in a urine culture in the absence of clinical symptoms) is a common finding. The significance of asymptomatic bacteriuria in patients with indwelling urinary catheters remains a matter of debate [72,82]. Recent guidelines from the Infectious Disease Society of America (IDSA) recommend that cultures be performed to detect asymptomatic bacteriuria in pregnant women and individuals about to undergo a urologic procedure [83]; however, screening urine cultures should not be obtained in asymptomatic catheterized patients [83]. Furthermore, the goal of therapy of asymptomatic catheter-associated bacteriuria remains poorly defined with bacteriuria recurring shortly after cessation of antimicrobial therapy [83].

As noted previously, the vast majority of documented health care–acquired UTIs are associated with use of a urinary catheter. As such, efforts to prevent health care–acquired UTIs have focused primarily on optimizing use of catheters when they are medically necessary and eliminating unnecessary use of catheters. The use of a closed sterile drainage system with indwelling catheters provides a significant short-term reduction in infection related to this device [84]. Breaks in aseptic technique in placement, and disruption and entry of pathogens into the closed system are the most significant factors in the development of catheter-related UTI [85]. Thus, appropriate care in the placement and maintenance of these devices is also essential to their success in preventing infection [77,86]. Use of alternative types of catheters (eg, suprapubic catheters, condom catheters) may be associated with a lower rate of infection, although rigorous comparative data are lacking [87]. Recent attention has also been paid to the role of urinary catheters coated with antimicrobial substances. A systematic review summarized the results of studies performed to date evaluating nitrofurazone-coated or silver alloy–coated urinary catheters [86]. Both types of antimicrobial-coated catheters can prevent bacteriuria during short-term catheterization in hospitalized patients. Evaluation of the impact of coated catheters on symptomatic UTI was not assessed in any of the reviewed studies [86].

Despite the clear risk, catheters are often overused and unnecessary, placing patients at needless risk of contracting infection [75,88]. Indeed, it has been noted that 38% of attending physicians were unaware as to whether a hospitalized patient under their care had a urinary catheter in place [88]. Better methods of monitoring catheter use and reducing the inappropriate use of urinary catheters can translate into reduced rates of nosocomial UTIs [89]. Guidelines for the control of health care–acquired UTIs have been developed in the past [90]. New IDSA guidelines are expected in early 2008.

Prevention of *Clostridium difficile*

Clostridium difficile is the most frequently identified cause of health care–acquired diarrhea [91]. It results in considerable morbidity and is associated with prolonged lengths of stay [92,93]. One group conservatively estimated that the annual cost associated with *C difficile* in the United States is $1.1 billion [92]. Between 1996 and 2003, the rate of *C difficile* in US hospitals nearly doubled from 31 to 61 per 100,000 discharges [94]. In recent years, large outbreaks have been reported that have been associated with unexpectedly high morbidity and mortality [95–98]. Furthermore, there have been reports of poor response rates to standard therapy and increasing rates of relapse and recurrence of infection [99]. Recently, a previously rare strain, B1/NAP1, has emerged as the cause of highly morbid geographically dispersed outbreaks [100].

The most important risk factors for *C difficile* include antibiotic use and hospitalization, but advanced age, severity of underlying illness, use of proton pump inhibitors, gastrointestinal surgery, and tube feeding have also been associated with increased risk of infection [101–104]. Infection usually occurs when an antibacterial agent disrupts the colonic flora, creating conditions that favor the acquisition or proliferation of *C difficile* [105]. Any antibacterial, including the drugs used to treat infection, metronidazole and vancomycin, can cause *C difficile* [91]. Clindamycin has been classically associated with *C difficile*, but amoxicillin and cephalosporins are more frequently implicated, and are more widely prescribed [91,106]. Recently, fluoroquinolone exposure has emerged as a major risk factor for infection, and was a particularly important contributor to outbreaks of *C difficile* caused by the epidemic strain, B1/NAP1 [96,98]. The importance of acquisition and spread in hospitals is evidenced by the clonality of several major outbreaks and by the 20% to 40% colonization rate in hospitalized adults compared with 2% to 3% rate in healthy adults [98,107,108]. Of note are recent reports of severe infection occurring in patients who received only a few doses of antibiotics or no antibiotics at all [109].

Given the pathogenesis of *C difficile*, judicious use of antimicrobials and strict infection control and environmental measures are keys to the prevention of disease. The implementation of antibiotic stewardship programs has been associated with decreased incidence of *C difficile* [110,111]. Aggressive restriction of antibiotics and hospital-wide formula changes may be required during epidemics [112–114]. To prevent spread, patients with *C difficile* infection should be isolated in a single room, on strict contact precautions (ie, gowns and gloves required for all persons entering the room), and rooms and equipment should be cleansed with a 1:10 dilution of bleach to kill spores that may be present [101,115]. Health care workers should wash their hands with soap and water, rather than alcohol hand rubs, especially in outbreak settings, because alcohol is not effective at killing clostridia spores [6]. Educational programs may also be of use in promoting practices that minimize spread [116].

Prevention of antimicrobial resistance

The emergence of antimicrobial resistance has threatened to render the existing antibiotic arsenal useless. Both the number of organisms exhibiting resistance, as well as the mechanisms of resistance have increased sharply in recent years [117]. The most common resistant gram-positive organisms encountered in the hospital setting are methicillin-resistant *Staphylococcus aureus* (MRSA) and vancomycin-resistant Enterococci (VRE). Among nosocomial gram-negative pathogens, extended-spectrum beta-lactamase (ESBL)-producing Enterobacteriaceae, multidrug-resistant *Pseudomonas aeruginosa*, and multidrug-resistant *Acinetobacter baumannii* are most prevalent [3]. As noted in data from the CDC's NNIS System, the prevalence of resistance for nearly all organisms studied increased substantially in recent years (Fig. 1) [3]. These trends are of particular concern given marked

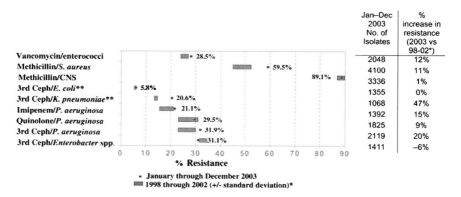

Fig. 1. Changes in antimicrobial-resistant pathogens associated with nosocomial infections in ICU patients. (*From* Weinstein RA. Controlling antimicrobial resistance in hospitals: infection control and use of antibiotics. Emerg Infect Dis 2001;7:188.)

slowing in development of new antimicrobial agents [118]. Indeed, Food and Drug Administration (FDA) approval of new antibacterial agents has decreased by 56% over the past 20 years (1998 to 2002 versus 1983 to 1987) [118].

Infections caused by antibiotic-resistant bacteria are associated with increased morbidity, mortality, and hospital costs [119–122]. Of note, expenditures due to antimicrobial resistance in the United States in 1995 were estimated to be $4 billion [123]. More recently, studies focusing on the impact of specific antimicrobial-resistant pathogens (eg, MRSA, VRE, and ESBL-producing Enterobacteriaceae) have also demonstrated significantly worse clinical outcomes in patients infected with resistant pathogens compared with patients infected with their susceptible counterparts [124–126].

The reason for the apparent relationship between resistant infection and negative clinical outcomes has not been fully elucidated. One possible explanation is that antibiotic-resistant organisms are more virulent than their antibiotic-susceptible counterparts. However, the limited existing data suggest the opposite: that virulence factors and invasive disease are more common among antibiotic-susceptible strains [127–129]. Another possible explanation of the association between resistant infection and negative outcomes is that resistance may result in a delay in initiation of adequate antimicrobial therapy. Recent studies of bloodstream infections suggest that a delay in effective antimicrobial therapy may result in poorer outcomes and that inadequate antimicrobial therapy is more likely to occur in resistant infections [130–132]. In a study of *Klebsiella* bacteremia, bloodstream infections that originated from blood-borne or respiratory infections had the highest mortality rate, whereas bacteremias that originated from a UTI had the lowest mortality rate [133]. In support, a recent cohort study of ESBL-producing Enterobacteriaceae noted that a delay in adequate antimicrobial therapy was strongly associated with mortality in non-urine infections (eg, blood, respiratory) but not in urine infections [134].

The continued emergence of antimicrobial resistance has been linked most closely to the selective pressure of the widespread use and misuse of antimicrobial agents [135,136]. Under pressure of antibiotic use, the environmental microbial flora of medical care institutions develops, increasing antibiotic resistance [62,137–140]. Patient acquisition of resistant microbial flora begins shortly after admission and is accelerated by antibiotic treatment [141]. This acquisition is paralleled by an increase in the prevalence of these bacteria as causative agents in health care infections.

Given the close relationship between antimicrobial use and antimicrobial resistance, efforts to optimize antimicrobial use in the hospital setting have received increased attention. To address this urgent need, antimicrobial stewardship programs have been developed at many institutions [142,143]. The exact components of such a program must be carefully tailored to the needs and resources of the institution, but may include education of prescribers regarding proper antimicrobial usage, creation of an antimicrobial formulary with restricted prescribing of targeted agents, and review of antimicrobial prescribing with feedback to prescribers [142]. Antibiotic stewardship programs should be administered by multidisciplinary teams composed of infectious diseases physicians, clinical pharmacists, clinical microbiologists, and infection control practitioners and should be actively supported by hospital administrators [142].

Another important component of the emergence of antimicrobial resistance is transmission of resistant organisms [135]. Spread of resistant organisms may occur directly from patient to patient or indirectly via health care workers or inanimate objects. The importance of transmission has been clearly demonstrated for several gram-positive nosocomial pathogens (ie, MRSA and VRE) [135]. Although genetic relatedness of hospital strains of some gram-negative organisms (eg, ESBL-producing Enterobacteriaceae, P aeruginosa, A baumannii) has been demonstrated, the relative contribution of person-to-person spread among gram-negative organisms remains controversial [126,144,145]. The goal of infection control isolation protocols is to prevent transmission of microorganisms from infected or colonized patients to other patients, hospital visitors, and health care workers. Personal protective equipment (eg, gloves, gowns), rigorous attention to hand hygiene, and isolation of persons infected or colonized with resistant organisms (for example, in private rooms) are essential to accomplishing this goal. Appropriate isolation remains the cornerstone of infection control and is assuming greater importance as the prevalence of multiply antibiotic-resistant organisms increases [135,146]. There are often marked differences across institutions with regard to the prevalence and epidemiology of particular resistant organisms. As such, it is critical that an infection-control approach suited to the unique needs of the institution be developed. Both the Society for Healthcare Epidemiology and HICPAC have published guidelines focusing on the prevention and management of health care–acquired multidrug-resistant organisms [135,147].

Summary

Health care–acquired infections present a tremendous challenge to the care of hospitalized patients. As these infections have continued to increase in recent years, strategies to limit these increases and lessen the impact of infections are urgently needed. These efforts will require both more rigorous evaluations of risk factors for infection as well as comprehensive assessments of the impact of intervention strategies. A coordinated approach between hospital physicians, nursing, infection control, and antimicrobial stewardship, is essential to addressing this critical issue.

References

[1] Haley RW, Culver DH, White JW, et al. The nationwide nosocomial infection rate. A new need for vital statistics. Am J Epidemiol 1985;121(2):159–67.
[2] Burke JP. Infection control—a problem for patient safety. N Engl J Med 2003;348(7): 651–6.
[3] National Nosocomial Infections Surveillance S. National Nosocomial Infections Surveillance (NNIS) System Report, data summary from January 1992 through June 2004, issued October 2004. Am J Infect Control 2004;32(8):470–85.
[4] Eggimann P, Pittet D. Infection control in the ICU. Chest 2001;120(6):2059–93.
[5] Mortimer E, Lipsitz P, Wolinsky E, et al. Transmission of staphylococci between newborns. Am J Dis Child 1962;104:289–95.
[6] Boyce JM, Pittet D. Healthcare Infection Control Practices Advisory C, Force HSAIHHT. Guideline for hand hygiene in health-care settings. Recommendations of the healthcare infection control practices advisory committee and the HIPAC/SHEA/APIC/IDSA hand hygiene task force. Am J Infect Control 2002;30(8):S1–46.
[7] Larson E. A causal link between handwashing and risk of infection? Examination of the evidence. Infect Control 1988;9(1):28–36.
[8] Pittet D. Improving compliance with hand hygiene in hospitals. Infect Control Hosp Epidemiol 2000;21(6):381–6.
[9] Boyce JM, Kelliher S, Vallande N. Skin irritation and dryness associated with two hand-hygiene regimens: soap-and-water hand washing versus hand antisepsis with an alcoholic hand gel. Infect Control Hosp Epidemiol 2000;21(7):442–8 [see comment].
[10] Voss A, Widmer AF. No time for handwashing!? Handwashing versus alcoholic rub: can we afford 100% compliance? Infect Control Hosp Epidemiol 1997;18(3):205–8.
[11] Boyce JM, Pittet D. Improving hand hygiene in healthcare settings. In: Lautenbach E, Woeltje K, editors. Practical handbook for healthcare epidemiologists. 2nd edition. Thorofare (NJ): SLACK Incorporated; 2004. p. 213–22.
[12] Pittet D, Wenzel RP. Nosocomial bloodstream infections. Secular trends in rates, mortality, and contribution to total hospital deaths. Arch Intern Med 1995;155(11):1177–84.
[13] Richards MJ, Edwards JR, Culver DH, et al. Nosocomial infections in combined medical-surgical intensive care units in the United States. Infect Control Hosp Epidemiol 2000; 21(8):510–5.
[14] Jarvis WR, Edwards JR, Culver DH, et al. Nosocomial infection rates in adult and pediatric intensive care units in the United States. National nosocomial infections surveillance system. Am J Med 1991;91(3B):185S–91S.

[15] Banerjee SN, Emori TG, Culver DH, et al. Secular trends in nosocomial primary blood-stream infections in the United States, 1980–1989. National nosocomial infections surveil-lance system. Am J Med 1991;91(3B):86S–9S.

[16] Mermel LA. Prevention of intravascular catheter-related infections. Ann Intern Med 2000;132(5):391–402 [see comment] [erratum appears in Ann Intern Med 2000 Sep 5;133(5):5].

[17] Raad I. Intravascular-catheter-related infections [see comment]. Lancet 1998;351(9106): 893–8.

[18] Miller PJ, Wenzel RP. Etiologic organisms as independent predictors of death and morbid-ity associated with bloodstream infections. J Infect Dis 1987;156(3):471–7.

[19] Setia U, Gross PA. Bacteremia in a community hospital: spectrum and mortality. Arch Intern Med 1977;137(12):1698–701.

[20] O'Grady NP, Alexander M, Dellinger EP, et al. Guidelines for the prevention of intravas-cular catheter-related infections. Centers for Disease Control and Prevention. MMWR Recomm Rep 2002;51(RR-10):1–29.

[21] Raad II, Hohn DC, Gilbreath BJ, et al. Prevention of central venous catheter-related infec-tions by using maximal sterile barrier precautions during insertion [see comment]. Infect Control Hosp Epidemiol 1994;15(4 Pt 1):231–8.

[22] Chaiyakunapruk N, Veenstra DL, Lipsky BA, et al. Chlorhexidine compared with povi-done-iodine solution for vascular catheter-site care: a meta-analysis. Ann Intern Med 2002;136(11):792–801 [see comment] [summary for patients in Ann Intern Med. 2002 Jun 4;136(11):I26; PMID: 12044142].

[23] Merrer J, De Jonghe B, Golliot F, et al. Complications of femoral and subclavian venous catheterization in critically ill patients: a randomized controlled trial [see comment]. JAMA 2001;286(6):700–7.

[24] Warren DK, Cosgrove SE, Diekema DJ, et al. A multicenter intervention to prevent cath-eter-associated bloodstream infections. Infect Control Hosp Epidemiol 2006;27(7):662–9.

[25] Eyer S, Brummitt C, Crossley K, et al. Catheter-related sepsis: prospective, randomized study of three methods of long-term catheter maintenance. Crit Care Med 1990;18(10): 1073–9.

[26] Raad I, Darouiche R, Dupuis J, et al. Central venous catheters coated with minocycline and rifampin for the prevention of catheter-related colonization and bloodstream infections. A randomized, double-blind trial. The Texas Medical Center Catheter Study Group [see com-ment]. Ann Intern Med 1997;127(4):267–74.

[27] Veenstra DL, Saint S, Saha S, et al. Efficacy of antiseptic-impregnated central venous cath-eters in preventing catheter-related bloodstream infection: a meta-analysis [see comment]. JAMA 1999;281(3):261–7.

[28] Safdar N. Bloodstream infection: an ounce of prevention is a ton of work [comment]. Infect Control Hosp Epidemiol 2005;26(6):511–4.

[29] Maki DG, Mermel LA, Klugar D, et al. The efficacy of a chlorhexidine-impregnanted sponge (Biopatch) for the prevention of intravascular catheter-related infection—a prospec-tive randomized controlled multicenter study [abstract 143C]. Presented at the Interscience Conference on Antimicrobial Agents and Chemotherapy. American Society for Microbiol-ogy. Toronto, Ontario, Canada. 2000.

[30] Rubinson L, Haponik EF, Wu AW, et al. Internists' adherence to guidelines for prevention of intravascular catheter infections. JAMA 2003;290(21):2802.

[31] Soifer NE, Borzak S, Edlin BR, et al. Prevention of peripheral venous catheter complica-tions with an intravenous therapy team: a randomized controlled trial. Arch Intern Med 1998;158(5):473–7.

[32] Berenholtz SM, Pronovost PJ, Lipsett PA, et al. Eliminating catheter-related bloodstream infections in the intensive care unit [see comment]. Crit Care Med 2004;32(10):2014–20.

[33] Pronovost P, Needham D, Berenholtz S, et al. An intervention to decrease catheter-related bloodstream infections in the ICU [see comment]. N Engl J Med 2006;355(26):2725–32.

[34] American Thoracic S, Infectious Diseases Society of A. Guidelines for the management of adults with hospital-acquired, ventilator-associated, and healthcare-associated pneumonia. Am J Respir Crit Care Med 2005;171(4):388–416 [see comment].

[35] Tablan OC, Anderson LJ, Besser R, et al. Guidelines for preventing health-care–associated pneumonia, 2003: recommendations of CDC and the Healthcare Infection Control Practices Advisory Committee. MMWR Recomm Rep 2004;53(RR-3):1–36.

[36] Hospital-acquired pneumonia in adults: diagnosis, assessment of severity, initial antimicrobial therapy, and preventive strategies. A consensus statement, American Thoracic Society, November 1995. Am J Respir Crit Care Med 1996;153(5):1711–25.

[37] Flanders SA, Collard HR, Saint S. Preventing nosocomial pneumonia. In: Lautenbach E, Woeltje K, editors. Practical handbook for healthcare epidemiologists. 2nd edition. Thorofare (NJ): SLACK Incorporated; 2004. p. 69–78.

[38] Rello J, Ollendorf DA, Oster G, et al. Epidemiology and outcomes of ventilator-associated pneumonia in a large US database. Chest 2002;122(6):2115–21 [see comment].

[39] Adair CG, Gorman SP, Feron BM, et al. Implications of endotracheal tube biofilm for ventilator-associated pneumonia. Intensive Care Med 1999;25(10):1072–6.

[40] Combes A, Figliolini C, Trouillet JL, et al. Incidence and outcome of polymicrobial ventilator-associated pneumonia. Chest 2002;121(5):1618–23 [see comment].

[41] Marik PE, Careau P. The role of anaerobes in patients with ventilator-associated pneumonia and aspiration pneumonia: a prospective study. Chest 1999;115(1):178–83 [see comment].

[42] Segal BH, Walsh TJ. Current approaches to diagnosis and treatment of invasive aspergillosis. Am J Respir Crit Care Med 2006;173(7):707–17.

[43] Horcajada JP, Pumarola T, Martinez JA, et al. A nosocomial outbreak of influenza during a period without influenza epidemic activity. Eur Respir J 2003;21(2):303–7.

[44] Brochard L, Mancebo J, Wysocki M, et al. Noninvasive ventilation for acute exacerbations of chronic obstructive pulmonary disease. N Engl J Med 1995;333(13):817–22 [see comment].

[45] Marelich GP, Murin S, Battistella F, et al. Protocol weaning of mechanical ventilation in medical and surgical patients by respiratory care practitioners and nurses: effect on weaning time and incidence of ventilator-associated pneumonia. Chest 2000;118(2):459–67.

[46] Torres A, Gatell JM, Aznar E, et al. Re-intubation increases the risk of nosocomial pneumonia in patients needing mechanical ventilation. Am J Respir Crit Care Med 1995;152(1): 137–41.

[47] Holzapfel L, Chastang C, Demingeon G, et al. A randomized study assessing the systematic search for maxillary sinusitis in nasotracheally mechanically ventilated patients. Influence of nosocomial maxillary sinusitis on the occurrence of ventilator-associated pneumonia. Am J Respir Crit Care Med 1999;159(3):695–701 [see comment].

[48] Craven DE, Goularte TA, Make BJ. Contaminated condensate in mechanical ventilator circuits. A risk factor for nosocomial pneumonia? Am Rev Respir Dis 1984;129(4): 625–8.

[49] Collard HR, Saint S, Matthay MA. Prevention of ventilator-associated pneumonia: an evidence-based systematic review. Ann Intern Med 2003;138(6):494–501 [see comment].

[50] Smulders K, van der Hoeven H, Weers-Pothoff I, et al. A randomized clinical trial of intermittent subglottic secretion drainage in patients receiving mechanical ventilation. Chest 2002;121(3):858–62 [see comment].

[51] Shorr AF, O'Malley PG. Continuous subglottic suctioning for the prevention of ventilator-associated pneumonia: potential economic implications. Chest 2001;119(1):228–35.

[52] Dezfulian C, Shojania K, Collard HR, et al. Subglottic secretion drainage for preventing ventilator-associated pneumonia: a meta-analysis. Am J Med 2005;118(1):11–8 [see comment].

[53] Orozco-Levi M, Torres A, Ferrer M, et al. Semirecumbent position protects from pulmonary aspiration but not completely from gastroesophageal reflux in mechanically ventilated patients. Am J Respir Crit Care Med 1995;152(4 Pt 1):1387–90.

[54] Drakulovic MB, Torres A, Bauer TT, et al. Supine body position as a risk factor for nosocomial pneumonia in mechanically ventilated patients: a randomised trial [see comment]. Lancet 1999;354(9193):1851–8.
[55] Byers JF, Sole ML. Analysis of factors related to the development of ventilator-associated pneumonia: use of existing databases [see comment]. Am J Crit Care 2000;9(5):344–9 [quiz 351].
[56] van Nieuwenhoven CA, Buskens E, van Tiel FH, et al. Relationship between methodological trial quality and the effects of selective digestive decontamination on pneumonia and mortality in critically ill patients [see comment]. JAMA 2001;286(3):335–40.
[57] Chlebicki MP, Safdar N. Topical chlorhexidine for prevention of ventilator-associated pneumonia: a meta-analysis [see comment]. Crit Care Med 2007;35(2):595–602.
[58] Yoneyama T, Yoshida M, Ohrui T, et al. Oral care reduces pneumonia in older patients in nursing homes [see comment]. J Am Geriatr Soc 2002;50(3):430–3.
[59] Cook D, Guyatt G, Marshall J, et al. A comparison of sucralfate and ranitidine for the prevention of upper gastrointestinal bleeding in patients requiring mechanical ventilation. Canadian Critical Care Trials Group [see comment]. N Engl J Med 1998;338(12):791–7.
[60] Heyland DK, Cook DJ, Schoenfeld PS, et al. The effect of acidified enteral feeds on gastric colonization in critically ill patients: results of a multicenter randomized trial. Canadian Critical Care Trials Group [see comment]. Crit Care Med 1999;27(11):2399–406.
[61] Tikhomirov E. WHO programme for the control of hospital infections. Chemioterapia 1987;6(3):148–51.
[62] Emori TG, Gaynes RP. An overview of nosocomial infections, including the role of the microbiology laboratory. Clin Microbiol Rev 1993;6(4):428–42.
[63] Wenzel RP, Osterman CA, Hunting KJ. Hospital-acquired infections. II. Infection rates by site, service and common procedures in a university hospital. Am J Epidemiol 1976;104(6):645–51.
[64] Stamm WE. Catheter-associated urinary tract infections: epidemiology, pathogenesis, and prevention. Am J Med 1991;91(3B):65S–71S.
[65] Rosenthal VD, Maki DG, Salomao R, et al. Device-associated nosocomial infections in 55 intensive care units of 8 developing countries. Ann Intern Med 2006;145(8):582–91.
[66] Hooton TM, Stamm WE. Diagnosis and treatment of uncomplicated urinary tract infection. Infect Dis Clin North Am 1997;11(3):551–81.
[67] Jarvis WR, Martone WJ. Predominant pathogens in hospital infections. J Antimicrob Chemother 1992;29(Suppl A):19–24.
[68] Stamm WE, Martin SM, Bennett JV. Epidemiology of nosocomial infection due to Gram-negative bacilli: aspects relevant to development and use of vaccines. J Infect Dis 1977;136(Suppl):S151–60.
[69] Bryan CS, Reynolds KL. Hospital-acquired bacteremic urinary tract infection: epidemiology and outcome. J Urol 1984;132(3):494–8.
[70] Krieger JN, Kaiser DL, Wenzel RP. Urinary tract etiology of bloodstream infections in hospitalized patients. J Infect Dis 1983;148(1):57–62.
[71] Weinstein MP, Towns ML, Quartey SM, et al. The clinical significance of positive blood cultures in the 1990s: a prospective comprehensive evaluation of the microbiology, epidemiology, and outcome of bacteremia and fungemia in adults. Clin Infect Dis 1997;24(4):584–602.
[72] Platt R, Polk BF, Murdock B, et al. Mortality associated with nosocomial urinary-tract infection. N Engl J Med 1982;307(11):637–42.
[73] Kunin CM, Douthitt S, Dancing J, et al. The association between the use of urinary catheters and morbidity and mortality among elderly patients in nursing homes. Am J Epidemiol 1992;135(3):291–301.
[74] Weinstein JW, Mazon D, Pantelick E, et al. A decade of prevalence surveys in a tertiary-care center: trends in nosocomial infection rates, device utilization, and patient acuity. Infect Control Hosp Epidemiol 1999;20(8):543–8.

[75] Saint S, Kaufman SR, Thompson M, et al. A reminder reduces urinary catheterization in hospitalized patients. Jt Comm J Qual Patient Saf 2005;31(8):455–62.
[76] Martin MA, Reichelderfer M. APIC guidelines for infection prevention and control in flexible endoscopy. Association for Professionals in Infection Control and Epidemiology, Inc. 1991, 1992, and 1993 APIC Guidelines Committee [see comment]. Am J Infect Control 1994;22(1):19–38.
[77] Garibaldi RA, Burke JP, Dickman ML, et al. Factors predisposing to bacteriuria during indwelling urethral catheterization. N Engl J Med 1974;291(5):215–9.
[78] Riley DK, Classen DC, Stevens LE, et al. A large randomized clinical trial of a silver-impregnated urinary catheter: lack of efficacy and staphylococcal superinfection. Am J Med 1995;98(4):349–56.
[79] Haley RW, Hooton TM, Culver DH, et al. Nosocomial infections in U.S. hospitals, 1975-1976: estimated frequency by selected characteristics of patients. Am J Med 1981;70(4):947–59.
[80] Soto SM, Smithson A, Horcajada JP, et al. Implication of biofilm formation in the persistence of urinary tract infection caused by uropathogenic Escherichia coli. Clin Microbiol Infect 2006;12(10):1034–6.
[81] Nickel JC, Ruseska I, Wright JB, et al. Tobramycin resistance of Pseudomonas aeruginosa cells growing as a biofilm on urinary catheter material. J Antimicrob Chemother 1985;27(4):619–24.
[82] Boscia JA, Abrutyn E, Kaye D. Asymptomatic bacteriuria in elderly persons: treat or do not treat? Ann Intern Med 1987;106(5):764–6.
[83] Nicolle LE, Bradley S, Colgan R, et al. Infectious Diseases Society of America guidelines for the diagnosis and treatment of asymptomatic bacteriuria in adults. Clin Infect Dis 2005;40(5):643–54 [erratum appears in Clin Infect Dis. 2005 May 15;40(10):1556].
[84] Kunin CM, McCormack RC. Prevention of catheter-induced urinary-tract infections by sterile closed drainage. N Engl J Med 1966;274(21):1155–61.
[85] Warren JW, Platt R, Thomas RJ, et al. Antibiotic irrigation and catheter-associated urinary-tract infections. N Engl J Med 1978;299(11):570–3.
[86] Johnson JR, Kuskowski MA, Wilt TJ. Systematic review: antimicrobial urinary catheters to prevent catheter-associated urinary tract infection in hospitalized patients. Ann Intern Med 2006;144(2):116–26.
[87] Shapiro J, Hoffmann J, Jersky J. A comparison of suprapubic and transurethral drainage for postoperative urinary retention in general surgical patients. Acta Chir Scand 1982;148(4):323–7.
[88] Saint S, Wiese J, Amory JK, et al. Are physicians aware of which of their patients have indwelling urinary catheters? Am J Med 2000;109(6):476–80.
[89] Huang WC, Wann SR, Lin SL, et al. Catheter-associated urinary tract infections in intensive care units can be reduced by prompting physicians to remove unnecessary catheters. Infect Control Hosp Epidemiol 2004;25(11):974–8.
[90] Wong ES. Guideline for prevention of catheter-associated urinary tract infections. Am J Infect Control 1983;11(1):28–36.
[91] Bouza E, Munoz P, Alonso R. Clinical manifestations, treatment and control of infections caused by Clostridium difficile. Clin Microbiol Infect 2005;11(Suppl 4):57–64.
[92] Kyne L, Hamel MB, Polavaram R, et al. Health care costs and mortality associated with nosocomial diarrhea due to Clostridium difficile. Clin Infect Dis 2002;34(3):346–53.
[93] Olson MM, Shanholtzer CJ, Lee JT Jr, et al. Ten years of prospective Clostridium difficile-associated disease surveillance and treatment at the Minneapolis VA Medical Center, 1982-1991 [see comment]. Infect Control Hosp Epidemiol 1994;15(6):371–81.
[94] McDonald LC, Owings M, Jernigan DB. Clostridium difficile infection in patients discharged from US short-stay hospitals, 1996-2003. Emerg Infect Dis 2006;12(3):409–15.
[95] Pepin J, Valiquette L, Alary ME, et al. Clostridium difficile-associated diarrhea in a region of Quebec from 1991 to 2003: a changing pattern of disease severity [see comment]. CMAJ 2004;171(5):466–72.

[96] Muto CA, Pokrywka M, Shutt K, et al. A large outbreak of *Clostridium difficile*-associated disease with an unexpected proportion of deaths and colectomies at a teaching hospital following increased fluoroquinolone use. Infect Control Hosp Epidemiol 2005;26(3): 273–80.

[97] Pepin J, Valiquette L, Cossette B. Mortality attributable to nosocomial *Clostridium difficile*-associated disease during an epidemic caused by a hypervirulent strain in Quebec [see comment]. CMAJ 2005;173(9):1037–42.

[98] Loo VG, Poirier L, Miller MA, et al. A predominantly clonal multi-institutional outbreak of *Clostridium difficile*-associated diarrhea with high morbidity and mortality. N Engl J Med 2005;353(23):2442–9 [see comment] [erratum appears in N Engl J Med. 2006 May 18;354(20):2200].

[99] Pepin J, Alary ME, Valiquette L, et al. Increasing risk of relapse after treatment of *Clostridium difficile* colitis in Quebec, Canada [see comment]. Clin Infect Dis 2005;40(11):1591–7.

[100] McDonald LC, Killgore GE, Thompson A, et al. An epidemic, toxin gene-variant strain of *Clostridium difficile* [see comment]. N Engl J Med 2005;353(23):2433–41.

[101] Bartlett JG. Narrative review: the new epidemic of *Clostridium difficile*-associated enteric disease. Ann Intern Med 2006;145(10):758–64.

[102] Kyne L, Sougioultzis S, McFarland LV, et al. Underlying disease severity as a major risk factor for nosocomial *Clostridium difficile* diarrhea. Infect Control Hosp Epidemiol 2002; 23(11):653–9.

[103] Bliss DZ, Johnson S, Savik K, et al. Acquisition of *Clostridium difficile* and *Clostridium difficile*-associated diarrhea in hospitalized patients receiving tube feeding. Ann Intern Med 1998;129(12):1012–9.

[104] Dial S, Alrasadi K, Manoukian C, et al. Risk of *Clostridium difficile* diarrhea among hospital inpatients prescribed proton pump inhibitors: cohort and case-control studies [see comment]. CMAJ 2004;171(1):33–8.

[105] Bartlett JG. Clinical practice. Antibiotic-associated diarrhea [see comment]. N Engl J Med 2002;346(5):334–9.

[106] Tedesco FJ, Barton RW, Alpers DH. Clindamycin-associated colitis. A prospective study. Ann Intern Med 1974;81(4):429–33.

[107] Viscidi R, Willey S, Bartlett JG. Isolation rates and toxigenic potential of *Clostridium difficile* isolates from various patient populations. Gastroenterology 1981;81(1):5–9.

[108] McFarland LV, Mulligan ME, Kwok RY, et al. Nosocomial acquisition of *Clostridium difficile* infection [see comment]. N Engl J Med 1989;320(4):204–10.

[109] Centers for Disease C, Prevention. Severe *Clostridium difficile*-associated disease in populations previously at low risk–four states. 2005. MMWR Morb Mortal Wkly Rep 2005; 54(47):1201–5.

[110] Carling P, Fung T, Killion A, et al. Favorable impact of a multidisciplinary antibiotic management program conducted during 7 years. Infect Control Hosp Epidemiol 2003;24(9): 699–706.

[111] Fishman N. Antimicrobial stewardship. Am J Med 2006;119(6 Suppl 1):S53–61 [discussion: S62–70].

[112] Gaynes R, Rimland D, Killum E, et al. Outbreak of *Clostridium difficile* infection in a long-term care facility: association with gatifloxacin use [see comment]. Clin Infect Dis 2004; 38(5):640–5.

[113] Thomas C, Riley TV. Restriction of third generation cephalosporin use reduces the incidence of *Clostridium difficile*-associated diarrhoea in hospitalised patients. Commun Dis Intell 2003;27(Suppl):S28–31.

[114] Johnson S, Samore MH, Farrow KA, et al. Epidemics of diarrhea caused by a clindamycin-resistant strain of *Clostridium difficile* in four hospitals. N Engl J Med 1999;341(22): 1645–51.

[115] Gerding DN, Johnson S, Peterson LR, et al. *Clostridium difficile*-associated diarrhea and colitis. Infect Control Hosp Epidemiol 1995;16(8):459–77.

[116] Zafar AB, Gaydos LA, Furlong WB, et al. Effectiveness of infection control program in controlling nosocomial *Clostridium difficile*. Am J Infect Control 1998;26(6):588–93.

[117] Tenover FC. Development and spread of bacterial resistance to antimicrobial agents: an overview [see comment]. Clin Infect Dis 2001;33(Suppl 3):S108–15.

[118] Spellberg B, Powers JH, Brass EP, et al. Trends in antimicrobial drug development: implications for the future. Clin Infect Dis 2004;38(9):1279–86.

[119] Cohen ML. Epidemiology of drug resistance: implications for a post-antimicrobial era [see comment]. Science 1992;257(5073):1050–5.

[120] Holmberg SD, Solomon SL, Blake PA. Health and economic impacts of antimicrobial resistance. Rev Infect Dis 1987;9(6):1065–78.

[121] Cosgrove SE. The relationship between antimicrobial resistance and patient outcomes: mortality, length of hospital stay, and health care costs. Clin Infect Dis 2006;42(Suppl 2):S82–9.

[122] Cosgrove SE, Carmeli Y. The impact of antimicrobial resistance on health and economic outcomes. Clin Infect Dis 2003;36(11):1433–7.

[123] US C, Office of Technology A. Impacts of antibiotic-resistant bacteria. Washington, DC: US Government Printing Office; 1995. OTA-H-629.

[124] Vergis EN, Hayden MK, Chow JW, et al. Determinants of vancomycin resistance and mortality rates in enterococcal bacteremia. a prospective multicenter study. Ann Intern Med 2001;135(7):484–92.

[125] Blot SI, Vandewoude KH, Hoste EA, et al. Outcome and attributable mortality in critically Ill patients with bacteremia involving methicillin-susceptible and methicillin-resistant *Staphylococcus aureus* [see comment]. Arch Intern Med 2002;162(19):2229–35.

[126] Lautenbach E, Patel JB, Bilker WB, et al. Extended-spectrum beta-lactamase-producing *Escherichia coli* and *Klebsiella pneumoniae*: risk factors for infection and impact of resistance on outcomes. Clin Infect Dis 2001;32(8):1162–71.

[127] Vila J, Simon K, Ruiz J, et al. Are quinolone-resistant uropathogenic *Escherichia coli* less virulent? J Infect Dis 2002;186(7):1039–42.

[128] Blazquez R, Menasalvas A, Carpena I, et al. Invasive disease caused by ciprofloxacin-resistant uropathogenic *Escherichia coli*. Eur J Clin Microbiol Infect Dis 1999;18(7):503–5.

[129] Maslow JN, Lautenbach E, Glaze T, et al. Colonization with extraintestinal pathogenic *Escherichia coli* among nursing home residents and its relationship to fluoroquinolone resistance. Antimicrob Agents Chemother 2004;48(9):3618–20.

[130] Kollef MH, Ward S, Sherman G, et al. Inadequate treatment of nosocomial infections is associated with certain empiric antibiotic choices. Crit Care Med 2000;28(10):3456–64.

[131] Lodise TP, McKinnon PS, Swiderski L, et al. Outcomes analysis of delayed antibiotic treatment for hospital-acquired *Staphylococcus aureus* bacteremia. Clin Infect Dis 2003;36(11):1418–23.

[132] Harbarth S, Garbino J, Pugin J, et al. Inappropriate initial antimicrobial therapy and its effect on survival in a clinical trial of immunomodulating therapy for severe sepsis [see comment]. Am J Med 2003;115(7):529–35.

[133] Paterson DL, Ko WC, Von Gottberg A, et al. International prospective study of *Klebsiella pneumoniae* bacteremia: implications of extended-spectrum beta-lactamase production in nosocomial infections. Ann Intern Med 2004;140(1):26–32 [summary for patients in Ann Intern Med. 2004 Jan 6;140(1):I43; PMID: 14706996].

[134] Hyle EP, Lipworth AD, Zaoutis TE, et al. Impact of inadequate initial antimicrobial therapy on mortality in infections due to extended-spectrum beta-lactamase-producing Enterobacteriaceae: variability by site of infection. Arch Intern Med 2005;165(12):1375–80.

[135] Muto CA, Jernigan JA, Ostrowsky BE, et al. SHEA guideline for preventing nosocomial transmission of multidrug-resistant strains of *Staphylococcus aureus* and *Enterococcus* [see comment]. Infect Control Hosp Epidemiol 2003;24(5):362–86.

[136] Safdar N, Maki DG. The commonality of risk factors for nosocomial colonization and infection with antimicrobial-resistant *Staphylococcus aureus, Enterococcus*, gram-negative bacilli, *Clostridium difficile*, and *Candida*. Ann Intern Med 2002;136(11):834–44.

[137] McGowan JE Jr. Antimicrobial resistance in hospital organisms and its relation to antibiotic use. Rev Infect Dis 1983;5(6):1033–48.
[138] Spach DH, Silverstein FE, Stamm WE. Transmission of infection by gastrointestinal endoscopy and bronchoscopy. Ann Intern Med 1993;118(2):117–28 [see comment].
[139] Donskey CJ. The role of the intestinal tract as a reservoir and source for transmission of nosocomial pathogens. Clin Infect Dis 2004;39(2):219–26.
[140] Donskey CJ, Chowdhry TK, Hecker MT, et al. Effect of antibiotic therapy on the density of vancomycin-resistant enterococci in the stool of colonized patients [see comment]. N Engl J Med 2000;343(26):1925–32.
[141] Selden R, Lee S, Wang WL, et al. Nosocomial *Klebsiella* infections: intestinal colonization as a reservoir. Ann Intern Med 1971;74(5):657–64.
[142] MacDougall C, Polk RE. Antimicrobial stewardship programs in health care systems. Clin Microbiol Rev 2005;18(4):638–56.
[143] John JF Jr, Fishman NO. Programmatic role of the infectious diseases physician in controlling antimicrobial costs in the hospital. Clin Infect Dis 1997;24(3):471–85.
[144] Paterson DL. The epidemiological profile of infections with multidrug-resistant *Pseudomonas aeruginosa* and *Acinetobacter* species. Clin Infect Dis 2006;43(Suppl 2):S43–8.
[145] Harris AD, McGregor JC, Furuno JP. What infection control interventions should be undertaken to control multidrug-resistant gram-negative bacteria? Clin Infect Dis 2006; 43(Suppl 2):S57–61.
[146] Garner JS. Guideline for isolation precautions in hospitals. The hospital infection control practices advisory committee. Infect Control Hosp Epidemiol 1996;17(1):53–80 [erratum appears in Infect Control Hosp Epidemiol 1996 Apr;17(4):214].
[147] Siegel J, Rhinehart E, Jackson M, et al. Committee tHICPAC. Management of multidrug-resistant organsims in healtcare settings. Available at: http://www.cdc.gov/ncidod/dhqp/pdf/ar/mdroGuideline2006.pdf, 2006. Accessed June 2, 2007.

THE MEDICAL
CLINICS
OF NORTH AMERICA

Med Clin N Am 92 (2008) 315–324

Care Transitions for Hospitalized Patients

Vineet M. Arora, MD, MA[a],*, Jeanne M. Farnan, MD[b]

[a]Department of Medicine, University of Chicago, 5841 South Maryland Avenue, MC 2007,
AMB W216, Chicago, IL 60637, USA
[b]Department of Medicine, University of Chicago, 5841 South Maryland Avenue, MC 2007,
AMB B226A, Chicago, IL 60637, USA

The development of safe care transitions has grown in importance with shortened hospital lengths of stay and with discontinuity of care related to multiple clinicians and hand-offs of care responsibility. These transitions can have detrimental effects on the quality and safety of health care delivery. Patients and their families entering the realm of inpatient care may be surprised by the rapid pace of care delivery and confused about the membership of the health care team that increasingly does not include a patient's primary care physician. Similarly, when patients leave the acute-care hospital and are discharged to an ambulatory setting or other facility, patients, their caregivers, and their ambulatory physicians may not be aware of new diagnoses or changes to their treatment plan, such as new or changed medications. These transitions become especially difficult for patients who have complex comorbidities, advanced age, and low health literacy.

The transition from inpatient hospitalization to outpatient care is not the only transition that plagues the care of hospitalized patients. In-hospital care also is characterized by many transitions between providers to ensure around-the-clock coverage by hospital-based physicians. This process, often known as the hand-off, is complicated further in academic teaching hospitals because of resident work-hour regulations. Often, competing priorities and time constraints can hamper an effective hand-off, potentially resulting in failures of communication, such as content omissions, which can have a negative impact on patient care [1]. It is during these times of transition, admission, hospitalization, and discharge that patients' vulnerability is

Dr. Vineet Arora is supported by Hartford Geriatrics Health Outcomes Research Award.
* Corresponding author.
 E-mail address: varora@medicine.bsd.uchicago.edu (V.M. Arora).

revealed and patient safety may be compromised. This article discusses the types of care transitions that hospitalized patients face, the importance of effective communication among providers to ensure patient safety, and strategies to promote safe and high-quality care transitions.

Barriers to inpatient-outpatient transitions

Patients experience many transitions and hand-offs as they navigate an increasingly complex health care system. Physician specialization, patient complexity, and the distributed nature of health care services have created a need for additional communication and coordination of care. With the increasing number of hospitalists in this country, physicians who care for patients during hospitalization often are not patients' primary care physicians. As a result, no single physician supervises the transition from outpatient to inpatient care and back again. Therefore, effective communication and coordination is important particularly at times of inpatient-outpatient transition, such as admission to and discharge from the hospital, and during major decision points within the hospital course [1–3].

Although it generally is agreed that effective communication is essential to safe patient care, health care providers continue to be challenged to design communication strategies that are consistent and reliable. As a result, communication issues frequently are cited as major contributors to adverse events. The Joint Commission [4] reports communication failures as the root cause of more than 70% of sentinel events. Not surprisingly, because of the complexity and volume of the interventions performed in the inpatient setting, communication failures can be major threats to ensuring patient safety during transitions from an inpatient to outpatient setting.

One of the primary goals of a hospital medicine program is to deliver quality inpatient care to patients who are hospitalized for an acute complaint. The success of a hospital care plan, however, is dependent on critical communication between a hospital-based physician and a patient's primary care physician [5]. Ensuring that a patient's hospital course and treatment, addition of new medications, and follow-up planning are relayed to a primary care physician establishes continuity of care between the inpatient and outpatient arenas. This is important particularly because primary care physicians often wish to remain involved in patients hospital care but lack the systems within which to interact effectively with a hospital care team [6].

Effective communication of information is important particularly to prevent gaps in clinical knowledge that may occur during transition into and out of the hospital. More specifically, lack of a structured approach to relaying information during admission and discharge and absence of reliable systems to ensure the transmission of such information can prevent the delivery of vital information to those assuming care of a patient. For example, in one study, medication issues at the time of hospital admission were a common source of error, with more than 40% of patients having an omission of a regularly used medication [7]. Approximately 38% of discrepancies were judged to be serious or have the potential to cause moderate to severe harm. Similar problems occur during discharge. In addition to medication problems, many patients are discharged from hospitals with test results pending, and physicians often are unaware of potentially actionable test results returning after discharge [8]. These problems reflect the need for systems-level solutions to track information and help facilitate communication during these transition points.

The growth of the hospitalist model in the context of management of older, sicker patients who have more comorbidities and therapies suggests that efforts to address inpatient-ambulatory transitions will become increasingly important [5]. Preliminary survey work with primary care physicians indicates that the majority believe hospitalists are a good idea (68%), but only 56% were satisfied with communication with hospitalists and only one third believed that they had received discharge summaries in a timely fashion that facilitated safe and effective management of patients on return to their practice [6]. The increasing use of hospitalists heralds the need for improved skills and competencies in the care of hospitalized patients and the transit of patients from the ambulatory setting into and throughout their hospitalization until discharge. Recognizing this, the Society of Hospital Medicine has included care transitions as critical to the core competencies for hospitalists [9]. Hospitalists also must demonstrate the ability to communicate effectively with patients and collaborating physicians, most importantly patients' primary care physicians.

Transitions of care at admission and discharge are fraught with fragmented and incomplete information transfer and represent points of patient vulnerability. Several factors that contribute to the risks of these care transitions include inefficient and unstructured systems for communication of important clinical data, such as medication changes or tests that are pending; lack of a longitudinal patient relationship; and standardized follow-up procedures. The infrequency of hospitalist-primary care physician communication and omission of details of patients' hospital course have further adverse impacts on patient care [10].

Strategies to improve inpatient–outpatient transitions

There are several strategies that may be used to counteract many common barriers to the delivery of coordinated patient care (Table 1). Ensuring that a patient's hospital course and treatment and information about any medication changes and specific follow-up needs are relayed to the primary care physician establishes continuity of care between the inpatient and outpatient arenas. The maintenance of open lines of communication between inpatient and outpatient physicians should occur at several points within

Table 1
Inpatient-outpatient transitions

Transition	Participants	Barriers	Successful strategies
Admission (outpatient to inpatient)	Admitting physicians (emergency department, PCP)	Perception of PCPs' suggestions as "intrusive"; PCP assuming managerial role in plan of care	Formal system for communication between PCP and hospital physician
	Inpatient physicians (nocturnists, other hospitalists, house staff)	Inpatient physicians' lack of personal and longitudinal relationship with patient	Patient empowerment or other adjunct transition coach
Discharge (inpatient to outpatient)	Home health service organizations/ professionals, including nurses, physical therapists	Timely transmission of accurate information related to the hospitalization	Process for medication reconciliation during transitions
	Primary care physician Hospitalist Family/primary caregivers	Involving PCP only at discharge without relaying information during hospitalization	System for follow-up of tests and other laboratory results that may be pending

a patient's hospital course, including admission, discharge, and times of critical decision making or major change in status during a hospitalization. This collaborative approach allows inpatient physicians to relay the trajectory of the hospital course as opposed to a single snapshot at the moment of discharge. In addition, the established relationship between patients and their primary care physicians may inform critical decisions to be made by the inpatient team and facilitate patient-centered care [11].

Initiatives that involve patients in their own care during the inpatient to outpatient transition show improved outcomes [12]. Coleman and colleagues [12] demonstrated lower readmission rates and lower hospital costs for older patients who received a "care transitions intervention," which encouraged patients to take a more active role in their care and provided tools and guidance from a "transition coach" to promote communication across transitions.

The use of a standardized approach to medication reconciliation or ensuring the appropriate addition, continuation, and discontinuation of medications from the inpatient to ambulatory transition can be an important strategy to facilitate communication regarding medication changes with patients' primary care physicians and with patients. When patients move from one setting to another, medication reconciliation ensures that an accurate, up-to-date list of medications is maintained and consistent with the plan of care. Not surprisingly, medication reconciliation is the subject of the 2005 National Patient Safety Goal from the Joint Commission [13]. The Institute of Healthcare Improvement, as part of its 100,000 Lives

Campaign, and the Massachusetts Coalition for the Prevention of Medical Errors have developed tools to assist in the medication reconciliation process [13,14].

Finally, as patients are discharged and returned to the care of their ambulatory physician, accurate and complete communication of a patient's hospital course, medication changes, and required follow-up are essential for maintaining continuity of care. Successful strategies for improving the coordination of care during this transition include standardizing the type of content that is relayed to primary care physicians via a specific content checklist [15] or via computerized documentation of patients' hospital stay and follow-up [10]. The Society of Hospital Medicine has developed a discharge checklist that can be used for this purpose [1]. In addition, the implementation of a postdischarge clinic, one structured for interim visits after hospital discharge should patients be unable to obtain timely visits with a primary care physician, are effective in reducing postdischarge emergency department visits [16].

Barriers to in-hospital hand-offs

An increased focus on the vulnerability of in-hospital transitions or patient hand-offs has occurred for a variety of reasons. These include implementation of restricted resident duty hours by the Accreditation Council of Graduate Medical Education [17] and the demand for in-hospital 24-hour coverage by various groups, such as Leapfrog Group. Poor communication at the time of hand-offs is implicated in near misses and adverse events in a variety of health care contexts, including nursing hand-over, physician sign-out of patients, and emergency medicine shift changes [18,19]. Despite the increased focus on the vulnerability of hand-offs, few medical trainees or hospitalists receive formal education on how to perform effective hand-offs.

Two types of in-hospital transition occur: shift change and service change (Table 2). Shift change involves the temporary change in responsibility as a primary provider or team transfers care to an evening or night shift. Patients often are moved from an active period of therapeutic management to a "holding phase" until the return of the regular provider or clinical team [20]. Physicians accepting a hand-off have a mandate to deal with emergencies, but planning, communication of care plans to patients and families, and nonurgent diagnostic testing usually are suspended.

Service change involves a more long-term change in responsibility, in which a physician or team of providers who has been caring for a group of patients for an extended period, usually a week or greater, changes, such that a new physician or team of providers assumes control of patient care. This service hand-off, unlike the shift change that anticipates potential overnight emergencies, involves the relay of a patients' acute needs for hospitalization, the hospital course to date, current health status, and overall continued plan of care. Often used synonymously with hand-off, sign-out

Table 2
In-hospital transitions

Transition	Participants	Barriers	Successful strategies
Shift change	Hospitalist/attending physician Midlevel clinician Nocturnist (night-covering physician) House staff	Competing time pressures, distractions, and interruptions leading to ineffective hand-off of patient information, resulting in breakdowns of communication (ie, omissions), lack of professional responsibility	Ensure verbal (preferably face-to-face) exchange with interactive questioning and limited interruptions Standard template or technology solution to facilitate accurate and up-to-date information
Service change	Hospitalist/attending physician Midlevel clinician House staff	Lack of continued interaction with patient and feedback, snapshot of patient's entire hospital course, competing time pressures	Use of structured language (ie, read-back or SBAR) Creation of standard hand-off protocol (process map and customized checklist) Training for frontline users

can refer to the written vehicle (eg, document or electronic file), the transfer of patient information during a hand-off, or the verbal communication that takes place at the time of any of these hand-offs [21].

Shift and service changes represent transitions within patients' hospital course in which the transfer of patient care responsibility may contribute to near-miss or adverse events. The shift change occurs more frequently, usually on a nightly basis, and the potential for harm frequently revolves around the lack of a personal relationship between covering physicians and patients and the resulting absence of the acknowledgment of professional responsibility. Covering physicians are expected to be prepared to manage patient emergencies that may arise; however, detailed information about patients and all facets of their medical history often is omitted. As such, these covering physicians often are equipped to manage critical illness but not the nuances of patients' chronic medical illnesses.

Unfortunately, the barriers present in this transition include accepting physicians' limited knowledge of the service of patients, which includes the lack of an a priori personal relationship with patients and entry into the care plan during a potentially difficult time. It also is possible that out-going physicians, or those who have completed their required service time, no longer may be invested in the ongoing care of this group of patients, especially those who have been passed from physician to physician in multiple service changes.

Several studies have demonstrated that ineffective physician-physician hand-offs during shift change can harm patients. Arora and colleagues [1] have used critical incident technique to interview internal medicine interns regarding communication failures during the verbal and written sign-out of patients. They found that communication failures during patient sign-out are characterized by omissions of content or failure-prone communication processes, which often lead to uncertainty in patient care decisions, resulting in unnecessary or repeat work. In addition, Solet and colleagues [3] reviewed the hand-offs at three Indiana hospitals and identified common reasons for poor information transmittal. These included noisy, distracting physical settings that impede conversation; the hierarchic nature of medicine (which can discourage open discussion between health professionals); language barriers among doctors; lack of face-to-face communication; and time pressures. To date, no controlled interventions evaluating the effect of a service change or shift change on patient outcomes have been performed. In one observational study, patients were more likely to suffer from a preventable adverse event (26% compared with 12% [odds ratio 3.5; $P = .01$]) when the cross-covering physician (not a physician on their primary team) was responsible for their care [22].

Often hospitalists work schedules of 8- to 12-hour shifts, which involve transfer of care between physicians, as individuals completing their shift relay the plan of care to those reporting for duty. Ensuring that pertinent and accurate information, including medications and their dosages, plans for diagnostic testing, and code status, is transmitted to these covering physicians improves the quality of care delivered. Often, competing priorities and time constraints can hamper an effective hand-off, potentially resulting in failures of communication, such as content omissions, which can have a negative impact on patient care [1]. An effective hand-off includes the transfer of critical patient information needed to continue care for a patient and the acceptance of the professional responsibility of continued care for a patient [23].

Strategies to improve in-hospital hand-offs

In the effort to improve in-hospital transitions, it is important to review the effect of interventions targeted at these hand-offs. Unfortunately, unlike inpatient-outpatient transitions, fewer controlled interventions exist to guide improvements in inpatient transitions. Nevertheless, the Joint Commission has made standardized hand-off communications the subject of a 2006 National Patient Safety Goal [2]. The goal requires hospitals to "implement a standardized approach to hand-off communications, including an opportunity to ask and respond to questions." The implementation expectations are focused on a hand-off process that is interactive, allows for the communication of up-to-date information that includes recent changes and anticipated events, facilitates verification or read-back as appropriate, and contains minimal interruptions. Support for these goals is found in reviewing the standards for hand-offs developed by other high-risk non–health care industries.

Patterson and colleagues [24] have conducted direct observations of hand-offs in other 24-hour, high-risk industries, such as aviation, transportation, and nuclear power. From this work, they derived as series of effective strategies that could be applied to health care. The use of standardization and a face-to-face verbal update with interactive questioning emerged as a key strategies from these observations. In addition, use of a written summary, access to updated information, limited interruptions, and the unambiguous transfer of professional responsibility were cited as key components of an effective and safe hand-off strategy.

The situational briefing model (Situation, Background, Assessment, Recommendation [SBAR]) is a technique that originated in the Navy to communicate critical content. This model has been used by Leonard and colleagues [25] to improve nurse communication of critical information to physicians. More recently, hospitals have been adopting the SBAR model as a way to meet the Joint Commission goal for standardized hand-offs for physician-physician communication and nursing shift change [26]. SBAR includes the activity of reading back the information or specific instruction. During requested read-back of 822 laboratory results, it reduced the number of errors [27]: in addition to detection and correction of all 29 errors, use of a read-back was cost effective. Although it has been adopted widely, it is important that the SBAR model be customized for frontline users.

Structured templates, in particular computer-aided sign-outs, have been used at several institutions with success. Van Eaton and colleagues [28] implemented and studied the University of Washington homegrown electronic sign-out system, known as UW Computerized Rounding and Sign-out (UW Cores). This system enhances patient care by decreasing patients missed on resident rounds and improving resident-reported quality of sign-out and continuity of care. Some outcomes of its use include a decrease—by up to 3 hours per week (range 1.5 to 3 hours)—in the time used by residents to complete rounds and a decrease in time spent recopying data during prerounding. Petersen and colleagues [29] demonstrated a trend toward a reduction of preventable adverse events after the implementation of a computerized sign-out system. Lee and colleagues [30] demonstrated in a randomized controlled trial that a standard sign-out card with set fields resulted in higher quality sign-outs with improved data recording.

In addition to strategies to improve communication during in-hospital transitions, formal training is needed. Horwitz and colleagues [31] in a national mail survey to chief residents in internal medicine demonstrated that most programs do not have formal education for sign-outs. Given the focus on meeting the Joint Commission goal, formal training for frontline clinicians in the use of standard hand-off protocols is a priority. Creating hand-off process maps and customized checklists can facilitate the creation and implementation of a standard hand-off protocol [23]. These documents then can be used to educate new users and obtain buy-in about the hand-off protocol. Finally, any sign-out or hand-off program must include an evaluation strategy to determine its effectiveness and help shape future changes or revisions to training or the hand-off process itself.

Summary

Ensuring safe care transitions is a core part of hospital medicine. These transitions include inpatient-outpatient transitions and in-hospital transitions. To ensure safe care during these transitions, clinicians should be aware of the types of transitions and the way in which these transitions can impede safe patient care. With this knowledge, strategies to ensure patient safety during care transitions can be adopted, and training directed at teaching physicians safe hand-off practices could be developed and supported.

Acknowledgments

We are grateful for the input and support of Julie Johnson, MSPH, PhD, in addition to the assistance of Megan Tormey in manuscript preparation.

References

[1] Arora V, Johnson J, Lovinger D, et al. Communication failures in patient sign out and suggestions for improvement: a critical incident analysis. Qual Saf Health Care 2005;14: 401–7.

[2] Cook R, Render M, Woods D. Gaps in the continuity of care and progress on patient safety. BMJ 2000;320(7237):791–4.

[3] Solet D, Norvell J, Rutan G, et al. Lost in translation: challenges and opportunities in physician-to-physician communication during patient hand-offs. Acad Med 2005;80(12): 1094–9.

[4] The Joint Commission: sentinel event statistics. Available at: www.jcaho.org/accredited+ organizations/sentinel+events+statistics.html. Accessed April 2007.

[5] Goldman L, Panilat S, Whitcomb W. Passing the clinical baton: 6 principles to guide hospitalists. Am J Med 2001;111(9B):36S–9S.

[6] Pantilat S, Lindenauer P, Katz P, et al. Primary care physicians attitudes regarding communication with hospitalists. Am J Med 2001;111(9B):15S–20S.

[7] Cornish P, Knowles S, Marchesano R, et al. Unintended medication discrepancies at the time of hospital admission. Arch Intern Med 2005;165(4):424–9.

[8] Roy C, Poon E, Karson A, et al. Patient safety concerns arising from test results that return after hospital discharge. Ann Intern Med 2005;143(2):121–31.

[9] Dressler DD, Pistoria MJ, Budnitz TL, et al. Core competencies in hospital medicine: development and methodology. J Hosp Med 2006;1(1):48–56.

[10] Kripalani S, LeFevre F, Phillips C, et al. Deficits in communication and information transfer between hospital-based and primary-care physicians: implications for patient safety and continuity of care. JAMA 2007;297(8):831–41.

[11] Coleman E, Berenson R. Lost in transition: challenges and opportunities for improving the quality of transitional care. Ann Intern Med 2004;140:533–6.

[12] Coleman E, Parry C, Chalmers S, et al. The care transitions intervention: results of a randomized controlled trial. Arch Intern Med 2006;166:1822–8.

[13] The Joint Commission: 2005 hospital national patient safety goals. Available at: http://www.jointcommission.org/PatientSafety/NationalPatientSafetyGoals/05_hap_npsgs.htm. Accessed April 2007.

[14] Institute for Healthcare Improvement: medication systems. Available at: http://www.ihi.org/IHI/Topics/PatientSafety/MedicationSystems/. Accessed April 2007.

[15] Halasyamani L, Kripilani S, Coleman E, et al. Transition of care for hospitalized elderly patients: development of a discharge checklist for hospitalists. J Hosp Med 2006;1(6): 354–60.

[16] Diem S, Prochazka A, Meyer T, et al. Effects of a postdischarge clinical on housestaff satisfaction and utilization of hospital services. J Gen Intern Med 1996;11(3):179–81.

[17] Accreditation Council for Graduate Medical Education. Available at: http://www.acgme.org/DutyHours/dutyHrsLang.pdf. Accessed April 2007.

[18] Beach C, Croskerry P, Shapiro M. Center for safety in emergency care. Profiles in patient safety: emergency care transitions. Acad Emerg Med 2003;10:364–7.

[19] Lally S. An investigation into the functions of nurses' communication at the inter-shift handover. J Nurs Manag 1999;7:29–36.

[20] Philibert I, Leach D. Re-framing continuity of care for this century. Qual Saf Health Care 2005;14(6):394–6.

[21] Vidyarthi A, Arora V, Schnipper J, et al. Managing discontinuity in academic medical centers: strategies for a safe and effective resident sign-out. J Hosp Med 2006;1(4):257–66.

[22] Petersen LA, Brennan TA, O'Neil AC, et al. Does housestaff discontinuity of care increase the risk for preventable adverse events? Ann Intern Med 1994;121(11):866–72.

[23] Arora V, Johnson J. A model for building a standardized hand-off protocol. Jt Comm J Qual Patient Saf 2006;32(11):645–55.

[24] Patterson E, Roth E, Woods D, et al. Hand-off strategies in settings with high consequences for failure: lessons for health care operations. Int J Qual Health Care 2004;16:125–32.

[25] Leonard M, Graham S, Bonacum D. The human factor: the critical importance of effective teamwork and communication in providing safe care. Qual Saf Health Care 2004; 13(Suppl 1):i85–90.

[26] Haig K, Sutton S, Whittington J. SBAR: a shared mental model for improving communication between clinicians. Jt Comm J Qual Patient Saf 2006;32(3):167–75.

[27] Barenfanger J, Sautter R, Lang D, et al. Improving patient safety by repeating (read-back) telephone reports of critical information. Am J Clin Pathol 2004;121(6):801–3.

[28] Van Eaton E, Horvath K, Lober W, et al. A randomized, controlled trial evaluating the impact of a computerized rounding and sign-out system on continuity of care and resident work hours. J Am Coll Surg 2005;200:538–45.

[29] Petersen L, Orav E, Teich J, et al. Using a computerized sign-out program to improve continuity of inpatient care and prevent adverse events. Jt Comm J Qual Improv 1998;24:77–87.

[30] Lee L, Levine J, Schultz H. Utility of a standardized sign-out card for new medical interns. J Gen Intern Med 1996;11(12):753–5.

[31] Horwitz L, Krumholz H, Green M, et al. Transfers of patient care between house staff on internal medicine wards: a national survey. Arch Intern Med 2006;166(11):1173–7.

ELSEVIER
SAUNDERS

THE MEDICAL
CLINICS
OF NORTH AMERICA

Med Clin N Am 92 (2008) 325–348

Perioperative Medicine
for the Hospitalized Patient

Paul J. Grant, MD*, David H. Wesorick, MD

*University of Michigan Medical School, Division of General Medicine,
Department of Internal Medicine, 3119 Taubman Center, Box 5376, 1500
East Medical Center Drive, Ann Arbor, MI 48109-5376, USA*

In many medical centers, hospitalists have become an important resource for providing inpatient preoperative evaluations. Given the increasing complexity of hospitalized patients and the increasing specialization among surgeons, there is greater reliance on hospitalists for preoperative assessment. Several institutions have developed surgery/medicine comanagement teams that jointly care for patients in the perioperative setting. Despite a growing body of evidence, it is important to recognize there are many gaps in the perioperative literature. This has led to considerable dependence on consensus statements and expert opinion when evaluating patients perioperatively.

This review focuses on the preoperative cardiovascular and pulmonary evaluation of the hospitalized patient: the two systems responsible for the greatest morbidity and mortality. Prevention of postoperative venous thromboembolism and management of perioperative hyperglycemia will also be discussed.

Clinical vignette

A 70-year-old female presents to the emergency department with a hip fracture after a fall. She has a history of chronic obstructive pulmonary disease (COPD), hypertension, type 2 diabetes treated with insulin, and chronic kidney disease with a baseline creatinine of 2.2 mg/dL. Her medications include aspirin, ramipril, hydrochlorothiazide, 70/30 insulin twice daily, and inhaled ipratropium. She has no complaints except those related to her hip, and denies all cardiopulmonary symptoms on a complete review

* Corresponding author.
  E-mail address: paulgran@umich.edu (P.J. Grant).

0025-7125/08/$ - see front matter © 2008 Elsevier Inc. All rights reserved.
doi:10.1016/j.mcna.2007.10.003   *medical.theclinics.com*

of symptoms. Her functional capacity has been limited to ambulating within her home but avoiding stairs. Her blood pressure is 134/86 and heart rate is 82. The remainder of her physical exam is normal. Should the medical consultant recommend stress testing before surgery for this patient? Are there any interventions that could be employed to reduce the patient's perioperative cardiac or pulmonary risk?

Cardiovascular evaluation

In 2004, there were approximately 35 million noncardiac inpatient surgical procedures performed in the United States [1]. To determine the risk of major perioperative cardiac events for noncardiac surgery, Devereaux and colleagues [2] pooled results from prospective studies that assessed patients who either had or were at risk for cardiac disease. They found that 3.9% of patients experienced a major cardiac event defined as cardiac death, nonfatal myocardial infarction, and nonfatal cardiac arrest. There are many reasons why the perioperative period poses an increased risk for cardiovascular complications. Operative stresses such as anesthesia, intubation/extubation, pain, fasting, stress steroid surges (eg, catecholamines and cortisol), blood loss, thrombophilia, and hypothermia may all increase the risk for a perioperative cardiovascular event [2].

We recommend a step-wise approach to preoperative cardiac assessment and risk reduction (Fig. 1). Although there are many areas of uncertainty within this approach, we feel that it represents a clinically useful synthesis of the available knowledge related to the subject.

Step 1. Determine if the patient has recently undergone a cardiac evaluation or revascularization procedure

Although limited to retrospective data, studies indicate that a previous revascularization procedure such as coronary artery bypass grafting (CABG) or percutaneous transluminal coronary angioplasty (PTCA) offers a protective benefit with respect to future surgical risk [3–7]. This is best demonstrated in a retrospective analysis of 1600 patients in the Coronary Artery Surgery Study (CASS) registry [3]. The operative mortality for patients without significant coronary artery disease (CAD) undergoing noncardiac surgery (0.5%) was not significantly different from those with CAD having had CABG before surgery (0.9%). However, in patients with considerable CAD without prior CABG, the operative mortality was significantly higher (2.4%). Extrapolating from these data, the American College of Cardiology/American Heart Association (ACC/AHA) guidelines on perioperative cardiovascular evaluation for noncardiac surgery suggest that coronary revascularization within 5 years, and a stable clinical status without signs or symptoms of ischemia, precludes the need for any further

Step 1. Determine if the patient has recently undergone a cardiac evaluation or revascularization procedure.

- Revascularization in the last 5 years usually precludes stress testing unless the patient presents with new signs or symptoms.
- Favorable results of non-invasive testing in the last 2 years usually make additional testing unnecessary.

Step 2. Assess for any signs or symptoms of active cardiac disease.

- Undiagnosed or unstable cardiac signs or symptoms require additional evaluation and/or risk stratification before surgery.

Step 3. Determine the patient's functional capacity.

- An assessment of functional capacity provides a context in which to view any reported symptoms.
- Extremes of functional capacity (eg. very good or very poor) may influence decision-making.

Step 4. Estimate cardiac risk using an objective measure.

- The Revised Cardiac Risk Index provides an objective measure of perioperative cardiovascular risk that can aid in decision-making (see tables 1 and 2).

Step 5. Determine the urgency of the surgery.

- Emergent surgery should not be delayed to allow for preoperative assessment.
- In urgent surgery, the main objective is to identify unstable cardiac conditions which may require urgent treatment. Noninvasive testing is rarely indicated prior to urgent surgery.

Step 6. Determine if additional testing is needed.

- We usually reserve preoperative noninvasive stress testing for the following situations:
    o patients with signs or symptoms of undiagnosed or unstable cardiac disease, or
    o patients with 3 or more of the RCRI undergoing intermediate- or high-risk surgery (see table 2).

Step 7. Incorporate appropriate risk reduction strategies.

- Coronary revascularization is only rarely indicated in the preoperative setting
- We recommend prophylactic perioperative beta-blockers for patients who are undergoing intermediate- or high-risk surgery with 2 or more of the RCRI predictors (see tables 1 and 2).

Fig. 1. A stepwise approach to perioperative cardiovascular assessment and risk reduction.

cardiac testing [8]. These guidelines also state that patients who have undergone a coronary evaluation with favorable results within the past 2 years (such as a cardiac stress test or diagnostic cardiac catheterization) do not require further testing, unless there are new signs or symptoms of ischemic heart disease.

Step 2. Assess for any signs or symptoms of active cardiac disease

The preoperative evaluation also provides an opportunity to unmask any cardiovascular conditions that have gone undiagnosed, or identify worsening of any preexisting conditions. A careful review of systems may reveal concerning signs and/or symptoms, such as chest pain or pressure, shortness of breath, orthopnea, lower extremity edema, unexplained syncope, palpitations, or focal neurologic deficits. The physical exam may also reveal signs that require further evaluation. Patients with clinical signs concerning undiagnosed or unstable cardiac disease (eg, angina, heart failure, valvular heart disease, arrhythmia) often require additional testing for diagnosis and/or risk stratification.

Step 3. Determine the patient's functional capacity

An accurate assessment of the patient's functional capacity is an important component of the preoperative evaluation. Patients who are able to achieve a high functional capacity may experience fewer perioperative complications [9,10]. One study included 600 preoperative patients who self-estimated the number of blocks they could walk and flights of stairs they could climb without experiencing symptomatic limitation [9]. Patients who reported poor exercise tolerance (defined as the inability to walk 4 blocks and climb 2 flights of stairs) had significantly more perioperative complications overall (20.4% versus 10.4%, $P < .001$); however, the difference in cardiovascular complications was not significantly different between the groups when adjusted for age.

A physical activity questionnaire can be a useful tool to assess a patient's functional capacity by asking if a patient can perform various tasks or activities [11]. The ACC/AHA perioperative guidelines indicate that the ability to perform four metabolic equivalents (METS) or greater is reflective of at least fair functional capacity [8]. These guidelines also recommend that many patients who are unable to perform four METS should undergo noninvasive cardiac testing, a recommendation that is based on expert opinion. We believe that strict adherence to this recommendation will result in overtesting. While self-reported functional capacity that is either extremely high or low may influence decision making, the existing data suggest that the assessment of functional capacity is most useful in creating a context for understanding a patient's symptoms (or lack thereof). More reliable predictors of risk should form the foundation for perioperative assessment.

Step 4. Estimate cardiac risk using an objective measure

For patients who lack signs or symptoms of undiagnosed or unstable cardiac disease, an objective estimate of perioperative cardiovascular risk can be made by employing a clinical assessment tool. Objectively estimating risk in this manner assists in making decisions about further testing and applying risk reduction interventions. Well-known examples of risk indices include those by Goldman [12], Detsky [13], and Lee [14] in addition to the clinical predictors used in the ACC/AHA perioperative guidelines [8]. Lee's Revised Cardiac Risk Index (RCRI) is a modern, simple, and prospectively validated system that was developed after studying 4315 patients aged 50 years or older undergoing elective major noncardiac surgery [14]. The authors identified six independent predictors of cardiac complications, as shown in Table 1. By simply summing these criteria, patients can be stratified into low (zero to one risk factor), intermediate (two risk factors), or high risk (three or more risk factors). When compared with other risk assessment models using receiver operating characteristic curve analysis, the RCRI proved to be the most accurate [14].

Table 1
The revised cardiac risk index (RCRI) as a predictor of major cardiac event rates[a] for noncardiac surgery

- Ischemic heart disease
  - defined as having any of the following: history of myocardial infarction, history of a positive stress test, current complaint of chest pain considered to be secondary to myocardial ischemia, use of nitrite therapy, or ECG with pathologic Q waves. Note that a history of percutaneous coronary intervention or CABG was not used as criteria for ischemic heart disease unless accompanied by any of the other criteria listed above.
- Congestive heart failure
  - defined by having any of the following: history of congestive heart failure, pulmonary edema, paroxysmal nocturnal dyspnea, bilateral rales or S3 gallop on physical examination, or chest radiograph showing pulmonary vascular redistribution.
- Cerebrovascular disease
  - defined as either stroke or transient ischemic attack.
- Diabetes mellitus requiring preoperative treatment with insulin
- Serum creatinine > 2.0 mg/dL
- High-risk surgery
  - defined as intraperitoneal, intrathoracic, or suprainguinal vascular.

RCRI classification	Event rate (95% confidence interval)	
	Derivation cohort	Validation cohort
Low risk		
• 0 risk factors	0.5 (0.2–1.1)	0.4 (0.05–1.5)
• 1 risk factor	1.3 (0.7–2.1)	0.9 (0.3–2.1)
Intermediate risk		
• 2 risk factors	3.6 (2.1–5.6)	6.6 (3.9–10.3)
High risk		
• ≥ 3 risk factors	9.1 (5.5–13.8)	11.0 (5.8–18.4)

Abbreviations: CABG, coronary artery bypass graft; ECG, electrocardiogram.

[a] Major cardiac events were defined as myocardial infarction, pulmonary edema, ventricular fibrillation or primary cardiac arrest, and complete heart block.

Data from Lee TH, Marcantonio ER, Mangione CM, et al. Derivation and prospective validation of a simple index for prediction of cardiac risk of major noncardiac surgery. Circulation 1999;100:1043–9.

Step 5. Determine the urgency of the surgery

When a hospitalized patient is to undergo surgery, it is usually emergent or urgent in nature. A formal preoperative evaluation before emergent surgery is unnecessary since there is no time for additional testing or therapeutic interventions. Urgent surgery can be described as surgery that needs to be performed during the same hospitalization, although a delay of a few days may be appropriate. In urgent surgical cases, identification of unstable cardiac conditions may influence management, but there is no role for testing to identify occult cardiac disease even when patients have significant risk factors. This is because there is neither time for, nor data to support, more extensive interventions (such as coronary revascularization) for stable patients in this setting. Hip fracture repair, as in our vignette, is a good example of an urgent procedure as studies have shown optimal outcomes when performed within 24 to 72 hours [15,16].

For elective procedures, the preoperative evaluation is usually performed under lesser time constraints. This allows for consideration of revascularization strategies if indicated for long-term benefit.

Step 6. Determine if additional testing is needed

The vast majority of pertinent clinical information will be acquired from the history and physical examination. Although an electrocardiogram (ECG) is usually obtained preoperatively, data to support this practice are limited [17]. An ECG is recommended for patients with known cardiac disease or significant risk factors, and the presence of pathologic Q-waves represents ischemic heart disease according to the RCRI.

The utility of noninvasive cardiac stress testing preoperatively is debated. Given recent evidence, there has been a trend toward less preoperative stress testing in favor of increased use of prophylactic pharmacologic interventions to decrease cardiovascular risk. It should also be emphasized that no testing should be performed if the results will not alter patient management. For example, a preoperative stress test would be inappropriate for patients who are poor candidates for coronary revascularization.

The ACC/AHA perioperative guidelines nicely summarize the trials that used stress testing for preoperative cardiac risk assessment [8]. Stress myocardial perfusion testing demonstrated a positive predictive value of 4% to 20% for cardiac ischemia, while the negative predictive value of a normal scan was approximately 99% for myocardial infarction and/or cardiac death. Similarly, trials employing dobutamine stress echocardiography (DSE) for preoperative risk assessment established a positive predictive value of myocardial infarction or death of 7% to 25%, with a negative predictive value ranging from 93% to 100%. These numbers illustrate that, although a negative stress test result can be reassuring, a positive test is poorly predictive of perioperative cardiovascular events and thus unhelpful in the large majority of patients.

There are circumstances, however, when the results of a preoperative stress test may provide useful risk-stratification. Among high-risk patients, noninvasive testing may help distinguish those whose perioperative risk might be acceptable from those whose risk will remain very high, even if treated with perioperative beta-blockers. This was demonstrated in a study by Boersma and colleagues [18], who examined the cardiac event rate in patients undergoing major vascular surgery in relation to clinical risk factors, DSE results, and beta-blocker therapy. The clinical risk factors used in this study were very similar to Lee's RCRI. The authors found that in patients with less than three risk factors, DSE offered minimal prognostic benefit. This was particularly true in patients receiving beta-blocker therapy. However, in patients with three or more risk factors, DSE did provide prognostic value. A normal DSE in this group was predictive of a relatively low postoperative event rate, while extensive reversible ischemia detected on DSE correlated with a high rate of cardiac death or nonfatal myocardial infarction, even for patients treated with beta-blockers. A more recent trial demonstrated that preoperative cardiac testing did not alter outcomes in intermediate-risk patients undergoing vascular surgery with tight heart rate control using beta-blockers [19].

Some authors have published preoperative approaches using the RCRI as the primary decision tool for determining if noninvasive cardiac testing is indicated [20–22]. Following these strategies, in contrast to the 2002 ACC/AHA perioperative guidelines, would lead to a significant reduction in the number of noninvasive cardiac stress tests performed. We generally reserve preoperative noninvasive testing for patients with signs or symptoms of undiagnosed or unstable cardiac disease, or patients with an RCRI score of three or more (Table 2). One might have a lower threshold for noninvasive testing in cases where the surgical risk is very high, the functional capacity is very low, or the patient is unable to tolerate beta-blocker medications.

Step 7. Incorporate appropriate risk-reduction strategies

Revascularization

The literature has consistently shown that coronary revascularization should almost never be performed simply to improve the odds of a favorable surgical outcome. The Coronary Artery Revascularization Prophylaxis (CARP) trial is the only prospective study to date that has assessed long-term mortality in high-risk patients who were randomized to either revascularization (percutaneous coronary intervention or CABG) or no revascularization before elective major vascular surgery [23]. Patients were included if they had significant but stable coronary artery disease (at least one coronary artery with a stenosis of 70% or more by angiogram). Exclusion criteria consisted of a stenosis of 50% or more in the left main coronary artery, left ventricular ejection fraction of less than 20%, and severe aortic stenosis. The results revealed no significant difference between the two

Table 2
A preoperative approach using the RCRI for determining when to use beta-blockers and/or noninvasive cardiac testing

RCRI score	Recommendations
0	Neither prophylactic beta-blockers nor noninvasive cardiac testing are recommended for these patients.
1	Prophylactic beta-blockers are generally not recommended but may be considered if surgery type is high-risk and/or functional capacity is very poor. Noninvasive stress testing is not recommended.
2	Prophylactic beta-blockers are recommended for these patients. Noninvasive stress testing is not recommended but may be considered if surgery type is high risk and/or functional capacity is very poor.
3 or more	Prophylactic beta-blockers are highly recommended for these patients. Noninvasive stress testing is reasonable for most of these patients but may be omitted if surgery type is low risk, functional capacity is very good, or surgery is urgent.

Abbreviation: RCRI, revised cardiac risk index.

Data from Wesorick DH, Eagle KA. The preoperative cardiovascular evaluation of the intermediate-risk patient: new data, changing strategies. Am J Med 2005;118:1413.

groups with respect to mortality at 2.7 years, or postoperative myocardial infarction at 30 days. Not surprisingly, there was a significant delay in surgery for the revascularization group. The authors concluded that preoperative revascularization before elective vascular surgery should not be recommended in this patient population.

Although the CARP trial was an intervention trial, it does raise questions about the utility of using noninvasive cardiac testing for the purpose of identifying asymptomatic coronary disease in preoperative patients. This is particularly true for situations involving urgent surgeries, such as those most commonly encountered in the hospitalized patient.

Antiplatelet management for patients with a recent coronary artery stent

Although preoperative coronary revascularization is very rarely indicated, it is not uncommon for patients to develop a need for surgery after having a coronary stent placed. This scenario warrants special attention from the evaluating clinician. The placement of a stent in a coronary artery increases the likelihood of a coronary thrombotic event. The duration of that increased risk remains uncertain, and probably correlates with the period of time before the stent is endothelized. This increased thrombotic risk is generally combated with dual antiplatelet therapy (aspirin and clopidogrel), which effectively reduces this risk. Therefore, in patients with recent coronary stents who are to undergo surgery, the decision to discontinue this therapy must be made with careful consideration of the risks and benefits to the patient.

Bare-metal stents endothelialize more rapidly than drug-eluting stents and thus require a shorter course of dual antiplatelet therapy. Current data indicate that patients who discontinue antiplatelet therapy soon after stent placement may be at increased risk of stent thrombosis [24–27]. The American College of Cardiology, the American Heart Association, and the Society for Cardiovascular Angiography and Interventions (ACC/AHA/SCAI) suggest that patients with bare-metal stents be treated with dual antiplatelet therapy with aspirin and clopidogrel for at least 1 month after stent implantation [28].

Dual antiplatelet therapy is required for a longer period after the implantation of drug-eluting stents. The ACC/AHA/SCAI guidelines recommend that dual antiplatelet therapy be continued for 1 year after implantation of drug-eluting stents in patients who are not at high risk for bleeding (and, at minimum, 3 months for sirolimus-eluting stents, and 6 months for paclitaxel-eluting stents) [28]. In studies examining stent thrombosis, the most powerfu predictor of this often-catastrophic event is the discontinuation of antiplatelet therapy. One study examining 2229 patients after stent implantation found that 5 of 17 patients who prematurely discontinued antiplatelet therapy suffered this complication [29]. Furthermore, the extended use of clopidogrel in patients with drug-eluting stents appears to be protective [30].

An advisory document, written by a multidisciplinary panel (including the ACC/AHA/SCAI, American College of Surgeons, and American Dental Society), provides specific recommendations about how to proceed when a patient with a recently placed coronary stent faces surgery [31]. These recommendations include the following:

- Elective procedures with significant perioperative bleeding risk should be delayed until patients have completed an appropriate course of thienopyridine (ie, clopidogrel) therapy.
- For patients treated with drug-eluting stents who are to undergo subsequent procedures that require discontinuation of thienopyridine therapy, aspirin should be continued if at all possible and the thienopyridine restarted as soon as possible postoperatively.
- For patients undergoing percutaneous coronary intervention who are likely to have a surgical procedure within the next 12 months, balloon angioplasty or implantation of a bare metal stent should be considered instead of a drug-eluting stent.

The true balance between risk and benefit of continuing antiplatelet therapy perioperatively remains uncertain. Although antiplatelet therapy is routinely held in this setting, there are many surgeries that can be safely completed while the patient is taking these medications [32]. Any recommendations to continue antiplatelet therapy through the perioperative period should be discussed directly with the referring surgeon. These discussions usually result in an acceptable plan for managing the antiplatelet agents.

Beta-blockers

The decision about which patients should receive perioperative beta-blocker therapy is not straightforward. The theory that beta-blockers can reduce demand ischemia and lower perioperative risk has not been consistently shown in the published literature. Study results have greatly varied demonstrating (1) extraordinary benefit in high-risk vascular surgery patients [33], (2) no significant benefit for low-risk diabetic patients [34], (3) delayed 2-year postoperative mortality reduction [35], and (4) no benefit in lower-risk vascular surgery patients [36]. Key factors that appear to influence trial outcomes include the degree of patient risk, type of surgery, duration of beta-blocker therapy, and whether the drug was titrated to a target heart rate.

More recent publications have attempted to clarify the role of perioperative beta-blockers. A meta-analysis of all randomized trials found that, although beta-blockers may reduce cardiac events, this benefit has only been demonstrated in a small number of trials encompassing few cardiac events [37]. Also, treatment with beta-blockers is associated with an increased risk of perioperative bradycardia and hypotension requiring treatment [37,38]. Another study used an administrative database of almost 800,000 patients to assess the effect of perioperative beta-blockers on in-hospital mortality [39]. Using propensity-score matching, a direct relationship was found corresponding to the patient's cardiac risk. In patients with an RCRI score of 0 or 1, beta-blocker use was associated with no benefit and possible harm. In patients with an RCRI score of 2 or more, the use of beta-blockers was associated with decreased in-hospital mortality. The ACC/AHA published a focused update on perioperative beta-blocker therapy in 2006 [40] that describes certain patient populations that may benefit from this therapy. According to these guidelines, beta-blockers are recommended for the following: patients already taking beta-blockers for a valid indication (eg, ischemic heart disease or hypertension), patients with coronary artery disease or findings of ischemia undergoing vascular surgery, and patients with multiple clinical risk factors undergoing intermediate- or high-risk procedures.

As described above, there is now evidence to suggest that beta-blockers may reduce perioperative cardiac risk in a subset of patients who are at higher baseline cardiac risk. However, more research is needed to more clearly delineate which patients will benefit from perioperative beta-blockade. The ongoing PeriOperative Ischemic Evaluation (POISE) trial plans to randomize 10,000 patients to metoprolol versus placebo before noncardiac surgery [41]. In the meantime, we believe there is sufficient evidence to recommend prophylactic perioperative beta-blockers to patients who are undergoing intermediate- or high-risk surgery with two or more of the RCRI predictors (see Table 2). Initiating beta-blockers should also be considered for patients who have a preexisting indication such as uncontrolled hypertension, congestive heart failure, or history of myocardial infarction. It should be noted that cardioselective beta-blockers are considered a safe intervention for patients with mild to moderate reactive airway disease or COPD as demonstrated in a meta-analysis [42] and Cochrane review [43].

Alpha-2 adrenergic agonists

Another class of medication that has been evaluated for perioperative cardiovascular risk reduction is the alpha-2 adrenergic agonists. A meta-analysis including 23 trials and 3395 patients demonstrated a significant reduction in mortality and ischemia in those receiving alpha-2 agonist therapy [44]. Among those undergoing vascular surgery, these agents achieved a significant reduction in mortality and myocardial infarction. A systematic review involving fewer trials established a significant reduction in cardiac mortality in patients with alpha-2 agonist exposure during noncardiac surgery [38]. It should be noted, however, that the benefits of alpha-2 agonists in these trials appeared to be influenced by a single large trial that used intravenous mivazerol—an alpha-2 agonist not available in the United States.

A large randomized trial of prophylactic alpha-2 agonists is needed to better determine the role of these agents in perioperative cardiovascular risk reduction. A head-to-head trial of perioperative alpha-2 agonists and beta-blockers is also required. For now, alpha-2 agonists should be considered for higher risk patients who have a contraindication to beta-blockers.

HMG-CoA reductase inhibitors (statins)

Recent observational trials have demonstrated reduced perioperative cardiovascular event rates in patients on statin therapy [45–49]. Despite this suggestive evidence, there has only been one randomized controlled trial assessing the effect of statin exposure on perioperative cardiovascular events in noncardiac surgery [50]. At present, we recommend that patients who are taking statins continue them in the perioperative period, although we currently do not initiate statins specifically for perioperative risk reduction. The ongoing Dutch Echocardiographic Cardiac Risk Evaluation Applying Stress Echo-IV (DECREASE-IV) trial [51] should clarify the role of perioperative statins.

Clinical vignette continued

This 70-year-old hip fracture patient has multiple cardiovascular risk factors and has not had a recent cardiac evaluation. She does not have any signs or symptoms suggestive of active cardiac disease, albeit in the setting of a poor functional capacity. Using the RCRI to estimate cardiac risk, this patient would score 2, indicating intermediate risk. This surgery would be classified as intermediate risk and urgent, ideally performed within 24 to 72 hours for optimal surgical outcome. Additional cardiac testing would not be recommended for this patient given her intermediate risk profile, the lack of undiagnosed or unstable cardiac symptoms, and the urgency of surgery. With respect to perioperative beta-blockers, the RCRI score of 2 suggests this patient is a reasonable candidate. A beta-blocker should be initiated, titrated to a goal heart rate of 50 to 65 beats per minute, and continued for at least 7 but up to 30 days postoperatively.

Pulmonary evaluation

Perioperative pulmonary complications are similar in prevalence to cardiac complications. In a prospective study of 3970 patients undergoing major noncardiac surgery, the frequency of cardiac complications was 1% for myocardial infarction and 1% for pulmonary edema, while pulmonary complications had a frequency of 2% for respiratory failure and 1% for bacterial pneumonia [52]. Furthermore, it has been shown that perioperative pulmonary complications lead to longer hospital lengths of stay when compared with cardiac complications [53]. Given these findings, it is important to fully assess a patient's pulmonary status during the preoperative evaluation (Fig. 2).

Step 1. Determine if the patient has known pulmonary disease

For patients with existing lung disease, it is important to determine the severity of the disease and the effectiveness of current management. Reports of recent pulmonary evaluations or testing may be helpful. Also, having the patient describe their perceived satisfaction of disease management is often useful in determining whether further evaluation or intervention is indicated.

Step 2. Assess for any signs or symptoms of active lung disease

Similar to the cardiovascular evaluation, the preoperative encounter is an opportunity to discover undiagnosed conditions. With appropriate questioning, the patient may report symptoms such as breathlessness, wheezing, cough, or sputum production. The patient's smoking history is also important to ascertain. If an undiagnosed pulmonary disease is suspected, additional evaluation may be appropriate.

Step 3. Recognize markers of increased perioperative pulmonary risk

Perioperative pulmonary complications are typically defined as any of the following: atelectasis, pneumonia, respiratory failure, exacerbation of a chronic lung disease, and bronchospasm. Pulmonary edema and pulmonary embolism are not considered pulmonary complications. To estimate the likelihood of developing a perioperative pulmonary complication, risk factors are categorized as patient-related and surgery-related.

Evidence-based guidelines for perioperative pulmonary evaluation were recently published [54] and accompanied by a systematic review on pulmonary risk stratification for noncardiothoracic surgery [55]. This analysis concluded that advanced age, an American Society of Anesthesiologists (ASA) class of greater than or equal to 2, congestive heart failure, functional dependence, and COPD were all strong indicators of patient-related risk for developing a perioperative pulmonary complication. Cigarette use is associated with a modest increase in risk, while obesity and asthma are

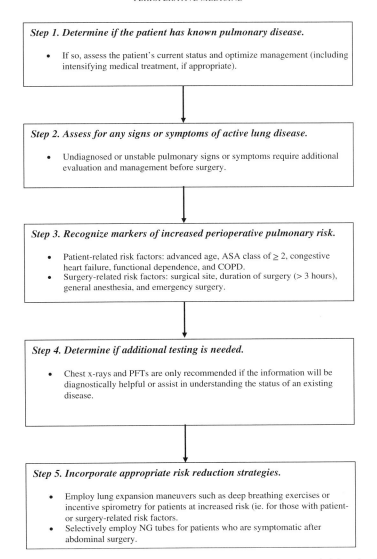

Step 1. Determine if the patient has known pulmonary disease.

- If so, assess the patient's current status and optimize management (including intensifying medical treatment, if appropriate).

Step 2. Assess for any signs or symptoms of active lung disease.

- Undiagnosed or unstable pulmonary signs or symptoms require additional evaluation and management before surgery.

Step 3. Recognize markers of increased perioperative pulmonary risk.

- Patient-related risk factors: advanced age, ASA class of ≥ 2, congestive heart failure, functional dependence, and COPD.
- Surgery-related risk factors: surgical site, duration of surgery (> 3 hours), general anesthesia, and emergency surgery.

Step 4. Determine if additional testing is needed.

- Chest x-rays and PFTs are only recommended if the information will be diagnostically helpful or assist in understanding the status of an existing disease.

Step 5. Incorporate appropriate risk reduction strategies.

- Employ lung expansion maneuvers such as deep breathing exercises or incentive spirometry for patients at increased risk (ie. for those with patient- or surgery-related risk factors.
- Selectively employ NG tubes for patients who are symptomatic after abdominal surgery.

Fig. 2. A stepwise approach to perioperative pulmonary assessment and risk reduction.

not associated with increased risk. There was insufficient evidence to determine if obstructive sleep apnea is a risk factor.

Surgery-related risk factors are likely more important than patient-related risk factors for predicting perioperative pulmonary complications. The surgery-related risk factors include surgical site, duration of surgery (> 3 hours), type of anesthesia (general), and emergency surgery [55]. The surgical site is by far the most significant risk, with aortic aneurysm repair, thoracic, and abdominal surgery posing the greatest risk [56,57]. The higher risk surgical sites can be remembered by the "closest to the diaphragm" rule, as diaphragmatic dysfunction and splinting secondary to pain can lower vital capacity and functional reserve capacity, increasing the risk for pulmonary complications.

Step 4. Determine if additional testing is needed

The history and physical examination will usually provide all of the information needed to complete the preoperative pulmonary evaluation. On occasion, additional testing may be indicated, most commonly when new symptoms are reported, a previous diagnosis is unclear, or the patient's presentation suggests worsening clinical status.

A preoperative chest radiograph is commonly ordered despite insufficient data showing clinical utility. Although an abnormal chest radiograph has been shown to be predictive of postoperative pulmonary complications [58], it is felt this imaging rarely provides any additional information beyond what can be determined by the history and physical examination. This was shown in a meta-analysis of 21 studies involving 14,390 patients where abnormalities were present in 10% of preoperative chest radiographs, but only 1.3% showed unexpected abnormalities and only 0.1% influenced management [59]. A more recent review demonstrated similar findings [60]; however, neither of these studies assessed for postoperative pulmonary complications. Despite the limited evidence, the recent guidelines from the American College of Physicians state that a preoperative chest radiograph may be helpful for patients older than 50 with known cardiopulmonary disease who are undergoing upper abdominal, thoracic, or abdominal aortic aneurysm surgery [54]. In our practice, we order chest radiographs for diagnostic indications or to better understand the status of an existing disease. We do not order this test for the purpose of preoperative "screening."

Pulmonary function tests (PFTs) are rarely indicated before surgery. PFTs have not been shown to predict perioperative risk more accurately than clinical assessment alone. A nested case-control trial of 2291 patients undergoing abdominal surgery sought to identify risk indicators for perioperative pulmonary complications [58]. Although variables including an abnormal chest radiograph and abnormal findings on lung physical examination were found to be independent risk factors, no components of PFTs were predictive of perioperative pulmonary complications. Furthermore, there is no established spirometry value cutoff for which noncardiac surgery should be denied [61].

Alternatively, preoperative PFTs can be diagnostically useful in the assessment of unexplained symptoms. In addition, they are sometimes helpful in assessing the status of known lung disease, especially when the history and physical exam do not lead to a firm conclusion. Last, PFTs are always obtained for patients scheduled for lung reduction surgery.

Step 5. Incorporate appropriate risk-reduction strategies

Despite fairly robust risk stratification data, strategies to reduce risk for perioperative pulmonary complications are limited. The initial approach for patients with chronic lung disease is to optimize their management. For example, in patients with respiratory symptoms such as chest tightness or wheezing, aggressive bronchodilator therapy with the option of preoperative systemic steroid therapy is recommended. Although physicians may fear that steroid exposure will increase perioperative infection risk and hinder wound healing, the limited evidence available suggests this is not the case [62].

The type of anesthesia is another potentially modifiable factor that may influence perioperative pulmonary complication risk. A large meta-analysis showed a significant reduction in pneumonia, respiratory depression, and overall mortality in patients allocated to neuraxial blockade, compared to those receiving general anesthesia [63]. However, this topic remains controversial and decisions about the specific type of anesthesia to be employed are usually made in consultation with an anesthesiologist.

The greatest reduction in postoperative pulmonary complications can be achieved by implementing lung expansion modalities. These include deep-breathing exercises, incentive spirometry, intermittent positive-pressure breathing, and continuous positive airway pressure. A meta-analysis of 14 randomized controlled trials of patients undergoing upper abdominal surgery demonstrated a significant reduction in postoperative pulmonary complications of approximately 50% among patients treated with these modalities [64]. Other strategies that have been shown to reduce the risk of pulmonary complications include postoperative epidural pain control [65] and selective use of nasogastric decompression for symptomatic patients following abdominal surgery [66].

Clinical vignette continued

Our patient has a history of COPD, but is not exhibiting any signs or symptoms related to this disease. Despite her perioperative pulmonary risk factors of advanced age, ASA class $\geq$ 2, and history of COPD, she does not require any preoperative testing such as chest radiography or PFTs. Postoperative lung expansion maneuvers are highly recommended for this patient.

Venous thromboembolism (VTE) prevention

The need for VTE prophylaxis in the surgical patient is undisputed. Given the high incidence of VTE, its significant morbidity and mortality, and the effective prevention strategies available, VTE prophylaxis must be a priority when managing patients in the postoperative setting [67]. The risk of developing DVT among surgical patients without prophylaxis is striking, with estimates of 15% to 30% in general surgery patients [68], 40% to 60% in lower extremity orthopedic patients [67], and greater than

60% in trauma patients [69]. Although mechanical forms of VTE prevention such as intermittent pneumatic compression devices and graduated compression stockings are available, the vast majority of hospitalized surgical patients will require pharmacologic prevention. Internists who manage perioperative patients should feel comfortable with the timing and duration of prophylactic anticoagulation. Low-dose unfractionated heparin (LDUH), low molecular weight heparin (LMWH), fondaparinux, and warfarin have all been shown to be efficacious for VTE prevention in surgical patients. The preferred agent and dosing regimen often depend on the level of VTE risk and the type of surgery (Table 3). The American College of Chest Physicians (ACCP) has published detailed guidelines for perioperative VTE prophylaxis [67].

Lower extremity orthopedic surgery is associated with a very high risk of VTE. In hip fracture patients, the risk for VTE starts at the time of injury as opposed to the time of surgery [70,71]. Therefore, prophylaxis should be initiated as soon as possible in the preoperative period and continued until 12 to 24 hours before surgery. For hip fracture and total hip replacement surgery, extended VTE prophylaxis is recommended for a total of 28 to 35 days, while total knee replacement surgery should receive prophylaxis for at least 10 days postoperatively [67].

The timing of prophylactic anticoagulation is further complicated when neuraxial anesthesia is employed. The delivery of anesthetic to the neuraxis requires insertion of a needle or catheter into the epidural space, and the concomitant use of prophylactic anticoagulation may increase the risk of paraspinal hematomas. Both the ACCP and the American Society of Regional Anesthesiology (ASRA) agree that pharmacologic VTE prophylaxis can still be used concomitant with neuraxial anesthesia, as long as precautions are taken to reduce bleeding risk [67,72]. These precautions are outlined in Table 4.

Since most hospitalized surgical patients are candidates for VTE prophylaxis, we believe that the approach should be standardized. Hospitals should have written protocols for VTE prophylaxis, and these protocols should be incorporated into order sets.

Clinical vignette continued

Hip fracture patients are at very high risk for VTE. Given our patient's chronic kidney disease, the choices for VTE prophylaxis become limited. Enoxaparin has an approved renal dosing of 30 mg subcutaneously daily, and should be started shortly after the patient's arrival to the hospital. The last dose should be given 24 hours before surgery, then restarted 12 to 24 hours postoperatively. Pharmacologic VTE prophylaxis should be continued for 4 weeks postoperatively, which can be achieved with enoxaparin or warfarin for this patient.

Table 3
Recommended VTE prophylaxis strategies for the surgical patient

Type of surgery	VTE prophylaxis options
Minor general, gynecologic, urologic, vascular, and arthroscopic surgical procedures without additional VTE risk factors[a]	• No routine pharmacologic prophylaxis recommended • Early mobilization
Minor general surgery with additional risk factors[a]	• LDUH 5000 U SC bid

Major general and gynecologic surgical procedures without additional risk factors[a]	• LMWH:
	  • enoxaparin 40 mg SC daily
	  • dalteparin 2500 U SC daily

Major gynecologic, vascular, urologic, and general surgical procedures with additional risk factors[a]	• LDUH 5000 U SC tid
	• LMWH:
	  • enoxaparin 40 mg SC daily
	  • dalteparin 5000 U SC daily

Lower extremity orthopedic surgery:
  • total hip arthroplasty
  • total knee arthroplasty
  • hip fracture surgery
	• LMWH:
	  • enoxaparin 40 mg SC daily or 30 mg SC bid starting 12–24 h postoperatively
	  • dalteparin 5000 U SC daily starting 12 h before surgery, or
	  • 2500 U SC starting 4–6 h postoperatively, then 5000 U SC daily
	  • fondaparinux 2.5 mg SC daily starting 6–8 h postoperatively
	  • warfarin starting the night before surgery or the evening after surgery adjusting to an INR goal of 2–3

Abbreviations: INR, international normalized ratio; LDUH, low dose unfractionated heparin; LMWH, low molecular weight heparin; SC, subcutaneous; VTE, venous thromboembolism.

[a] VTE risk factors include prior VTE, advancing age, malignancy, trauma, immobility, inherited or acquired thrombophilia, pregnancy, estrogen therapy, obesity, smoking, and varicose veins.

Data from Geerts WH, Pineo GF, Heit JA, et al. Prevention of venous thromboembolism: the seventh ACCP conference on antithrombotic and thrombolytic therapy. Chest 2004;126(suppl 3):338S–400S.

Glycemic management

Optimal glycemic control in the perioperative period can be challenging for many reasons. Hyperglycemia often results from physiologic stress, infection, reduced activity, total parenteral nutrition, and the modification of the patient's usual diabetes medications. Hypoglycemia is also common, largely due to patient anorexia or fasting (NPO) status.

Achievement of euglycemia in the postoperative setting appears to be beneficial. Basic science research has shown that hyperglycemia is associated with an increased risk of thrombosis, reversible immune dysfunction, inflammatory marker elevation, and dysfunction of vascular endothelium

Table 4
VTE prophylaxis management for patients receiving neuraxial anesthesia/analgesia

	Before neuraxial technique	Before catheter removal	After catheter removal
LDUH	No contraindication	No contraindication	No contraindication
LMWH			
• single daily dosing	Wait 10–12 hours after last dose	Wait 10–12 hours after last dose	Wait 2 hours before resuming
• twice daily dosing	Wait 10–12 hours after last dose	Not recommended for use while catheter in place	Wait 2 hours before resuming
Warfarin	INR < 1.5	INR ≤ 1.5	Resume therapy to INR goal
Fondaparinux	Currently not recommended in conjunction with neuraxial anesthesia/analgesia		

Abbreviations: INR, international normalized ratio; LDUH, low-dose unfractionated heparin; LMWH, low molecular-weight heparin; VTE, venous thromboembolism.

Data from Horlocker TT, Wedel DJ, Benzon H, et al. Regional anesthesia in the anticoagulated patient: defining the risks (the second ASRA consensus conference on neuraxial anesthesia and anticoagulation). Reg Anesth Pain Med 2003;28:172–97.

[73]. Moreover, the benefits of euglycemia in surgical patients have been recently demonstrated in clinical trials. The strongest evidence comes from a prospective trial involving 1548 patients admitted to a surgical intensive care unit who were randomized to intensive (intravenous) insulin therapy versus conventional treatment [74]. Intensive care unit mortality was reduced by 42% and overall in-hospital mortality was reduced by 34% in the group receiving intensive insulin treatment. In addition, postoperative hyperglycemia is associated with increased infection rates [75] and studies have shown that aggressive blood sugar control decreases the risk of deep sternal wound infections [76] and mortality [77] in diabetic patients undergoing cardiac surgical procedures.

Guidelines set forth by the American Diabetes Association [78] recommend a glycemic target for hospitalized patients in the intensive care unit between 80 and 110 mg/dL. For non–critical care patients, the preprandial goal is 90 to 130 mg/dL and the postprandial or random blood glucose target is less than 180 mg/dL.

Scientific evidence supports using intravenous insulin to control hyperglycemia in critically ill postoperative patients. However, the current best practice for insulin in the non–critically ill postoperative patient is based primarily on expert opinion. Oral antidiabetic agents are sometimes contraindicated in the perioperative patient, and these agents are difficult to rapidly titrate to effect. In addition, using "sliding-scale insulin" as the sole means of glycemic control is ineffective for most patients, and potentially harmful [79,80]. Therefore, to achieve optimal glycemic targets, hospitalists must become comfortable using subcutaneous insulin in an anticipatory and physiologic manner [73].

The best practice for glycemic control in non–critically ill hospitalized patients is sometimes referred to as "basal-bolus" subcutaneous insulin delivery [73,81], with insulin divided into its physiologic components: basal insulin (longer-acting, nonpeaking insulin), nutritional insulin (short- or rapid-acting insulin provided as boluses with meals), and correctional insulin (additional boluses of short- or rapid-acting insulin given to correct hyperglycemia). This approach allows clinicians to provide basal insulin to patients continuously, and to provide nutritional insulin that best matches the patient's actual nutritional intake.

To effectively use insulin regimens in perioperative patients, hospitalists must be able to estimate a patient's total daily dose of insulin (TDD), and understand how that dose should be divided into the physiologic components. There are several ways to estimate the TDD. For patients on insulin, the easiest way is to simply add up how much insulin the patient takes at home. However, for patients who are not on full insulin regimens at home, the TDD can be estimated based on the patient's weight. A total daily dose of 0.4 units/kg is a reasonable starting place for most patients. One half of this dose can be provided to cover basal insulin needs, and continued even when the patient is fasting perioperatively. Basal insulin is best supplied as a low- or nonpeaking insulin, such as glargine or detemir. The other half of the TDD can be given as divided doses to cover the patient's nutritional needs, once nutrition is resumed. Nutritional insulin is usually provided as rapid-acting or regular insulin, and must be matched, in real time, to the patient's nutritional intake. When the patient is fasting perioperatively, the nutritional insulin is held. A small amount of correctional insulin should be given in addition to the basal and nutritional insulin, if hyperglycemia occurs. Many institutions are now using standardized subcutaneous insulin order sets to promote this physiologic use of insulin. Although a complete discussion of insulin management in the hospital is outside the scope of this article, there are several resources available to help clinicians learn and employ these principles [82].

Clinical vignette continued

This patient has type 2 diabetes mellitus and uses 60 units/day of mixed insulin at home. To facilitate perioperative management, we would recommend changing to an insulin regimen that provides separate basal and nutritional insulin for this patient. For basal insulin coverage, we would initiate glargine insulin 30 units subcutaneously daily, which can be given even if the patient is NPO (nothing by mouth) for surgery. We would recommend 10 units of rapid-acting insulin to be given with each of her three daily meals, and held when the patient is fasting. A small amount of correctional insulin can be given in addition to the basal and nutritional components if the patient experiences hyperglycemia.

References

[1] DeFrances CJ, Podgornik MN. 2004 National hospital discharge survey. Advance data from vital and health statistics. National center for health statistics 2006;371:1–20.

[2] Devereaux PJ, Goldman L, Cook DJ, et al. Perioperative cardiac events in patients undergoing noncardiac surgery: a review of the magnitude of the problem, the pathophysiology of the events and methods to estimate and communicate risk. CMAJ 2005;173(6):627–34.

[3] Foster ED, Davis KB, Carpenter JA, et al. Risk of noncardiac operation in patients with defined coronary disease: The Coronary Artery Surgery Study (CASS) registry experience. Ann Thorac Surg 1986;41:42–50.

[4] Mahar LJ, Steen PA, Tinker JH, et al. Perioperative myocardial infarction in patients with coronary artery disease with and without aorta-coronary artery bypass grafts. J Thorac Cardiovasc Surg 1978;76:533–7.

[5] Nielsen JL, Page CP, Mann C, et al. Risk of major elective operation after myocardial revascularization. Am J Surg 1992;164:423–6.

[6] Gottlieb A, Banoub M, Sprung J, et al. Perioperative cardiovascular morbidity in patients with coronary artery disease undergoing vascular surgery after percutaneous transluminal coronary angioplasty. J Cardiothorac Vasc Anesth 1998;12:501–6.

[7] Hassan SA, Hlatky MA, Boothroyd DB, et al. Outcomes of noncardiac surgery after coronary bypass surgery or coronary angioplasty in the bypass angioplasty revascularization investigation (BARI). Am J Med 2001;110:260–6.

[8] Eagle KA, Berger PB, Calkins H, et al. ACC/AHA guideline update for perioperative cardiovascular evaluation for noncardiac surgery: a report of the American College of Cardiology/American Heart Association Task Force on Practice Guidelines. 2002. American College of Cardiology Web site. Available at: http:/www.acc.org/clinical/guidelines/perio/dirIndex.htm. Accessed October 18, 2007.

[9] Reilly DF, McNeely MJ, Doerner D, et al. Self-reported exercise tolerance and the risk of serious perioperative complications. Arch Intern Med 1999;159:2185–92.

[10] Girish M, Trayner E, Dammann O, et al. Symptom-limited stair climbing as a predictor of postoperative cardiopulmonary complications after high-risk surgery. Chest 2001;120:1147–51.

[11] Hlatky MA, Boineau RE, Higginbotham MB, et al. A brief self-administered questionnaire to determine functional capacity (the Duke activity status index). Am J Cardiol 1989;64:651–4.

[12] Goldman L, Caldera DL, Nussbaum SR, et al. Multifactorial index of cardiac risk in noncardiac surgical procedures. N Engl J Med 1977;297:845–50.

[13] Detsky AS, Abrams HB, Forbath N, et al. Cardiac assessment for patients undergoing noncardiac surgery. A multifactorial clinical risk index. Arch Intern Med 1986;146:2131–4.

[14] Lee TH, Marcantonio ER, Mangione CM, et al. Derivation and prospective validation of a simple index for prediction of cardiac risk of major noncardiac surgery. Circulation 1999;100:1043–9.

[15] Bottle A, Aylin P. Mortality associated with delay in operation after hip fracture: observational study. BMJ 2006;332:947–50.

[16] McLaughlin MA, Prosz GM, Magaziner J, et al. Preoperative status and risk of complications in patients with hip fracture. J Gen Intern Med 2006;21:219–25.

[17] Pasternak LR, Arens JF, Caplan RA, et al. Practice advisory for preanesthesia evaluation: a report by the American Society of Anesthesiologists Task Force on Preanesthesia evaluation. Anesthesiology 2002;96:485–96.

[18] Boersma E, Poldermans D, Bax JJ, et al. Predictors of cardiac events after major vascular surgery: role of clinical characteristics, dobutamine echocardiography, and B-blocker therapy. JAMA 2001;285:1865–73.

[19] Poldermans D, Bax JJ, Schouten O, et al. Should major vascular surgery be delayed because of preoperative cardiac testing in intermediate-risk patients receiving beta-blocker therapy with tight heart rate control? J Am Coll Cardiol 2006;48:964–9.

[20] Auerbach A, Goldman L. Assessing and reducing the cardiac risk of noncardiac surgery. Circulation 2006;113:1361–76.

[21] Wesorick DH, Eagle KA. The preoperative cardiovascular evaluation of the intermediate-risk patient: new data, changing strategies. Am J Med 2005;118:1413.

[22] Grayburn PA, Hillis LD. Cardiac events in patients undergoing noncardiac surgery: shifting the paradigm from noninvasive risk stratification to therapy. Ann Intern Med 2003;138:506–11.

[23] McFalls EO, Ward HB, Moritz TE, et al. Coronary-artery revascularization before elective major vascular surgery. N Engl J Med 2004;351:2795–804.

[24] Kaluza GL, Joseph J, Lee JR, et al. Catastrophic outcomes of noncardiac surgery soon after coronary stenting. J Am Coll Cardiol 2000;35:1288–94.

[25] Wilson SH, Fasseas P, Orford JL, et al. Clinical outcomes of patients undergoing non-cardiac surgery in the two months following coronary stenting. J Am Coll Cardiol 2003;42:234–40.

[26] Sharma AK, Ajani AE, Hamwi SM, et al. Major noncardiac surgery following coronary stenting: when is it safe to operate? Catheter Cardiovasc Interv 2004;63:141–5.

[27] Reddy PR, Vaitkus PT. Risks of noncardiac surgery after coronary stenting. Am J Cardiol 2005;95:755–7.

[28] Smith Jr SC, Feldman TE, Hirschfeld JW, et al. ACC/AHA/SCAI 2005 guideline update for percutaneous coronary intervention: a report of the American College of Cardiology/American Heart Association Task Force on Practice Guidelines (ACC/AHA/SCAI Writing Committee to Update the 2001 Guidelines for Percutaneous Coronary Intervention) American Heart Association Web Site. Available at: http://www.americanheart.org. Accessed October 18, 2007.

[29] Iakovou I, Schmidt T, Bonizzoni E, et al. Incidence, predictors, and outcome of thrombosis after successful implantation of drug-eluting stents. JAMA 2005;293:2126–30.

[30] Eisenstein EL, Anstrom KJ, Kong DF, et al. Clopidogrel use and long-term clinical outcomes after drug-eluting stent implantation. JAMA 2007;297:159–68.

[31] Grines CL, Bonow RO, Casey DE, et al. Prevention of premature discontinuation of dual antiplatelet therapy in patients with coronary artery stents: a science advisory from the American Heart Association, American College of Cardiology, Society for Cardiovascular Angiography and Interventions, American College of Surgeons, and American Dental Association, with representation from the American College of Physicians. J Am Coll Cardiol 2007;49:734–9.

[32] Burger W, Chemnitius JM, Kneissl GD, et al. Low-dose aspirin for secondary cardiovascular prevention—cardiovascular risks after its perioperative withdrawal versus bleeding risks with its continuation—review and meta-analysis. J Intern Med 2005;257:399–414.

[33] Poldermans D, Boersma E, Bax JJ, et al. The effect of bisoprolol on perioperative mortality and myocardial infarction in high-risk patients undergoing vascular surgery. Dutch Echocardiographic Cardiac Risk Evaluation Applying Stress Echocardiography Study Group. N Engl J Med 1999;3431:1789–94.

[34] Juul AB, Wetterslev J, Gluud C, et al. Effect of perioperative beta blockade in patients with diabetes undergoing major noncardiac surgery: randomised placebo controlled, blinded multicentre trial. BMJ 2006;332:1482.

[35] Mangano DT, Layug EL, Wallace A, et al. Effect of atenolol on mortality and cardiovascular morbidity after noncardiac surgery. Multicenter Study of Perioperative Ischemia Research Group. N Engl J Med 1996;335:1713–20.

[36] Brady AR, Gibbs JS, Greenhalgh RM, et al. Perioperative beta-blockade (POBBLE) for patients undergoing infrarenal vascular surgery: results of a randomized double-blind controlled trial. J Vasc Surg 2005;41:602–9.

[37] Devereaux PJ, Beattie WS, Choi PTL, et al. How strong is the evidence for the use of perioperative β blockers in non-cardiac surgery? Systematic review and meta-analysis of randomised controlled trials. BMJ 2005;331:313–21.

[38] Stevens RD, Burri H, Tramer MR. Pharmacologic myocardial protection in patients undergoing noncardiac surgery: a quantitative systematic review. Anesth Analg 2003;97:623–33.

[39] Lindenauer PK, Pekow P, Wang K, et al. Perioperative beta-blocker therapy and mortality after major noncardiac surgery. N Engl J Med 2005;353:349–61.

[40] Fleisher LA, Beckman JA, Brown KA, et al. ACC/AHA 2006 guideline update on perioperative cardiovascular evaluation for noncardiac surgery: focused update on perioperative beta-blocker therapy. A report of the ACC/AHA task force on practice guidelines (Writing committee to update the 2002 guidelines on perioperative cardiovascular evaluation for noncardiac surgery). J Am Coll Cardiol 2006;47:2343–55.

[41] POISE Trial Investigators, Devereaux PJ, Yang H, et al. Rationale, design, and organization of the PeriOperative Ischemic Evaluation (POISE) Trial: a randomized controlled trial of metoprolol versus placebo in patients undergoing noncardiac surgery. Am Heart J 2006; 152:223–30.

[42] Salpeter SR, Ormiston TM, Salpeter EE. Cardioselective beta-blockers in patients with reactive airway disease: a meta-analysis. Ann Intern Med 2002;136:715–25.

[43] Salpeter S, Ormiston T, Salpeter E. Cardioselective beta-blockers for chronic obstructive pulmonary disease. Cochrane Database Syst Rev 2005;4:CD003566.

[44] Wijeysundera DN, Naik JS, Beattie WS. Alpha-2 adrenergic agonists to prevent perioperative cardiovascular complications: a meta-analysis. Am J Med 2003;114:742–52.

[45] Poldermans D, Bax JJ, Kertai MD, et al. Statins are associated with a reduced incidence of perioperative mortality in patients undergoing major noncardiac vascular surgery. Circulation 2003;107:1848–51.

[46] Lindenauer PK, Pekow P, Wang K, et al. Lipid-lowering therapy and in-hospital mortality following major noncardiac surgery. JAMA 2004;291:2092–9.

[47] O'Neil-Callahan K, Katimaglis G, Tepper MR, et al. Statins decrease perioperative cardiac complications in patients undergoing noncardiac vascular surgery. J Am Coll Cardiol 2005; 45:336–42.

[48] McGirt MJ, Perler BA, Brooke BS, et al. 3-Hydroxy-3-methylglutaryl coenzyme A reductase inhibitors reduce the risk of perioperative stroke and mortality after carotid endarterectomy. J Vasc Surg 2005;42:829–36.

[49] Ward RP, Leeper NJ, Kirkpatrick JN, et al. The effect of preoperative statin therapy on cardiovascular outcomes in patients undergoing infrainguinal vascular surgery. Int J Cardiol 2005;104:264–8.

[50] Durazzo AE, Machado FS, Ikeoka DT, et al. Reduction in cardiovascular events after vascular surgery with atorvastatin: a randomized trial. J Vasc Surg 2004;39:967–76.

[51] Schouten O, Poldermans D, Visser L, et al. Fluvastatin and bisoprolol for the reduction of perioperative cardiac mortality and morbidity in high-risk patients undergoing non-cardiac surgery: Rationale and design of the DECREASE-IV study. Am Heart J 2004;148:1047–52.

[52] Fleischmann KE, Goldman L, Young B, et al. Association between cardiac and noncardiac complications in patients undergoing noncardiac surgery: outcomes and effects on length of stay. Am J Med 2003;115:515–20.

[53] Lawrence VA, Hilsenbeck SG, Mulrow CD, et al. Incidence and hospital stay for cardiac and pulmonary complications after abdominal surgery. J Gen Intern Med 1995;10:671–8.

[54] Qaseem A, Snow V, Fitterman N, et al. Risk assessment for and strategies to reduce perioperative pulmonary complications for patients undergoing noncardiothoracic surgery: a guideline from the American College of Physicians. Ann Intern Med 2006;144:575–80.

[55] Smetana GW, Lawrence VA, Cornell JE. Preoperative pulmonary risk stratification for noncardiothoracic surgery: systematic review for the American College of Physicians. Ann Intern Med 2006;144:581–95.

[56] Arozullah AM, Daley J, Henderson WG. Multifactorial risk index for predicting postoperative respiratory failure in men after major noncardiac surgery. The National Veterans Administration Surgical Quality Improvement Program. Ann Surg 2000;232:242–53.

[57] Arozullah AM, Khuri SF, Henderson WG, et al. Development and validation of a multifactorial risk index for predicting postoperative pneumonia after major noncardiac surgery. Ann Intern Med 2001;135:847–57.

[58] Lawrence VA, Dhanda R, Hilsenbeck SG, et al. Risk of pulmonary complications after elective abdominal surgery. Chest 1996;110:744–50.

[59] Archer C, Levy AR, McGregor M. Value of routine preoperative chest x-rays: a meta-analysis. Can J Anaesth 1993;40:1022–7.

[60] Smetana GW, Macpherson DS. The case against routine preoperative laboratory testing. Med Clin North Am 2003;87:7–40.

[61] Kroenke K, Lawrence VA, Theroux JF, et al. Operative risk in patients with severe obstructive pulmonary disease. Arch Intern Med 1992;152:967–71.

[62] Pien LC, Grammer LC, Patterson R. Minimal complications in a surgical population with severe asthma receiving prophylactic corticosteroids. J Allergy Clin Immunol 1988;82: 696–700.

[63] Rodgers A, Walker N, Schug S, et al. Reduction of postoperative mortality and morbidity with epidural or spinal anesthesia: results from overview of randomised trials. BMJ 2000; 321:1493.

[64] Thomas JA, McIntosh JM. Are incentive spirometry, intermittent positive pressure breathing, and deep breathing exercises effective in the prevention of postoperative pulmonary complication after upper abdominal surgery? A systematic overview and meta-analysis. Phys Ther 1994;74:3–16.

[65] Ballantyne JC, Carr DB, deFerranti S, et al. The comparative effects of postoperative analgesic therapies on pulmonary outcome: cumulative meta-analysis of randomized, controlled trials. Anesth Analg 1998;86:598–612.

[66] Cheatham ML, Chapman WC, Key SP, et al. A meta-analysis of selective versus routine nasogastric decompression after elective laparotomy. Ann Surg 1995;221:469–76.

[67] Geerts WH, Pineo GF, Heit JA, et al. Prevention of venous thromboembolism: the seventh ACCP conference on antithrombotic and thrombolytic therapy. Chest 2004;126(Suppl 3): 338S–400S.

[68] Clagett GP, Reisch JS. Prevention of venous thromboembolism in general surgical patients: results of meta-analysis. Ann Surg 1988;208:227–40.

[69] Kudsk KA, Fabian TC, Baum S, et al. Silent deep vein thrombosis in immobilized multiple trauma patients. Am J Surg 1989;158:515–9.

[70] Hefley FG Jr, Nelson CL, Puskarich-May CL. Effect of delayed admission to the hospital on the preoperative prevalence of deep-vein thrombosis associated with fractures about the hip. J Bone Joint Surg Am 1996;78:581–3.

[71] Zahn HR, Skinner JA, Porteous MJ. The preoperative prevalence of deep vein thrombosis in patients with femoral neck fractures and delayed operation. Injury 1999;30:605–7.

[72] Horlocker TT, Wedel DJ, Benzon H, et al. Regional anesthesia in the anticoagulated patient: defining the risks (the second ASRA consensus conference on neuraxial anesthesia and anticoagulation). Reg Anesth Pain Med 2003;28:172–97.

[73] Clement S, Baithwaite SS, Magee MF, et al. Management of diabetes and hyperglycemia in hospitals. Diabetes Care 2004;27:553–91.

[74] Van den Berghe G, Wouters P, Weekers F, et al. Intensive insulin therapy in critically ill patients. N Engl J Med 2001;345:1359–67.

[75] Pomposelli JJ, Baxter JK 3rd, Babineau TJ, et al. Early postoperative glucose control predicts nosocomial infection rates in diabetic patients. J Parenter Enter Nutr 1998;22: 77–81.

[76] Furnary AP, Zerr KJ, Grunkemeier GL, et al. Continuous intravenous insulin infusion reduces the incidence of deep sternal wound infection in diabetic patients after cardiac surgical procedures. Ann Thorac Surg 2000;69:667–8.

[77] Furnary AP, Gao G, Grunkemeier GL, et al. Continuous insulin infusion reduces mortality in patients with diabetes undergoing coronary artery bypass grafting. J Thorac Cardiovasc Surg 2003;125:985–7.

[78] The American Diabetes Association. Standards of medical care in diabetes—2006. Diabetes Care 2006;29(Suppl 1):4–9.

[79] Knecht LAD, Gauthier SM, Castro JC, et al. Diabetes care in the hospital: is there clinical inertia? J Hosp Med 2006;1:151–60.

[80] Queale WS, Seidler AJ, Brancati FL. Glycemic control and sliding scale insulin use in medical inpatients with diabetes mellitus. Arch Intern Med 1997;157:545–52.

[81] Inzucchi SE. Management of hyperglycemia in the hospital setting. N Engl J Med 2006;355: 1903–11.

[82] Society of Hospital Medicine. The Society of Hospital Medicine Glycemic Control Resource Room. Available at: http://www.hospitalmedicine.org/AM/Template.cfm?Section=Quality_Improvement_Resource_Rooms&;Template=/CM/HTMLDisplay.cfm&ContentID=11585. Accessed October 18, 2007.

ELSEVIER
SAUNDERS

THE MEDICAL
CLINICS
OF NORTH AMERICA

Med Clin N Am 92 (2008) 349–370

End-of-Life Care for the Hospitalized Patient

Steven Z. Pantilat, MD[a],*, Margaret Isaac, MD[b]

[a]Department of Medicine, UCSF Medical Center, 521 Parnassus Avenue, Suite C-126,
Box 0903, University of California, San Francisco, San Francisco, CA 94143-0903, USA
[b]University of Washington School of Medicine, Harborview Medical Center,
Box 359892, 325 9th Avenue, Seattle, WA 98104-2499, USA

The end of life

Contrary to the ideal vision of death—dying at home, surrounded by loved ones, and free from pain—most Americans die in hospitals, in pain, and alone [1]. Although death always will be a sad event, there is a great deal that physicians can do to relieve as much suffering as possible at the end of life. Because so many people die in hospitals, and many more are hospitalized in their last year of life, hospitalists and other hospital-based physicians have a unique opportunity to improve end-of-life care.

Patients and their families are clear about what they want and need from the health care system at the end of life: freedom from distressing symptoms, such as pain and dyspnea; the opportunity to communicate with physicians and others about death and dying; and the knowledge that they will be attended to and comforted by their physicians as they approach death [2]. These goals form the basis of comprehensive palliative care. Palliative care is the medical field focused on improving quality of life for people living with serious, chronic, and life-threatening illness irrespective of prognosis. Palliative care can be provided at any stage of illness and should be provided, in particular, simultaneously with all other appropriate medical treatments. Patients approaching the end of life certainly need palliative care but so do other patients who have acute exacerbations of chronic illness, such as heart failure, chronic obstructive pulmonary disease (COPD), cirrhosis, dementia, and cancer.

Because the end of life is an especially trying time for patients and families, the discontinuity between the inpatient and outpatient settings inherent in hospitalist systems imparts special challenges. It is critical for hospitalists

* Corresponding author.
  E-mail address: stevep@medicine.ucsf.edu (S.Z. Pantilat).

and primary care physicians (PCPs) to communicate clearly about treatment and to create opportunities for PCPs to visit patients and provide input regarding their care [3].

Symptom management

Patients who die in hospitals needlessly suffer a great deal. The Study to Understand Prognoses and Preferences for Outcomes and Risks of Treatments (SUPPORT), which enrolled more than 9000 seriously ill adults at five medical centers across the United States, documented the high prevalence of symptoms, such as pain, dyspnea, and delirium, in dying patients [4]. Treatments exist to relieve all of these symptoms.

Pain

Pain is one of the most common end-stage symptoms for hospitalized patients. SUPPORT found that 40% of dying patients had moderate to severe pain in the last 3 days of life. These patients include not only those who had lung and colon cancer, in whom pain might be expected, but also patients who had congestive heart failure and COPD, typically not associated with pain. Pain control often is insufficient, in part because physicians are poor at assessing pain, are overly concerned with side effects and addiction, and fear legal consequences from prescribing opioids [5].

Because pain inherently is subjective, the only way to know if patients are in pain is to ask. There are no objective measures for pain, and patients who have chronic pain may not exhibit the typical physiologic signs of tachycardia, hypertension, diaphoresis, and crying. Fortunately, pain scales offer a reliable, quantitative, and reproducible way to assess pain in individual patients [6]. The 0 to 10 numeric rating scale offers a quick assessment tool. Patients can be asked, "On a scale of 0 to10, with 0 being no pain and 10 being the worst pain you can imagine, how much pain are you having now?" Scores of 1 to 3 indicate mild pain, 4 to 6 moderate pain, and 7 to 10 severe pain. When physicians believe their patients' self-assessment of pain, strive for total pain relief, and prescribe pain medications more liberally, patients receive better pain control. Assessing pain in patients who have cognitive impairment presents particular challenges. A variety of standardized rating scales have been developed focusing on behavioral cues, such as appetite, posture, interactivity, facial expression, and vocalizations [7].

Hospitalized patients often are admitted for management of severe pain and many physicians still associate dying with the need for a "morphine drip." For patients who have mild or moderate pain, however, acetaminophen, aspirin, and nonsteroidal anti-inflammatory drugs (NSAIDs) can be helpful. NSAIDs can precipitate exacerbations of congestive heart failure and, therefore, should be used cautiously in patients who have this condition [8,9].

Moderate or severe pain often requires opioids. For acute, severe pain the intravenous or subcutaneous routes provide the most rapid relief. Although not used routinely in hospitals, the subcutaneous route of administration of opioids is effective and doses of opioids are the same as for intravenous use. For patients who are opioid naïve, morphine sulfate, 2 to 4 mg intravenously every 3 hours as needed, is an appropriate starting dosage. For patients who have been using opioids at home, physicians should continue the same regimen or escalate the dose if the pain is not well controlled. Dose escalation is accomplished best using a percentage increase. For unrelieved moderate pain, consider increasing the dose of opioid by 25% to 50%. For severe pain, increase the dose by 50% to 100%. Equianalgesic dosing charts help convert between agents and across routes of administration (Table 1). Once pain is controlled, it is helpful to switch to oral medications, which are cheaper, easier to administer at home, and prevent infectious risk from needles.

If pain is constant, control must be continuous. Once pain control is achieved using short-acting oral, intravenous, or subcutaneous opioids, it is appropriate to transition to long-acting oral or transdermal opioids. Because their long half-life makes titration impractical, these formulations are appropriate only when a patient's pain is well controlled. For hospitalized patients approaching the end of life who experience constant pain, physicians can use repeated intravenous boluses of opioids or a continuous intravenous or subcutaneous infusion of opioids to control pain rapidly.

Table 1
Equianalgesic dosing table

	Equianalgesic dose (mg)	
Opioid analgesic	Oral	Parenteral
Morphine (Roxanol, MS Contin)	30	10
Hydromorphone (Dilaudid)	7.5	1.5
Oxymorphone[c]	10	
Oxycodone (Percocet, OxyContin)	20	—
Hydrocodone (Vicodin, Lortab, Norco)	30	—
Codeine (Tylenol #2 = 15 mg, #3 = 30 mg, #4 = 60 mg; each with acetaminophen 300 mg)	180–200	130
Fentanyl		0.1 (100 μg)
Fentanyl transdermal[a] (Duragesic)	2:1 rule[b]	—

[a] The onset of analgesia is delayed 8 to 12 hours, so continue to treat pain for the first 12 hours with other medication; there is a residual effect after patch is removed; do not use in opioid-naïve patients. Use only for chronic stable pain.

[b] The 2:1 rule: divide the total 24-hour dose of oral morphine by 2 to get the dose of transdermal fentanyl in μg/h.

[c] Data from Hale ME, Ahdieh H, Ma T, et al. Efficacy and safety of OPANA ER (oxymorphone extended release) for relief of moderate to severe chronic low back pain in opioid-experienced patients: a 12-week, randomized, double-blind, placebo-controlled study. J Pain 2007;8(2):175–84; and the Palliative care pocket consult guide, UCSF Palliative Care Service.

Frequent assessment by physicians or nurses ensures that medication doses are escalated in response to poorly controlled pain. Once controlled, doses of opioids for breakthrough pain should be equal to the total daily dose of opioid divided into equal doses based on the half-life of the medication. For example, for a patient well controlled with morphine (3 mg per hour) by continuous intravenous or subcutaneous infusion (72 mg per day), an appropriate bolus for breakthrough pain is morphine (9 mg intravenously or subcutaneously every 3 hours).

The side effects associated with opioid use, such as sedation, respiratory depression, and constipation, can be managed easily and effectively. Sedation typically resolves after 2 to 3 days at the same dose of opioid. If necessary, physicians can treat persistent sedation with methylphenidate or dextroamphetamine (2.5 mg orally in the morning and at noon). The dose can be titrated upward, by 2.5 mg in the morning and at noon every 2 to 3 days. A usual dose is 5 to 15 mg per day and should not exceed 30 mg per day [10]. Although respiratory depression can occur with opioid use, it is uncommon when low doses are used and the medication is titrated slowly. Patients who have pulmonary disease can tolerate low-dose opioids if monitored carefully and should not be denied opioids for pain.

Constipation is one side effect of opioids that does not resolve with time. In addition, it is a side effect for which prevention is better and easier than treatment. It is critical to prescribe a bowel regimen, such as senna, a laxative that stimulates the bowel (at doses of two tablets or 10 to 15 mL of syrup orally twice a day [not to exceed eight tablets or 30 mL per day]), or docusate sodium, a stool softener (250 mg orally twice a day). If this regimen fails, bisacodyl tablets (10 to 15 mg orally or 10 mg rectally twice a day) or lactulose (15 to 30 g or sorbitol 30 g once or twice a day) is likely to help. Some patients may develop nausea, pruritus, or urinary retention with a particular opioid. Decreasing the dose or changing opioids often relieves these symptoms.

Physicians should understand the cause of pain to direct specific treatment. For example, neuropathic pain, commonly described as burning, shooting, or electrical in quality, and often associated with numbness or paresthesias, responds well to tricyclic antidepressants, serotonin-noradrenergic reuptake inhibitors, opioids, transdermal lidocaine patches, tramadol [11], and anticonvulsants, such as gabapentin (Table 2). The tricyclic antidepressants in this setting work more quickly and at lower dosages than typically used for treatment of depression. Bone pain from metastases may respond to a variety of agents, including NSAIDs, whose anti-inflammatory properties make them useful in this setting. Additionally, steroids, radiation therapy, and radiopharmaceuticals can be helpful. Bisphosphonates are useful in preventing pain by reducing risk for pathologic fracture in patients who have metastatic cancer and seem to have a modest effect on metastatic bone pain independent of fracture prevention [12].

Table 2
Treatment of neuropathic pain

Drug	Dosage
Tricyclic antidepressants[a]	
Nortriptyline	10–150 mg orally at bedtime
Desipramine	10–200 mg orally at bedtime
Anticonvulsants	
Gabapentin	300–900 mg orally 3 times a day
Pregabalin	75 mg by mouth twice a day[b]
Serotonin-noradrenergic reuptake inhibitor antidepressants	
Duloxetine	60 mg/d to 60 mg twice a day
Venlafaxine	150–225 mg/d (extended release)
Lidocaine patch 5%[c]	≤3 patches at a time, 12 hours on, 12 hours off
Tramadol[d]	50–100 mg by mouth every 4–6 h as needed for pain[e]

[a] Begin with a low dose. Pain relief often can be achieved at doses far below antidepressant doses, thereby minimizing side effects.

[b] Start at 75 mg by mouth every night; if well tolerated, titrate to 75 mg by mouth twice a day after 7 days. Likewise, when discontinued, should be tapered over 7 days. Maximum dosage 300 mg per day. Dose adjustment required for renal failure.

[c] Use if pain is localized or on most painful area.

[d] Generally it is not advisable to use tramadol in conjunction with opioids.

[e] Maximum 400 mg per day; 300 mg per day if > 75 years old, per manufacturer.

Adapted from Rowbotham MC, Goli V, Kunz NR, et al. Venlafaxine extended release in the treatment of painful diabetic neuropathy: a double-blind, placebo-controlled study. Pain 2004;110(3):697–706.

In addition to pharmaceuticals, certain nonpharmacologic interventions, such as radiation therapy, can provide pain relief in specific clinical settings. Procedures, such as celiac plexus nerve blocks for patients who have pancreatic cancer, sometimes are helpful [13,14]. Complementary therapies, such as acupuncture, may be beneficial, although a recent systematic review found a paucity of data supporting the efficacy of acupuncture for the treatment of cancer pain [15]. Modalities, such as guided imagery and meditation, also can be considered.

"Double effect"

In most circumstances, the amount of opioids required to treat symptoms adequately is not enough to affect survival [16,17]. Rarely, in an attempt to relieve patient suffering, physicians may need to prescribe opioids at doses that might suppress respiration and hasten death. As long as the ultimate goal is to provide comfort, such actions are acceptable morally under the ethical concept of "double effect" [17]. This concept provides that known but unintended consequences of opioids, such as respiratory suppression and sedation, are acceptable even if they hasten death, because the primary intent of the treatment is the relief of suffering. In such circumstances, ethical practice requires that physicians and nurses document that increases in doses of opioids are in response to specific symptoms.

Dyspnea

Dyspnea refers to the subjective sensation of difficulty breathing [18]. This extremely distressing symptom occurs in nearly 90% of patients dying of COPD, in more than 60% of patients dying of congestive heart failure or lung cancer, and in more than 30% of patients dying of colon cancer [4]. The key to the management of dyspnea in dying patients is its rapid alleviation, followed by a determination as to whether or not patients desire a work-up to discover an underlying cause. If patients desire a work-up, treatment often can be targeted at the underlying cause, such as pneumonia, pleural or pericardial effusion, asthma or COPD exacerbation, congestive heart failure, anemia, or pneumothorax.

In the setting of end-of-life care, opioids and oxygen are appropriate first steps in relieving the sensation of shortness of breath. Although most studies of opioids for treatment of dyspnea have been conducted with cancer patients, experience suggests that opioids also can be effective in relieving dyspnea in many patients, often at lower doses than needed for pain relief [18]. Many patients who are not hypoxemic, and even some who are, also may find relief from fresh air or a fan.

Nausea and vomiting

Nausea and vomiting are other common symptoms at the end of life, experienced by up to 68% of people dying of cancer, 46% percent of patients who have end-stage AIDS, and 30% to 43% of patients dying of renal failure [19]. In approaching the management of nausea and vomiting, it is helpful to group the causes by mechanism because treatment is targeted best at underlying mechanisms and pathways (Table 3). Drugs, toxins, and metabolic derangements can stimulate the chemoreceptor trigger zone in the brain, leading to nausea and vomiting. In addition to eliminating the possible offending agent, prochlorperazine (10 mg orally or intravenously or 25 mg rectally every 8 hours) or haloperidol (0.5–2 mg orally or intravenously every 6–8 hours) can provide relief by blocking

Table 3
Mechanisms and causes of nausea and vomiting

Mechanism/pathway	Cause
Chemoreceptor trigger zone	Drugs: opioids, digoxin, antibiotics, NSAIDs; metabolic derangements: hypercalcemia; uremia; chemotherapeutic agents
Vagal afferent nerve	Mucosal irritation (candidiasis); gastrointestinal stretch or enlargement due to constipation, gastroparesis, gastric outlet obstruction, or bowel obstruction; viscus enlargement
Higher cortical structures	Increased intracranial pressure from tumor, bleed, or infection; anxiety
Vestibular apparatus	Movement

the chemoreceptor trigger zone's dopamine, serotonin, and histamine receptors. Additionally, if an opioid is the suspected cause of the nausea and vomiting, changing to another opioid may provide relief, as this side effect often is unique to a particular opioid in particular patients and not a generalized class effect.

Vagal afferent nerve stimulation by mucosal irritation, such as stretching of the bowel from constipation, obstruction, or gastroparesis; or viscus enlargement, such as hepatomegaly, can trigger vomiting directly. Treatment is directed best at relieving the underlying cause, such as constipation or a bowel obstruction. Promethazine, diphenhydramine, and hydroxyzine (12.5–25 mg orally every 6 hours) are good choices for treatment, as histamine receptors also play a role in this mechanism of nausea. On their own, benzodiazepines are poor antiemetics and may increase the risk for aspiration by causing sedation. They may be helpful, however, in preventing anticipatory nausea associated with chemotherapy. The serotonin antagonists, such as ondansetron and granisetron, are most efficacious in chemotherapy-induced and postoperative nausea and vomiting but also may relieve nausea and vomiting caused by other stimuli. Practical approaches, such as well presented, small meals of favorite foods; cold, carbonated drinks; and the avoidance of strong odors, also can help reduce nausea and vomiting. In addition, all medications except antiemetics should be given after meals to minimize the risk for nausea.

Delirium

Delirium is defined as a state of waxing and waning levels of consciousness combined with confusion, agitation, disturbance of the sleep-wake cycle, anxiety, and disorders of memory, cognition, and behavior. It is seen in up to 40% of hospitalized elders [20] and up to 75% of terminally ill patients who have cancer. Common causes of delirium include drugs, metabolic derangements, organ failure, and infections. If desired by a family, physicians can try to identify and resolve delirium by treatment of specific causes, including by changing medications. Other interventions, such as maintaining a well-lit environment and providing reassuring words from loved ones, can be effective in mild cases. If a cause cannot be found or reversed, physicians can treat delirium with haloperidol (starting dose of 0.5–1 mg, titrated to a maximum dose of 10 mg orally, subcutaneously, or intravenously, each given every 6 hours). Benzodiazepines should be avoided as they often precipitate delirium [21] and are ineffective at treating it [22].

Death rattle

Patients who are dying imminently may develop "death rattle," the sound made by air passing over the thin layer of saliva and mucus that forms in the back of the throat when secretions no longer can be cleared. Although it is impossible to know how disturbing this phenomenon is to patients, the sound can be distressing to families and loved ones [23]. Deep suctioning can increase discomfort, so pharmacologic treatment is preferred using atropine ophthalmic solution (1%, at a dose of 1–2 drops sublingually every hour) or, in awake patients, glycopyrrolate (0.1–0.2 mg intravenously every 4 hours as needed). Because atropine crosses the blood-brain barrier, it can cause more mental status changes than glycopyrrolate and, therefore, should be reserved for use only in obtunded patients.

Palliative sedation

In the setting of severe symptoms, when even expert management is not sufficient, physicians may consider palliative sedation. Palliative sedation therapy is described as "the use of specific sedative medications to relieve intolerable suffering from refractory symptoms by a reduction in patient consciousness, using appropriate drugs carefully titrated to the cessation of symptoms" [24]. Appropriate treatments usually include sedatives, such as benzodiazepines, barbiturates, or propofol. Palliative sedation can be considered an appropriate treatment strategy if three conditions are met: (1) standard treatments prove ineffective at managing symptoms or confer unbearable side effects; (2) the purpose of sedative treatment is to alleviate suffering, not hasten death; and (3) a patient is moribund, making it unlikely that death will be hastened [25].

A full discussion of palliative sedation is beyond the scope of this article. Before considering palliative sedation, however, physicians should insure that they have taken all reasonable steps to alleviate suffering. Consultation with a palliative care specialist strongly is encouraged. If symptoms persist despite expert management and palliative sedation is considered, patients or their surrogate must be informed fully of the procedure and its implications.

Other issues in medical management at the end of life

Artificial nutrition and hydration

Ceasing to eat and drink is a normal part of dying, not its cause. Understandably, families often become distressed when their loved one refuses food, at least in part because feeding has great cultural significance. Families often request artificial nutrition and hydration in the mistaken hope that it will prolong life, promote comfort, or improve functional status and quality of life. Unlike in the setting of acute illness, where these interventions may play an important role in recovery, in end-stage dementia, stroke, and cancer, artificial nutrition and hydration typically do not confer clinical benefit and may pose risks [26,27]. For patients who are dying imminently, minimizing fluids may increase comfort by preventing and reducing pulmonary and peripheral edema, pleural effusions, ascites, and death rattle. Physicians play an important role in helping families understand the appropriate role of artificial nutrition and hydration. They also may direct families' desires to help away from feeding and toward more productive actions that promote patient comfort, such as moistening the mouth with a swab or putting petroleum jelly on dry lips.

Imminent death

As patients approach the final 24 to 48 hours of life, families may notice changes that, although normal, can be distressing if left unexplained. In addition to developing death rattle or dry mouth, patients may have Cheyne-Stokes breathing patterns, irregular breathing, or slow and gasping respirations. Breathing may pause for as long as 20 to 30 seconds. Urine output may fall, especially if patients are not drinking and not receiving artificial hydration, and patients may become incontinent of urine and stool. The extremities typically become cold, mottled, blue, and swollen. Patients often become progressively less responsive and many become completely unresponsive. In contrast to this gradual and peaceful decline, some patients experience distressing symptoms at the very end of life, including dyspnea, pain, and delirium. These symptoms must be treated aggressively, using the interventions described previously. In all cases, gentle reassurance that the changes the family is witnessing are a normal part of dying can ameliorate anxiety and fear. It can be comforting for families to know that physicians are aware of and anticipating these changes, and watching for specific signs and symptoms can assist clinicians with prognosis (Table 4).

Death in intensive care units

Approximately 20% of Americans die in intensive care units (ICUs) [28]. The focus on aggressive, life-saving, high-technology interventions in ICUs creates special challenges for providing high-quality end-of-life care. Nowhere is the mission to prolong life more pronounced than in this particular setting, even when the likelihood of success is small. Yet nearly 1 of 10 patients admitted to an ICU dies [29]. The ability to integrate palliative care to

Table 4
Signs and symptoms of impending death

Sign	Hours before death: mean/median (SD)
Retained respiratory secretions audible ("death rattle")	57/23 (82)
Respirations with mandibular movement	8/3 (18)
Cyanosis of extremities	5/1 (11)
No radial pulse	3/1 (4.2)

Data from Morita T, Ichiki T, Tsunoda J, et al. A prospective study on the dying process in terminally ill cancer patients. Am J Hosp Palliat Care 1998;15(4):217–22.

make the shift from curative to palliative care in ICUs is a vital skill that can help patients and families deal with death. To the extent possible, create a private, quiet space; liberalize visitation; turn off or remove monitors and machines; avoid laboratory or imaging studies; and remove all lines and drains that do not promote comfort [30,31]. Although it may be difficult to determine the severity of pain or dyspnea in patients in ICUs who already are sedated, physicians should look for and treat signs, such as grimacing, moaning, or tachypnea that typically reflect discomfort.

An increasing number of deaths in ICUs are preceded by withdrawing or withholding life-sustaining interventions [32], such as mechanical ventilation, vasopressors, dialysis, antibiotics, and nutrition and hydration. The following specific principles, adapted from Rubenfeld and Crawford [31], can help guide the withdrawal of life-sustaining interventions in ICUs:

1. Remove treatments that no longer are desired or do not provide comfort.
2. Focus on treatments that promote comfort.
3. Actions with the sole goal of hastening death are ethically and legally problematic.
4. Any treatment can be withheld or withdrawn.
5. After deciding to withhold or withdraw one medical treatment, strongly consider withdrawing other life sustaining interventions.

Withdrawal of mechanical ventilation is considered best as a procedure like any other, with specific steps to follow. Before beginning, ensure adequate sedation using opioids. Benzodiazepines can be added if needed. The goal is not to render patients silent and motionless, simply comfortable. Next, reduce inspired oxygen to room air, remove positive end-expiratory pressure and set the ventilator to an intermittent mandatory ventilation rate equal to the patient's spontaneous rate. These steps help determine a patient's underlying respiratory rate, allowing for treatment of tachypnea with opioids before proceeding to the next step. Once the physician, nurse, and respiratory therapist are convinced that the patient is comfortable, reduce the intermittent mandatory ventilation rate slowly to 0, increasing sedation as needed. At that point, the team can remove the endotracheal tube. Although the authors' routine practice is to remove the endotracheal tube, some physicians choose to leave it in place with a T-piece and humidified air for fear of precipitating choking. In the authors' experience, this is a rare event and one that can be managed with opioids and suctioning. One advantage of removing an endotracheal tube is that it makes it easier for loved ones to get close to a patient and allows a patient to appear more peaceful and comfortable. Informing families of what to expect allows them to anticipate possible outcomes, and staying at the bedside allows physicians to respond to any discomfort. It is important to switch off ventilator alarms and monitors during this process to reduce anxiety and concern. Families may be present during this procedure if they wish but should be forewarned that patients may demonstrate temporary increases in agitation or respiratory rate while sedation is titrated.

Physicians should discontinue pharmacologic paralysis before initiating the withdrawal of life-sustaining interventions, because paralysis masks patient discomfort and may hasten death without promoting comfort. In some circumstances, paralysis persists for many hours or days after medication is discontinued. In these situations, persistent paralysis is considered a complication of the medical illness and withdrawal of life-sustaining interventions can proceed. Throughout the process of withdrawing life-prolonging interventions, families must be reassured that palliation will continue. Phrases, such as "withdrawing care," should be avoided and emphasis placed on changing the focus of care to aggressive symptom management and preservation of dignity.

Psychosocial support and spiritual issues

The experience of the end of life encompasses the psychologic, social, spiritual, and the physiologic state of a patient. Providing comprehensive care to dying patients demands that physicians attend to these issues in addition to relieving distressing symptoms.

Grief

Elizabeth Kübler-Ross first described five stages of grief experienced by dying patients. Although often believed a linear progression, these stages—denial, anger, bargaining, depression, and acceptance—are viewed more appropriately as a range of responses that patients have in response to death [33]. Patients commonly move between stages, often exhibiting the coexistence of multiple stages at the same time. As patients deal with these sad and powerful emotions, physicians can help by listening, providing reassurance, and making appropriate referrals for psychotherapy and group support.

Depression

Depression at the end of life is not normal. Depression often is unrecognized and untreated and can lead to decreased quality of life, more severe pain, and even requests for hastened death [34–36]. Alternatively, sadness and grief are expected in dying patients. The challenge for hospitalists is to distinguish between the two in a patient a physician has just met. The typical vegetative symptoms of anhedonia, poor sleep, and decreased appetite are less helpful in making a diagnosis, as these symptoms may be related to the underlying illness and not to depression. More helpful diagnostic symptoms of depression at this stage are guilt, hopelessness, helplessness, and worthlessness. In difficult cases, psychiatric consultation can be helpful in diagnosis and treatment.

Even at the end of life, there are effective medicines for treating depression. The one caveat is that dying patients often cannot wait 4 to 6 weeks for medications to take effect. Although clinical trials are limited, expert recommendations for treating depression in the terminally ill include psychotherapy, patient and family education, and medications [34]. Stimulants, such as methylphenidate and dextroamphetamine (starting doses of 2.5 mg orally morning and noon) may elevate mood in as little as 1 to 2 days [34]. These medications can be titrated up by 2.5-mg intervals every 2 to 3 days as needed to achieve the desired effect (with maximum doses of 30 mg daily).

Psychosocial support

Patients who are dying sometimes fear that their physicians will abandon them [37]. This fear may be particularly acute for dying patients cared for by hospitalists. Patients may interpret hospitalist care as abandonment by their PCP and discharge as abandonment by the hospitalist. PCPs who do not visit their hospitalized patients routinely may consider doing so for the dying. Although hospitalists may not participate in care after discharge, in the case of imminently dying patients discharged home, hospitalists may fill an important role in the transition back to the PCP. In all settings, statements, such as, "I will make sure you get the best possible care, whatever happens," emphasize the caring and concern of physicians. Fulfilling this promise typically requires coordinated care and close communication between hospitalists and PCPs.

Physicians may pull away from dying patients to lessen their own sense of abandonment, grief, and loss. Hospitalists can counter this tendency by visiting their dying patients more frequently. These visits remind physicians of their commitment to patients and prevent the therapeutic nihilism to which physicians sometimes fall prey. There is much to be done for patients who are dying. The care may be less intensive technologically, but in relieving suffering, it is no less aggressive or effective. An approach that emphasizes what will be done sends a hopeful message to patients and families.

Physicians can help patients recognize the need and desire to bring closure to important relationships as the end of life approaches. Author and physician, Ira Byock, MD, suggests that to help achieve closure, patients make the following five statements to those they care about: "Forgive me," "I forgive you," "Thank you," "I love you," and "Good-bye" [38]. Physicians can suggest these phrases to patients and their families. Physicians also can encourage patients to complete important projects, such as writing a book, creating a work of art, or establishing a trust or foundation.

Spiritual issues

Many patients turn to spirituality for comfort and to cope with death and dying. Although physicians are not trained explicitly in spiritual matters, they can ask about them and encourage patients to consider talking about them [39,40]. Although physicians worry that they will unleash a torrent of questions for which they have no answers, exploration of spiritual issues may require no more than attentive listening. Referrals to a chaplain can be helpful for many patients. Hospital chaplains or a patient's own spiritual advisor are appropriate when patients have specific religious or spiritual questions or request specific guidance.

Cultural issues

Traditions surrounding and approaches to death vary across cultures. The desire for prognostic information and the locus of decision making are among the important issues influenced by a patient's background. Cultures are not monolithic and patients from the same culture may embrace different approaches to the end of life [41]. Curiosity, open-ended questions, and sensitivity to differences demonstrate physicians' respect for patients' desires and customs.

Many patients' families express a desire to shield their family member from bad news—information about a serious diagnosis or poor prognosis. In this situation, obtaining "informed refusal" is appropriate. Physicians can tell a patient, in front of the family, "I have information about your illness. Some patients want to hear from me directly and others prefer that I speak to someone else. How do you feel?" With this approach, physicians permit patients to decide how much information they want without making assumptions based on patients' ethnicity or cultural background.

Decision making at the end of life

Discussing end-of-life care with patients

For patients who have serious, chronic, and terminal illness, hospitalization typically signals an abrupt change in clinical status and affords inpatient physicians the opportunity to discuss end-of-life care. Physicians may worry that such discussions will upset patients or rob them of hope, yet studies demonstrate that patients welcome these discussions [35,42]. Explaining to patients that end-of-life care is a routine part of a hospitalist's discussions with inpatients may help alleviate concerns that such conversations reflect prognostic pessimism [43]. For patients who already have had such conversations with their PCP, hospitalists simply can confirm what has been discussed. When these issues have not been considered previously, the information elicited is critical to ensuring that patients receive the care they desire. Hospitalists can start by checking patients' understanding of his illness by asking, "Could you please tell me what you understand about your medical condition and what your doctors have told you about it?"

These discussions can be difficult because they involve emotionally laden issues, confront death explicitly, and may convey bad news. Furthermore, physicians often dominate the conversation, use jargon, fail to elicit patient values and goals of care, and miss opportunities for empathic connection [44]. Several straightforward strategies designed to overcome these common shortfalls may improve the quality of these discussions (Table 5). Sample phrases can be useful in getting started (Table 6).

First, physicians must listen to patients and encourage patients to share important information. Asking open-ended questions and allowing patients to complete their opening statements uninterrupted tells patients that a physician wants to listen. Physicians should avoid the tendency to use jargon. Physicians tend to focus on specific interventions, such as mechanical ventilation or vasopressors, but patients more often speak pragmatically of how they live. To elicit patients' values and goals of care rather than their preferences for specific treatments, physicians could say, "Mr. Johnston when you think about the future and the possibility of getting sicker, what worries you the most?" Finally, patients often express a great deal of emotion during such discussions [45]. In response to a patient's concern that he is a burden on his family, a physician might say, "It sounds like you are very worried about how much time and effort it takes for your family to care for you." This empathic response encourages patients to say more and reassures them that the physician is attuned to their emotional needs and can help identify important emotions. Finally, good communication signals to patients that he can rely on the physician as the end of life nears.

Advance directives

As patients approach the end of life, they often reach a point at which they no longer can participate in decision making about their care. In

Table 5
Communicating about end-of-life care

Technique	Description	Example
Listen	Sit silently, allowing the patient to finish his opening statement uninterrupted	Focus on the patient and sit quietly.
Avoid jargon	Use simple words and phrases that the patient or family member will understand	"The medicines we are using to raise your father's blood pressure are no longer working, telling me that he is getting even sicker."
Elicit values and goals of care	Ask patients what they fear most as they face the future or what they hope will happen	"When you think about getting sicker, what worries you the most?"
Make empathic statements	Listen for and respond to emotionally laden terms, phrases, or comments	"Sounds like you are really worried about being a burden on your family."

Table 6
Useful phrases in communicating with patients and families at the end of life

Getting started	"Can you tell me what your understanding is about your illness?"
	"As you think about what lies ahead, what concerns you the most?"
Continuing phrases	"What do you mean by... (futile, giving up, everything)?"
Talking about dying	"Many patients with x (cancer, heart disease) tell me they think about the possibility of dying. They have questions. How about you?"
Informed refusal	"I have information about your condition. Some patients want to know the details; other patients want me to talk to someone else. How do you feel?"
Surrogate	"If you were to get so sick that you couldn't talk to me directly, who should I talk to help me make decisions about your care?"
Other useful statements	"I wish there was something to make your cancer go away. Unfortunately, there isn't, but there are things we can do to help you feel better."
	"When you think about the future, what do you hope for?"
	"We will certainly do everything possible to make your father more comfortable and relieve his suffering."
Spirituality	"Do you have any spiritual beliefs or practices that are important to you? As your health care provider, I would like to be supportive of these."

Data from the Palliative care pocket consult guide, UCSF Palliative Care Service.

anticipation of such situations, physicians should encourage patients, while they still have capacity to make medical decisions, to make oral or written statements meant to guide their care in the future. In these statements, called advance directives, patients also can designate a surrogate decision maker to make decisions on their behalf, should they lose the ability to do so. These statements allow patients to project their autonomy into the future and are meant to guide care. Although written advance directives, such as a durable power of attorney for health care, typically are considered a more definitive reflection of patients' values and preferences, oral statements made to family, friends, or physicians also should be respected. Physicians should become familiar with the laws in their state or seek advice when conflicts arise between a patient's written or verbal wishes and family members' expressed desires.

Although patients want to discuss advance directives, few in the outpatient setting actually do [35]. A study of more than 100 oncology inpatients found that only 9% of patients had discussed advance care planning with their outpatient oncologists, and only 23% of the remaining patients wished to do so. In contrast, 58% of all patients interviewed supported establishment of a policy to make discussion of advance care planning part of the inpatient admission history [46]. For this reason, it is important for hospitalists to determine routinely at the time of admission whether or not these issues have been addressed previously, and if not, open the discussion of patient preferences [43]. Hospitalists should determine a patient's general values and goals, ask patients to appoint a surrogate, and ask the PCP about the patient's wishes. A nonthreatening way to initiate a discussion of advance directives and to elicit choice of a surrogate is to say, "I now want to talk with you about something I talk about with all the patients I care for in the hospital: if you were to get so sick that you could not talk to me directly, with whom should I speak to help me make decisions about your care?"

In addition to obtaining generally important information with a routine discussion of preferences at the time of admission, hospitalists can focus on specific issues that are likely to arise based on the clinical situation. For example, for patients admitted who have acute renal failure, a discussion of dialysis is appropriate, whereas in the outpatient setting, it may never have been a relevant issue.

Do not attempt resuscitation orders

On admission, it is important to ascertain a patient's wishes regarding cardiopulmonary resuscitation (CPR). Studies suggest that do not attempt resuscitation (DNAR) discussions occur infrequently, and even when patients want to be "no code," in half the cases, physicians fail to write the order [1]. Such data emphasize the need to initiate and properly document these discussions to implement patient preferences.

The term, DNAR, rather than do not resuscitate (DNR), is often used to emphasize that clinicians only can attempt CPR and that it usually is ineffective. It is important to inform patients of the likelihood of success of CPR, as such knowledge affects patient decisions. Overall survival to discharge for hospitalized patients who receive CPR is 14% [47]. Patients who have multisystem organ failure or metastatic cancer have a dramatically poorer chance of survival, less than 10% [48], whereas those who have had a myocardial infarction have a 25% to 40% chance of survival.

Because patients can be swayed by how physicians describe interventions, the description of CPR should be neutral but accurate. It is important for patients to understand that a decision about CPR is not just a decision about one intervention. Rather, it is a statement about how and in what circumstance a patient may die—amidst turmoil, in a room full of strangers, typically without family present.

Prognosis

Physicians find it difficult and anxiety provoking to discuss prognosis with patients [49]. Yet this information is important because patients make different treatment decisions when they understand prognosis. In one study of older patients, half as many respondents said they would want CPR in the event of cardiac arrest once researchers corrected their overly optimistic assumptions of its success [50]. Perhaps the most compelling reason to discuss prognosis is the recognition that most people say they would live their lives differently if they knew their life span was limited significantly.

One study found that physicians were overly optimistic in their predictions of survival for patients referred to hospice. Physicians who knew their patients well were more likely to be optimistic. These data suggest that hospitalists, by virtue of their shorter acquaintance, may provide more accurate prognoses. Indices, such as the Palliative Prognosis Score, Palliative Prognostic Index, and others, can help predict survival for hospitalized patients [51].

Physicians worry that patients have unrealistic expectations of their prognostic capabilities. Yet most patients can understand explanations of statistical probability and appreciate the limits of accuracy. Physicians can address their limitations explicitly by saying, "I am wrong as often as I am right but want to let you know my best guess for what the future holds." Physicians can convey prognostic information in a way that reflects the inherent uncertainty by speaking in terms of temporal ranges, such as "weeks to months," "days to weeks," and "hours to days."

Some fear that discussing prognosis robs patients of hope. In the absence of realistic discussions about prognosis, patients are likely to be overly optimistic and embrace false hopes for survival. A compassionate discussion of prognosis can help patients identify what is most important and realistic to achieve. Physicians can ask, "When you think about the future, what do you hope for?" [39].

Ethical and legal issues

Many ethical issues arise at the end of life. In caring for dying patients, physicians must be guided by the same ethical principles that guide all medical care: autonomy, beneficence, nonmaleficence, confidentiality, truth-telling, and justice. When difficult ethical issues arise, as when two or more ethical principles conflict, physicians should consult with colleagues, books, journals, and ethics committees from their institutions or professional organizations [52].

Futility

All commonly encountered ethical issues, such as confidentiality and decision-making capacity, arise in end-of-life care. Less frequently experienced issues, however, such as futility, also occur. The concept of futility is invoked when a physician judges that an intervention is unlikely to achieve the goal of care and on that basis refuses to provide an intervention that a patient or family requests. These conflicts often arise with CPR, mechanical ventilation, or hemodialysis. Despite its appeal to physicians, the concept of futility is difficult to implement fairly in clinical practice. First, there is little agreement as to how minimal a chance of success must be to be deemed futile [53]. Second, classifications of futility based on assessments of patient quality of life inherently are biased. Finally, physicians often invoke futility when they are frustrated by what they consider unrealistic patient or family requests and expectations. This frustration typically indicates a breakdown in communication. Satisfactory resolution is more likely to occur with good communication, perhaps involving other physicians, a palliative care team, or an ethics committee, rather than resorting to the futility argument.

Withholding and withdrawing life-sustaining interventions

The withholding and withdrawing of life-sustaining interventions represents another potentially confusing ethical issue at the end of life. Withdrawing mechanical ventilation, antibiotics, or nutrition and hydration may feel different from withholding them, but these actions ethically are equivalent [52]. They also are legally equivalent as established by the United States Supreme Court in the Cruzan decision [54]. By honoring wishes to withdraw or withhold interventions, physicians demonstrate their respect for patient autonomy.

Hospice

Dying patients often are hospitalized for management of a symptom or because the family becomes unable to care for them at home. Hospice can provide symptom management, communication, and psychosocial support that assist families as they care for their loved ones at home. In fact, although often believed a physical location, in the United States, hospice is a service provided most commonly to patients in their own homes. Enrollment in hospice requires (1) that a physician be willing to state that a patient has a 6-month prognosis and (2) that a patient has a designated physician of record. Despite the comprehensive set of services offered, only 36% of dying patients enroll in hospice [55]. In addition, patients enroll in hospice late in the course of illness with a median survival in hospice of only 3 weeks [56].

Although physicians may worry that a discussion of hospice leads patients to lose hope, there are ways of broaching the topic that may be less threatening. Hospice can be suggested in the context of getting patients and families more help at home: "It sounds like you think your husband could use more help caring for you at home. Have you considered hospice?" Hospitalists also may raise the possibility of hospice early in the course of illness by saying, "I realize this may not be right for you now, but I would like you to start thinking about hospice." In this role, hospitalists may increase the timeliness and number of hospice referrals. Because it may be difficult for a hospitalist to remain a physician of record for purposes of hospice enrollment, the hospitalist must work closely with a PCP or the hospice medical director to ensure continuity of care.

After death

The responsibility of physicians does not end when patients die. There are several tasks that a physician must complete after a patient's death. A licensed physician who attended the patient must complete the death certificate accurately. Discussing autopsy with families also is important. Over the past 30 years, despite increasingly sophisticated diagnostic tests and imaging, the usefulness of autopsy in determining the cause of death, confirming diagnoses, and uncovering unsuspected conditions has remained paramount. In up to 44% of cases, autopsies reveal previously unknown, potentially treatable conditions and, in 10% to 20% of cases, conditions that might have made a difference in patient survival had they been diagnosed during life [57].

Although less intense than the grief experienced by patients' loved ones, physicians do experience loss with the death of each patient. Talking with colleagues, friends, or partners; writing; and performing rituals can help. Physicians also may consider attending funerals or memorial services of patients with whom they developed close attachments.

Summary

Hospitalists frequently care for dying patients. There is much that hospitalists can do to provide high-quality care to patients approaching the end of life. By providing expert symptom management; discussing issues, such as prognosis and death sensitively and compassionately; and providing emotional, spiritual, psychologic, and social support, physicians can provide comfort and ease the suffering inherent in the end of life. In addition to the manifest rewards of promoting dignity and comfort to the dying, the greatest reward for physicians in caring for patients approaching the end of life may be the sense of clarity about personal priorities that derives from helping dying patients make the most of the time they have remaining.

Acknowledgments

The authors would like to thank Thomas Bookwalter, PharmD, for his help in editing the pain management section, and Emily Philipps and Salina Ng for their expert assistance in editing and preparing the manuscript.

References

[1] The SUPPORT Principal Investigators. A controlled trial to improve care for seriously ill hospitalized patients. The study to understand prognoses and preferences for outcomes and risks of treatments (SUPPORT). JAMA 1995;274(20):1591–8.
[2] Singer PA, Martin DK, Kelner M. Quality end-of-life care: patients' perspectives. JAMA 1999;281(2):163–8.

[3] Pantilat SZ, Lindenauer PK, Katz PP, et al. Primary care physician attitudes regarding communication with hospitalists. Am J Med 2001;111(98):155–205.

[4] Lynn J, Teno JM, Phillips RS, et al. Perceptions by family members of the dying experience of older and seriously ill patients. SUPPORT Investigators. Study to understand prognoses and preferences for outcomes and risks of treatments. Ann Intern Med 1997; 126(2):97–106.

[5] Von Roenn JH, Cleeland CS, Gonin R, et al. Physician attitudes and practice in cancer pain management. A survey from the Eastern Cooperative Oncology Group. Ann Intern Med 1993;119(2):121–6.

[6] Jacox A, Carr DB, Payne R. New clinical-practice guidelines for the management of pain in patients with cancer. N Engl J Med 1994;330(9):651–5.

[7] Herr K, Bjoro K, Decker S. Tools for assessment of pain in nonverbal older adults with dementia: a state-of-the-science review. J Pain Symptom Manage 2006;31(2):170–92.

[8] Page J, Henry D. Consumption of NSAIDs and the development of congestive heart failure in elderly patients: an underrecognized public health problem. Arch Intern Med 2000;160(6): 777–84.

[9] Bresalier RS, Sandler RS, Quan H, et al. Cardiovascular events associated with rofecoxib in a colorectal adenoma chemoprevention trial. N Engl J Med 2005;352(11):1092–102.

[10] Doyle D, Hanks G, Cherny N, et al, editors. Oxford textbook of palliative medicine. Oxford: Oxford University Press; 2005.

[11] Hollingshead J, Duhmke RM, Cornblath DR. Tramadol for neuropathic pain. Cochrane Database Syst Rev 2006;3:CD003726.

[12] Wong R, Wiffen PJ. Bisphosphonates for the relief of pain secondary to bone metastases. Cochrane Database Syst Rev 2002;2:CD002068.

[13] Wong GY, Schroeder DR, Carns PE, et al. Effect of neurolytic celiac plexus block on pain relief, quality of life, and survival in patients with unresectable pancreatic cancer: a randomized controlled trial. JAMA 2004;291(9):1092–9.

[14] Yan BM, Myers RP. Neurolytic celiac plexus block for pain control in unresectable pancreatic cancer. Am J Gastroenterol 2007;102(2):430–8.

[15] Lee H, Schmidt K, Ernst E. Acupuncture for the relief of cancer-related pain—a systematic review. Eur J Pain 2005;9(4):437–44.

[16] Sykes N, Thorns A. The use of opioids and sedatives at the end of life. Lancet Oncol 2003; 4(5):312–8.

[17] Forbes K, Huxtable R. Clarifying the data on double effect. Palliat Med 2006;20(4):395–6.

[18] Luce JM, Luce JA. Perspectives on care at the close of life. Management of dyspnea in patients with far-advanced lung disease: "once I lose it, it's kind of hard to catch it". JAMA 2001;285(10):1331–7.

[19] Solano JP, Gomes B, Higginson IJ. A comparison of symptom prevalence in far advanced cancer, AIDS, heart disease, chronic obstructive pulmonary disease and renal disease. J Pain Symptom Manage 2006;31(1):58–69.

[20] Inouye SK, Rushing JT, Foreman MD, et al. Does delirium contribute to poor hospital outcomes? A three-site epidemiologic study. J Gen Intern Med 1998;13(4):234–42.

[21] Pandharipande P, Shintani A, Peterson J, et al. Lorazepam is an independent risk factor for transitioning to delirium in intensive care unit patients. Anesthesiology 2006;104(1): 21–6.

[22] Breitbart W, Marotta R, Platt MM, et al. A double-blind trial of haloperidol, chlorpromazine, and lorazepam in the treatment of delirium in hospitalized AIDS patients. Am J Psychiatry 1996;153(2):231–7.

[23] Wee BL, Coleman PG, Hillier R, et al. The sound of death rattle I: are relatives distressed by hearing this sound? Palliat Med 2006;20(3):171–5.

[24] de Graeff A, Dean M. Palliative sedation therapy in the last weeks of life: a literature review and recommendations for standards. J Palliat Med 2007;10(1):67–85.

[25] Lo B, Rubenfeld G. Palliative sedation in dying patients: "we turn to it when everything else hasn't worked". JAMA 2005;294(14):1810–6.
[26] Finucane TE, Christmas C, Travis K. Tube feeding in patients with advanced dementia: a review of the evidence. JAMA 1999;282(14):1365–70.
[27] Dy SM. Enteral and parenteral nutrition in terminally ill cancer patients: a review of the literature. Am J Hosp Palliat Care 2006;23(5):369–77.
[28] Angus DC, Barnato AE, Linde-Zwirble WT, et al. Use of intensive care at the end of life in the United States: an epidemiologic study. Crit Care Med 2004;32(3):638–43.
[29] Prendergast TJ, Claessens MT, Luce JM. A national survey of end-of-life care for critically ill patients. Am J Respir Crit Care Med 1998;158(4):1163–7.
[30] Brody H, Campbell ML, Faber LK, et al. Withdrawing intensive life-sustaining treatment—recommendations for compassionate clinical management. N Engl J Med 1997;336(9): 652–7.
[31] Rubenfeld GD, Crawford SW. Principles and practice of withdrawing life-sustaining treatment in the ICU. In: Curtis JR, Rubenfeld GD, editors. Managing death in the ICU. New York: Oxford University Press; 2001. p. 127–47.
[32] Prendergast TJ, Luce JM. Increasing incidence of withholding and withdrawal of life support from the critically ill. Am J Respir Crit Care Med 1997;155(1):15–20.
[33] Kübler-Ross E. On death and dying. New York: Macmillan; 1969.
[34] Block SD. Assessing and managing depression in the terminally ill patient. ACP-ASIM End-of-Life Care Consensus Panel. American College of Physicians—American Society of Internal Medicine. Ann Intern Med 2000;132(3):209–18.
[35] Emanuel LL, Barry MJ, Stoeckle JD, et al. Advance directives for medical care—a case for greater use. N Engl J Med 1991;324(13):889–95.
[36] Bharucha AJ, Pearlman RA, Back AL, et al. The pursuit of physician-assisted suicide: role of psychiatric factors. J Palliat Med 2003;6(6):873–83.
[37] Quill TE, Cassel CK. Nonabandonment: a central obligation for physicians. Ann Intern Med 1995;122(5):368–74.
[38] Byock I. Dying well. New York: Riverhead Books; 1997.
[39] Pantilat SZ. Care of dying patients: beyond symptom management. West J Med 1999;171(4): 253–6.
[40] Sulmasy DP. Spiritual issues in the care of dying patients: "it's okay between me and god". JAMA 2006;296(11):1385–92.
[41] Volker DL. Control and end-of-life care: does ethnicity matter? Am J Hosp Palliat Care 2005;22(6):442–6.
[42] Lo B, McLeod GA, Saika G. Patient attitudes to discussing life-sustaining treatment. Arch Intern Med 1986;146:1613–5.
[43] Pantilat SZ, Alpers A, Wachter RM. A new doctor in the house: ethical issues in hospitalist systems. JAMA 1999;282(2):171–4.
[44] Tulsky JA, Fischer GS, Rose MR, et al. Opening the black box: how do physicians communicate about advance directives? Ann Intern Med 1998;129(6):441–9.
[45] Lo B, Quill T, Tulsky J. Discussing palliative care with patients. ACP-ASIM End-of-Life Care Consensus Panel. American College of Physicians-American Society of Internal Medicine. Ann Intern Med 1999;130(9):744–9.
[46] Lamont EB, Siegler M. Paradoxes in cancer patients' advance care planning. J Palliat Med 2000;3(1):27–35.
[47] Ebell MH, Becker LA, Barry HC, et al. Survival after in-hospital cardiopulmonary resuscitation. A meta-analysis. J Gen Intern Med 1998;13(12):805–16.
[48] Reisfield GM, Wallace SK, Munsell MF, et al. Survival in cancer patients undergoing in-hospital cardiopulmonary resuscitation: a meta-analysis. Resuscitation 2006;71(2):152–60.
[49] Christakis NA, Iwashyna TJ. Attitude and self-reported practice regarding prognostication in a national sample of internists. Arch Intern Med 1998;158(21):2389–95.

[50] Murphy DJ, Burrows D, Santilli S, et al. The influence of the probability of survival on patients' preferences regarding cardiopulmonary resuscitation. N Engl J Med 1994;330(8): 545–9.

[51] Maltoni M, Caraceni A, Brunelli C, et al. Prognostic factors in advanced cancer patients: evidence-based clinical recommendations—a study by the Steering Committee of the European Association for Palliative Care. J Clin Oncol 2005;23(25):6240–8.

[52] Meisel A, Snyder L, Quill T. Seven legal barriers to end-of-life care: myths, realities, and grains of truth. JAMA 2000;284(19):2495–501.

[53] Curtis JR, Park DR, Krone MR, et al. Use of the medical futility rationale in do-not-attempt-resuscitation orders. JAMA 1995;273(2):124–8.

[54] Annas GJ, Arnold B, Aroskar M, et al. Bioethicists' statement on the U.S. Supreme Court's Cruzan decision. N Engl J Med 1990;323(10):686–7.

[55] National Hospice and Palliative Care Organization. Fact and figures: hospice care in America, November 2007 edition. Available at: http://www.nhpco.org/files/public/statistics_research/nhpcd_facts-and-figures_nov2007.pdf. Accessed December 29, 2007.

[56] Lynn J. Serving patients who may die soon and their families: the role of hospice and other services. JAMA 2001;285(7):925–32.

[57] Roulson J, Benbow EW, Hasleton PS. Discrepancies between clinical and autopsy diagnosis and the value of post mortem histology; a meta-analysis and review. Histopathology 2005; 47(6):551–9.

THE MEDICAL
CLINICS
OF NORTH AMERICA

Med Clin N Am 92 (2008) 371–385

Pain Management in the Hospitalized Patient

Joseph Ming Wah Li, MD[a,b,*]

[a]Harvard Medical School, Boston, MA, USA
[b]Hospital Medicine Program, Beth Israel Deaconess Medical Center, 330 Brookline Avenue,
PBS 221, Boston, MA 02215, USA

The hospitalist's role

In 2006, the Society of Hospital Medicine described pain management as a hospitalist core competency [1]. "Hospitalists should be able to describe the symptoms and signs of pain; assess pain severity using validated measurement tools; formulate a pain management plan; determine appropriate route, dosing and frequency for pharmacologic agents; determine equianalgesic dosing and titrate narcotics to desired effect; anticipate and manage side effects of pain medications; discuss with patients the goals for pain management; employ a multidisciplinary approach to management of patients with pain; use evidence based recommendations; participate in development of pathways that facilitate effective pain management; and participate in efforts to measure quality of inpatient pain control." Alleviating pain is one of the basic tenets of being a doctor. The goal of alleviating pain is the responsibility of all health care providers, and as leaders of hospital care teams, hospitalists should be at the forefront of pain management.

Pain pathophysiology

The perception of pain begins at the site of perceived or real tissue injury. Injury stimulates nociceptors or free nerve endings to release neurotransmitters. The neurotransmitters activate firing of other nociceptors, which results in information being sent via afferent nerve fibers to the dorsal horn of the spinal cord. In the spinal cord, nociceptive information is sent via the spinothalamic tract to the thalamus. In the thalamus, information is sent to the

* Hospital Medicine Program, Beth Israel Deaconess Medical Center, 330 Brookline Avenue, PBS 221, Boston, MA 02215.
E-mail address: jli2@bidmc.harvard.edu

0025-7125/08/$ - see front matter © 2008 Elsevier Inc. All rights reserved.
doi:10.1016/j.mcna.2007.11.003　　　　　　　　　　　　　　　*medical.theclinics.com*

cortical areas of the brain, which processes the information. There are different areas of the brain involved in the modulation of pain information. These include the hypothalamus, pons, and somatosensory cortex. Stimulation of these areas causes analgesia.

Pain assessment

Any patient-doctor relationship is potentially fraught with personal bias. Participants carry their own personal baggage into each encounter. Encounters to discuss pain may be particularly problematic. For example, patients who view pain as a weakness may be more likely to suffer with pain and present with other somatic complaints. Providers who view pain as a weakness may be less likely to appreciate the extent of patients' pain. Pain is always subjective, can be very personal and thus, always requires a careful history for a reliable assessment.

Pain assessment tools should be simple, reliable, brief, and sensitive to any changes in pain intensity. Many hospitals commonly use numeric rating scales, where providers ask patients to rate their pain from 0 to 10. The endpoints represent the extremes, ranging from "no pain" to "worst pain possible." This tool is reasonably easy to administer but does require some abstract thought. For some patients, it may be easier to use a picture-based pain intensity assessment scale, like the Wong-Baker Faces Pain Rating Scale [2]. In this scale, a series of faces ranging from smiling face to a crying face correspond to the numbers on a numeric rating scale. This tool may be easier to use in situations where patients and providers don't speak the same language. Using the right tool is important because not all hospitalized patients may have the physical stamina or cognitive ability to participate in conversation or elaborate tests [3]. After any therapeutic intervention, a reassessment of the patient's pain allows providers to make adjustments in a rational manner.

As part of any pain history assessment, it is important to ask about the nature and quality of the patient's pain. Does the pain come in colicky waves or does it throb and ache? Where is the pain located? How often does the pain occur? When pain occurs, how long does it last? Is there anything that initiates or exacerbates the pain? What has the patient tried previously to alleviate the pain, with success or failure? What does pain mean to the patient? Does it bring back any memories? What is the patient's attitude toward the use of narcotics or anxiolytics? Is there any history of substance abuse? The patient's answers are not only important clues to the etiology of the pain, but can also guide the provider's examination and management decisions. Avoid the use of placebos as part of pain assessment. Deception is unethical and has no role in pain assessment or management.

Pharmacologic pain therapy

In 1986, the World Health Organization (WHO) developed the WHO Analgesic Ladder as a tool to address deficiencies in the management of cancer pain [4]. Despite the fact that no randomized, controlled trials have been conducted to validate its effectiveness, the WHO Analgesic Ladder is widely disseminated and commonly used to treat not only cancer pain but pain arising from any condition [5]. Three steps make up the WHO Analgesic Ladder (Fig. 1).

Step 1 recommends the use of nonopioid analgesics, with or without adjuvants for treatment of mild pain. In Step 2, the WHO advises adding weak opioids for treatment of moderate intensity pain, with or without non-opioid analgesics and with or without adjuvants. In Step 3, they recommend adding more potent opioids, in addition to those drugs recommended in Steps 1 and 2, for treatment of severe pain.

Nonopioid analgesics

Commonly used nonopioid analgesics include acetaminophen, salicylates, and nonsteroidal anti-inflammatory drugs (NSAIDs). Acetaminophen is an effective nonopioid analgesic with an average analgesic dose of 325 mg to 650 mg every 4 to 6 hours. At doses greater than 2 grams per day, patients on concurrent warfarin therapy may experience an increase in their prothrombin time. The maximum adult daily dose of acetaminophen is 4 grams, but adults with underlying liver disease should take no more than 2 grams daily. Acetaminophen over-dosage can result in fatal hepatotoxicity.

Discovered in 1897, aspirin (acetylsalicylic acid) remains the most commonly used drug in the salicylate drug class. Aspirin is similar to acetaminophen in its analgesic and antipyretic effects. But unlike acetaminophen, it has anti-inflammatory properties. Aspirin's usual analgesic adult dose is 325 mg to 650 mg, given once every 4 to 6 hours. The maximum adult analgesic dose is 4 grams daily. The most common side effects involve the gastrointestinal (GI) tract (eg, nausea, abdominal discomfort, dyspepsia, and peptic ulceration) and bleeding (caused by irreversible inhibition of platelet thromboxane production). Aspirin hypersensitivity may occur in association with asthma, urticaria, and angioneurotic edema. Children should

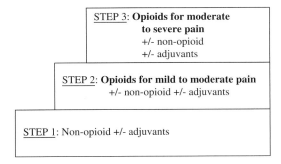

Fig. 1. WHO Analgesic Ladder.

not ingest aspirin because of concern for development of Reye's syndrome. Others salicylates include diflunisal and choline magnesium trisalicylate. Diflunisal has fewer GI effects than aspirin, and choline magnesium trisalicylate has minimal antiplatelet effects.

Patients with aspirin sensitivity may also be sensitive to some NSAIDs, which can also cause GI side effects. NSAIDs, like aspirin, also inhibit platelet aggregation, but unlike aspirin, the effect is reversible and lasts only for the duration of effective drug concentration. NSAIDs, despite their name, have efficacy for pain with and without associated inflammation [6]. Like acetaminophen and aspirin, NSAIDs offer the advantage of effective analgesia without the risk of physical or psychologic dependence associated with opioid therapy. There are numerous NSAIDs in a number of chemical classes (Box 1).

Unfortunately, there is insufficient data to clearly understand the differences between the NSAIDs. Ibuprofen is purported to have weaker antiinflammatory effects, but may have the lowest potential for GI side effects [7]. Indomethacin, naproxen, and sulindac present intermediate risks for GI side effects, while tolmetin, ketoprofen, and piroxicam may have the highest risk [8]. Endogenous prostaglandins are responsible for the body's

---

Box 1. NSAID chemical classes

Propionic acids
fenoprofen
flurbiprofen
ibuprofen
ketoprofen
naproxen
exazoprin

Acetic acids
diclofenac
etodolac
indomethacin
ketorolac
sulindac
tolmetin

Enolic acids
meloxicam
piroxicam

Anthranilic acids
mefenamic acid
nabumetone

inflammatory response. NSAID inhibition of the cyclo-oxygenase (COX) enzyme prevents the formation of prostaglandins, leading to NSAIDs' anti-inflammatory effects. NSAID activity in the brain and spinal cord contribute to their analgesic effects. There is a ceiling for analgesia but not for side effects, meaning administration of NSAIDs above recommended doses may increase toxicity without increasing analgesic efficacy [9].

NSAIDs have numerous potential side effects, usually because of inhibition of prostaglandins not involved in the inflammatory process [10,11]. The previously mentioned COX enzyme is expressed in tissue in at least two isoforms: COX-1 and COX-2. COX-1 is present in most tissues and is known to play an important role in the maintenance of the gastric mucosa, preservation of renal blood flow, and platelet function (the latter via production of a platelet enzyme called thromboxane). COX-2 is expressed only in the central nervous system (CNS) and kidneys. NSAIDs can cause renal side effects (via reduction of vasodilatory renal prostaglandins), hematologic side effects (via inhibition of platelet aggregation), CNS effects (via inhibition of central prostaglandin production), and GI side effects (via reduction of prostaglandin production in the gastric mucosa). The concurrent use of proton pump inhibitors or misoprostol (a prostaglandin analog) with NSAIDs may reduce the risk of peptic ulcer disease.

During the past decade, several NSAIDs that selectively block the COX-2 enzyme became commercially available. Selective inhibition of COX-2 with reduced inhibition of COX-1 was thought to offer the benefit of reduced GI, renal, and hematologic side effects. While studies show there may be some reduction in the incidence of GI side effects, the COX-2 inhibitors do not appear to offer any benefit of reduced renal side effects. After-market surveillance revealed that some selective COX-2 inhibitors may be associated with increased incidence of cardiac events. The proposed theory is that selective COX-2 inhibition prevents prostacyclin formation, leading to unopposed platelet thromboxane (a prothrombotic prostaglandin) effects. Celecoxib is the only COX-2 inhibitor which remains on the market in the United States. Its role in pain management is controversial.

Opioid analgesics

Opioids should be added to the analgesic regimen when nonopioids alone are insufficient for pain control. However, many hospitalized patients present with acute pain that is moderate to severe in intensity, and it would be inappropriate to initially withhold opioid analgesics pending the response to nonopioid therapies. On initial pain assessment, if the patient has moderate to severe acute pain, consider a pharmacologic regimen that includes both nonopioid and opioid analgesics, along with adjuvant analgesics and nonpharmacologic measures. Opioid agonists, unlike nonopioids, have no ceiling for analgesic effects. Providers should titrate up the opioid dose until there is sufficient analgesic effect or until side effects become intolerable.

Opioids bind to endogenous opioid receptors in several classes: delta, kappa, and mu. Opioids are classified as full agonists, partial agonists, or mixed agonist-antagonists. All available opioids are full agonists that act on the mu opioid receptor. Stimulation of the mu opioid receptor is responsible for the opioids' analgesic and adverse effects. Adverse effects include urinary retention, pruritis, sedation (typically dose-related), muscle rigidity (more common with higher doses of potent, rapidly acting drugs), respiratory depression (dose-dependent), bradycardia, decreased sympathetic tone, nausea (via stimulation of receptors in the chemoreceptor trigger zone), and constipation. There is significant individual variation in development of side effects, but sedation and constipation appear most frequently. Patients on chronic opioid therapy can develop tolerance to some side effects (eg, respiratory depression) but typically do not develop tolerance to other effects (eg, constipation). It is important to differentiate side effects from allergy. True allergy to opioids is rare but if allergy exists, one should switch patients to an opioid in a different chemical class [10].

Morphine is the standard against which all other opioids are compared. This does not mean morphine is the opioid of choice for all patients in all situations. Morphine, available for oral, parenteral, rectal, and intraspinal use, is effective for moderate to severe acute and chronic pain. It is renally excreted, so patients with renal failure may experience prolonged effects. Compared with other opioids, morphine is more likely to cause histamine release, which can increase the risk of vasodilation, flushing, and hypotension.

At equianalgesic doses, all opioid full agonists have similar efficacy. Providers should choose an opioid based on side-effect profiles. Clinicians should always use the equianalgesic conversion chart when transitioning from one opioid to another (Table 1).

Table 1 compares morphine 10-mg intramuscular injection with other opioids and alternative routes. Providers should recognize that the conversion

Table 1
Equivalent narcotic dosing chart[a]

Narcotic	IM / IV (Mg)	PO (Mg)	Duration (Hrs)
Codeine	120	200	4–6
Fentanyl	0.1	—	1–2
Hydromorphone	1.5	7.5	4–5
Meperidine	75	300	2–4
Methadone	10	20	4–6
Morphine	10	30–60	3–7
Oxycodone	—	15–30	4–6
Oxymorphone	1	—	3–6
Propoxyphene	—	130	4–6

Abbreviations: IM, intramuscularly; IV, intravenously; PO, by mouth.

[a] For treatment of ACUTE pain and not for chronic pain.

Data from World Health Organization. WHO Guidelines: Cancer Pain Relief. 2nd ed. Geneva: World Health Organization; 1996.

chart is based on limited data, and there is significant individual response to various opioids. The conversion process from one opioid to another involved five steps:

1) Calculate the total dose of the current opioid over the previous 24 hours.
2) Use the conversion chart to convert to the 24-hour total dose of the new drug or route.
3) Divide the 24-hour total dose into individual doses, based on the schedule.
4) For opioid-tolerant patients where cross-tolerance may not exist, consider reducing the calculated dose of the new drug by 33% to 50% [10].
5) Calculate a breakthrough dose of the new drug. This should be either 10% to 20% of the total daily dose or 25% to 30% of the single standing dose [10].

Meperidine is an opioid with a short duration of analgesic effects because of extensive first pass metabolism. Normeperidine, a meperidine metabolite that accumulates with repetitive dosing, causes numerous CNS side effects, including seizures. Patients who use meperidine for longer than 48 hours, patients who take doses greater than 600 mg per 24 hours, patients with underlying renal failure, or patients treated concurrently with monoamine oxidase inhibitors are all at increased risk for side effects. Naloxone does not reverse the meperidine CNS effects. Given meperidine's narrow therapeutic window and the availability of safer and more effective alternative agents, it is difficult to justify its use in clinical practice. The American Pain Society states it should not be used for acute or cancer pain [6].

Methadone is most commonly used in management of opioid addiction. Its role in acute pain is controversial. Proponents like its low cost, its effectiveness in neuropathic pain, and its long half-life, which make it an attractive agent to treat persistent pain. But methadone's pharmacokinetics pose a challenge for those unfamiliar with the drug. Methadone has a short-lasting analgesic effect but a long half-life, which can result in accumulation of the drug with repeated dosing. Because of this fact, it is reasonable to use other short-acting opioids and titrate to therapeutic effects and then transition to methadone using the equianalgesic table. It is important to understand that the equianalgesic table is designed for management of acute pain and not for long-term use. Conversion from other opioids to methadone using the equianalgesic table will result in an inappropriately high dose of methadone. If one is to use the equianalgesic table to convert from another opioid, the dose of methadone should be reduced by 50% or more. Rather than using an alternative opioid and transitioning to methadone, one can use methadone for acute pain by prescribing it initially every 2 to 3 hours for 2 to 5 days, at which point the blood levels will approach a steady state, then reduce the methadone dose by 50%. Without a dose reduction, there is a risk of methadone overdose. For providers unfamiliar with methadone, it may be reasonable to seek consultation with a pain specialist before using this drug.

Tramadol is a centrally acting synthetic analgesic classified as an opioid because it is a weak agonist at the mu opioid receptor. Unlike most opioids, it also appears to block the reuptake of serotonin and norepinephrine, so one would not expect naloxone to fully reverse its effects [6]. However, this activity on serotonin and norepinephrine makes it useful in neuropathic pain. Tramadol, unlike other opioids, is not a controlled substance in the United States. Tolerance and dependence is rare. At the usual prescribed dose of 50 mg by mouth every 4 to 6 hours, its analgesic effect is similar to acetaminophen 300 mg with codeine 30-mg [12]. Side effects, which can be ameliorated if the dose is gradually titrated over several weeks, include nausea, dizziness, dry mouth, sweating, and seizures. At doses greater than 400-mg daily, tramadol is associated with increased risk of seizures. Concurrent use with serotonin selective reuptake inhibitors or tricyclic antidepressants (TCAs) cannot only increase risk of seizures, but also risk the development of serotonin syndrome.

Patient-controlled analgesia

In patient-controlled analgesia (PCA), an infusion pump delivers opioids intravenously (IV). Patients push a button to activate IV opioid boluses. A preset dose of opioid is delivered as long as a predetermined amount of time (the lockout period) has elapsed since the previous dose. PCA is particularly useful in postoperative acute pain because it minimizes any delays in treating pain. Compared with patients who receive opioids for acute pain via other methods, patients on PCAs tend to use less total amounts of opioids because drug delivery more closely matches their pain pattern. When starting a PCA, set the hourly limit at three to five times the projected hourly requirement. For example, if you believe a patient will need 10 mg of a drug per hour, set the hourly limit at 30 mg to 50 mg. Observe the hourly consumption and adjust the hourly limit based on actual need. For opioid-naive patients with acute pain, the usual starting dose for morphine is 1 mg (range 0.5 mg–2.5 mg) with a usual lockout of 8 minutes (range 5–10 min). Setting a lockout time of 8 minutes means a patient would receive no more than one dose of narcotic every 8 minutes, regardless of how often they push the PCA button. The usual starting dose for fentanyl is 10 mcg (range 10 mcg–50 mcg), with usual lockout of 6 minutes (range 5–8 min). The usual starting dose of hydromorphone is 0.2 mg (range 0.05 mg–0.4 mg) with a lockout of 8 minutes (range 5–10 min) [6].

In addition to bolus dosing, clinicians can also administer a continuous (or basal) narcotic infusion. Basal infusions may be particularly useful in opioid-tolerant patients (eg, chronic cancer pain), but their use in opioid-naive patients with acute pain is controversial. Basal infusions increase the incidence and severity of opioid-related side effects and increase the risk of overdose. In opioid-naive patients, there is inconclusive data to support improved pain control [13]. When weaning patients off the PCA, it is important to start oral long-acting, controlled-release opioids (eg, morphine or oxycodone) at least 12 hours before discontinuation of the PCA. Start with a dose of long-acting opioid, which is equivalent to the amount of drug given by continuous infusion, plus one half of the total dosage given by intermittent boluses [14]. Over the next 24 hours, wean off the PCA by increasing the lockout period and decrease the dose of drug given by boluses. PCA is not appropriate for all patients. Patients who are unable to understand the principle or have altered mental status are not candidates because they may receive inappropriate amounts of drug.

Pain treatment principles

Make every effort to individualize analgesic dose, route, and schedule. There is significant individual variation in doses of opioids required to provide sufficient analgesia in individuals across all age groups, between genders, among ethnic groups, and in opioid-naive and opioid-experienced patients. Frequently re-evaluate patients, especially when one is beginning or changing analgesic regimens.

Route of delivery

Although the oral route of administration is typically most acceptable, IV bolus administration produces the most rapid onset of effect for patients in acute pain. Opioids given rectally or subcutaneously also provide rapid onset of action, but some patients may find the rectal route of administration unacceptable; only limited drug amounts can be delivered in the subcutaneous space. Intraspinal (epidural, intrathecal) administration of opioids is a more invasive route of administration but can produce analgesia with small doses of opioids, as the drug is being delivered directly to the spinal cord. Fentanyl is the only opioid which is also available in oral transmucosal and transdermal formulations. The fentanyl lozenge is indicated only for cancer-related breakthrough pain. Approximately 25% of the dose is absorbed via the buccal mucosa and the remainder of the drug is absorbed from the GI tract. Unlike the lozenge, the transdermal fentanyl patch is indicated for continuous analgesia. The onset of analgesia may occur in 12 to 16 hours but it often takes up to 48 hours to achieve steady-state blood levels [15]. Providers should titrate with short-acting opioids for analgesia before converting to the transdermal fentanyl patch. Unlike the patch, the fentanyl patient-controlled transdermal system (PCTS) is designed for management of acute pain. Similar to a PCA pump, the PCTS delivers fentanyl on demand but does so without an IV line. Unlike the patch, there is no passive absorption of drug. The credit card size PCTS delivers drug only when the patient pushes a button to activate the device. One disadvantage of the device is that it is preprogrammed to deliver a fixed dose of 40 mcg, which may not be appropriate for all patients.

Frequency of dosing

Regardless of the drug choice and route of administration, the frequency of administration is critical to achieving the analgesic effect. Providers should be familiar with each drug's recommended schedule. For example, short-acting oxycodone should be administered every 3 to 4 hours. Providers who want to decrease the total daily dose should decrease the drug dosage rather than increase the interval between doses. Less frequent administration would result in break-through pain. Whenever possible, providers should anticipate pain and treat it in a prophylactic manner. Give analgesics before procedures and never rely only on "as needed" dosing of analgesics when you know the patient can expect pain.

Managing side effects

Providers should also anticipate, recognize and treat side effects associated with analgesics. For example, respiratory depression, itching, sedation, constipation, nausea, and vomiting are frequent opioid side effects. When prescribing opioids, providers should discuss these potential side effects with patients. Providers can choose an opioid based on its potential side-effect profile. For example, morphine tends to release histamine more than other opioids, with resultant itching and flushing. Choose an alternative opioid if this side effect occurs. Another method to minimize side effects is to increase the frequency of opioid dosing, which will result in more constant blood levels. It is the peak serum drug levels that are often associated with side effects. Providers can also decrease the incidence of side effects without sacrificing analgesic relief by using combination pharmacotherapy. One can often use less opioids by adding nonnarcotic adjuvants to the regimen. To address the issue of opioid-induced constipation, providers should initiate routinely scheduled stool softeners and cathartics at the same time they initiate opioid therapy. There are also new peripheral opioid receptor antagonists (eg, methylnaltrexone) on the horizon that may help providers address this issue of opoioid-induced constipation.

Tolerance, withdrawal, and addiction

Providers must always monitor for opioid tolerance, expect physical dependence, and prevent withdrawal [6]. Within days of starting an opioid, expect some tolerance. Tolerance is the need to increase the amount of a drug to achieve the same effect. Tolerance occurs to some opioid-induced side effects, such as nausea, respiratory depression, and somnolence. Unfortunately tolerance to constipation does not occur. Tolerance to opioid-induced analgesia can also occur in the first 2 weeks of therapy but typically does not occur after that. Patients who experience increased pain after the first 2 weeks of opioid therapy should be evaluated for other causes of pain.

Physical dependence, which also occurs with drugs other than analgesics, is common in patients who take opioid analgesics. Patients with physical dependence develop withdrawal symptoms when a given medication is abruptly withdrawn. Symptoms of opioid withdrawal include anxiety, irritability, tachycardia, abdominal pain, nausea, and vomiting. The drug's half-life dictates the time course of the symptoms. To prevent withdrawal symptoms, wean patients, rather than abruptly discontinuing chronic opioid therapy. Do not confuse opioid dependence with opioid addiction. Opioid dependence can occur after just 2 weeks of opioid use. Addiction is an abnormal behavioral condition that may include compulsive use, impaired control over drug use, continued use despite harm, and craving [16]. The risk of iatrogenic opioid addiction is low and should not dissuade clinicians from using opioid analgesics to treat acute pain. "Pseudo-addiction" is a term that describes patient behavior when their pain is under-treated [6]. Patients with insufficiently controlled pain may seem focused on obtaining additional drugs. This may even include illicit drug use and deception as part of his or her efforts. If a patient has pseudo-addiction, rather than addiction, such behaviors will go away if the pain is appropriately treated.

Adjuvant analgesics

There are a number of drugs which, when given with narcotics or NSAIDs, can enhance the analgesic effects. These drugs are called adjuvants or coanalgesics. Drugs include the TCAs (eg, amitriptyline, imipramine, desipramine, and nortriptyline), antiepileptic drugs (eg, gabapentin, carbamazepine, topiramate, levetiracetam, oxycarbazapine, phenytoin, lamotrigine, zonisimade, and valproate), glucocorticoids, local anesthetics (eg, lidocaine), benzodiazepines (eg, diazepam, lorazepam, and clonazepam), skeletal muscle relaxants (eg, tizanidine), antihistamines (eg, hydroxyzine), antispasmodil agents (eg, baclofen), and caffeine. Many of these drugs are most effective when used in conjunction with opioid analgesics to treat specific types of pain. Their concurrent use can often result in improved pain control along with reduction in required doses of opioids. Most of these drugs are administered orally, but some are available by injection or topical formulations (eg, lidocaine). Each has potential advantages and possible side effects. For example, in patients with cancer-related pain, glucocorticoid administration cannot only relieve pain but also increase appetite and elevate mood. Glucocorticoids are particularly useful in alleviating pain related to headache caused by brain tumors, pain caused by spinal cord compression, or malignant infiltration of lumbar and brachial plexus. Chronic use, however, can lead to numerous side effects, including osteoporosis, Cushing's syndrome, and increased risk of GI bleeding. For the terminally ill, such chronic side effects should be of no concern. Care must be taken not to withdraw glucocorticoids rapidly as that can result in pain exacerbation.

Treating pain in the elderly

Elderly patients have an increased risk for complications related to treatment of pain. Analgesics may have prolonged effects caused by decreased elimination from the plasma [17]. For example, elderly patients may be twice as sensitive to parenteral fentanyl as compared with younger patients. When treating elderly patients with pain, consider initiation of opioids at dosage levels 25% to 50% lower than normal adults and titrate carefully. Close monitoring and careful titration can minimize adverse effects. Some drugs should be used with extreme caution or not used at all in the elderly. The Beers Criteria for potentially inappropriate medication use in older adults lists numerous analgesics [18]. Most of these drugs are listed because of narrow therapeutic windows or adverse CNS effects, which may contribute to falls or other adverse events. Drugs listed include the opioids propoxyphene, pentazocine, and meperidine. They discourage the long-term use of all NSAIDs and short-term use of indomethacin and ketorolac. They advise against the use of specific adjuvants, including long-acting benzodiazepines, higher doses of short-acting benzodiazepines, and TCAs.

Neuropathic pain

Neuropathic pain is relatively common. Causes include postherpetic neuralgia, diabetic neuropathy, chemotherapy-induced neuropathy, alcoholic polyneuropathy, spinal cord injury pain, and complex regional pain syndrome (reflex sympathetic dystrophy). The diagnosis of neuropathic pain is based primarily on the pain description. Patients with neuropathic pain are more likely to describe their pain as "burning, tingling, electric shock, cold, pricking and itching" [19]. Physical examination can reveal flushing, sweating, fasiculations, or atrophy. Unfortunately there is no single test that confirms neuropathic pain. Identification of pain as neuropathic is important because not all analgesics are effective in treatment of neuropathic pain. For example, topical lidocaine, antidepressants (TCAs, venlafaxine, duloxetine), antiepileptic drugs, tramadol, gabapentin, and pregabalin appear effective in managing neuropathic pain. NSAIDs can reduce pain in diabetic neuropathy and sciatica [20,21] but, like acetaminophen, appear less efficacious in treatment of other causes of neuropathic pain [22]. The role of capsaicin cream is uncertain and often produces pain when applied [23]. Noninvasive therapies, such as transcutaneous electrical nerve stimulation, can be effective in some patients with diabetic neuropathy and radicular pain [24,25]. Patients with recalcitrant neuropathic pain may benefit from a referral to a pain specialist to discuss more invasive therapy, such as sympathetic regional anesthetic blocks, intrathecal medication (opioids or baclofen), or spinal cord stimulation. The use of oral opioids in treatment of neuropathic pain often requires very high doses. In some patients, the development of side effects at high doses precludes their use. Intrathecal opioids require much smaller doses because the opioids are delivered directly to the dorsal horn of the spinal cord.

It is important to recognize that in some patients, neuropathic pain can coexist with nociceptive pain. For example, patients with radicular and low back pain may experience pain from both myofacial causes and from nerve root compression [22]. Up to one third of patients with cancer pain have a component of neuropathic pain in addition to their coexisting nociceptive pain [6].

Nonpharmacologic pain therapy

Physical measures, such as application of heat or cold, are often underutilized in management of pain in hospitalized patients. Applying heat or cold is easy and can be an effective way to minimize unnecessary escalating doses of pharmacologic therapy and their potential side effects.

Although providers often think of complementary and alternative therapies as outside the mainstream, their use is widespread among patients. These include mind-body therapies (eg, relaxation response, biofeedback, prayer, imagery, and meditation), manipulative therapies (eg, massage, chiropractic and osteopathic manipulation) and new-age therapies (eg, Qi Gong, Reiki). Surveys have demonstrated that physicians are often unaware of their patients' use of alternative therapies [26]. Not unlike asking about pain, it is important for providers to ask patients about their use of alternative therapies. These questions can be insightful, revealing a patient's thoughts on why they have pain and belief on whether traditional medicine can address their pain sufficiently.

Treating pain safely: Joint Commission's 2007 National Patient Safety Goals

The Joint Commission's latest National Patient Safety Goals include goals applicable to pain management [27]. Management of pain in the hospital is a complex system and dangerous medical errors can occur. For example, one Joint Commission on Accreditation of Healthcare Organization goal is to "standardize a list of abbreviations, acronyms, symbols and dose designations that are not to be used throughout the organization." For example, providers should never abbreviate morphine sulfate because "MSO4" can be confused for magnesium sulfate and vice versa. When writing drug dosages, always write a "zero" before any decimals and never write any "trailing zeros." Write morphine 0.3 mg and never write ".30". Another Joint Commission goal is to "identify and, at a minimum, annually review a list of look-alike/sound-alike drugs used by the organization." For example, some health care providers have mistaken immediate-release oxycodone with controlled-release oxycodone. Overdose or under dosing has occurred with adverse patient outcomes. One strategy to address this problem is to encourage brand name prescribing of controlled-release oxycodone. Another strategy is to stock the products in different locations away from one another.

Summary

Effective management of acute pain should be a primary goal of each health care provider. Acute pain is a complex medical problem with multiple possible etiologies. Management of acute pain requires providers to not only understand how to assess pain, but also how to apply pharmacologic and nonpharmacologic therapies to address pain. There are many barriers to the effective management of pain in the hospital. As leaders of the hospital care team, it is incumbent on hospitalists to overcome these barriers and address the challenge of acute pain in hospitalized patients.

References

[1] Pistoria MJ, Amin AN, Dressler DD, et al. The core competencies in hospital medicine: a framework for curriculum development. J Hosp Med 2006;1(Suppl 1):28–9.

[2] Wong DL, Baker CM. Pain in children: comparison of assessment scales. Pediatr Nurs 1998; 14:9–17.

[3] Hamill-Ruth R, Marohn M. Evaluation of pain in the critically ill patient. Crit Care Clin 1999;15(1):35–51.

[4] World Health Organization. WHO guidelines: cancer pain relief. 2nd edition. Geneva (IL): World Health Organization; 1996.

[5] Jadad A, Browman GP. The WHO analgesic ladder for cancer pain management: stepping up the quality of its evaluation. JAMA 1995;274:1870–3.

[6] Principles of analgesic use in the treatment of acute pain and cancer pain. 5th edition. Glenview (IL): American Pain Society; 2003.

[7] Henry D, Lim LL, Garcia Rodriguez LA, et al. Variability in risk of gastrointestinal complications with individual non-steroidal anti-inflammatory drugs: results of a collaborative meta-analysis. BMJ 1996;312:1563–6.

[8] McCarberg B, Passik S, editors. Pain management. The ACP Guide for Hospitalists August 2006;1:3–9.

[9] Eisenberg E, Berkey CS, Carr DB, et al. Efficacy and safety of nonsteroidal anti-inflammatory drugs for cancer pain: a meta-analysis. J Clin Oncol 1994;12:2756–65.

[10] McNicol E, Carr DB. Pharmacological treatment of pain. In: McCarberg B, Passik SD, editors. Expert guide to pain management. Philadelphia: American College of Physicians; 2005. p. 145–78.

[11] Graham DJ, Campen DH, Cheetham C, et al. Risk of acute myocardial infarction and sudden cardiac death with use of COX-2 selective and non-selective NSAIDs. Presented at 20th International Conference on Pharmacoepidemiology & Therapeutic Risk Management. Bordeaux, France, August 22–25, 2004.

[12] Rauck R, Ruoff G, McMillen J. Comparison of tramadol and acetaminophen with codeine for long-term pain management in elderly patients. Current Therapeutic Research 1994;55:1417–31.

[13] Parker R, Holtmann B, White P. Patient-controlled analgesia. Does a concurrent opioid infusion improve pain management after surgery? JAMA 1991;266:1947.

[14] Reuben SS, Connelly NR, Maciolek H. Postoperative analgesia with controlled-release oxycodone for outpatient anterior cruciate ligament surgery. Anesth Analg 1999;88:1286–91.

[15] Portenoy RK, Southam MA, Gupta SK, et al. Transdermal fentanyl for cancer pain. Repeated dose pharmacokinetics. Anesthesiology 1993;78:36–43.

[16] Savage S, Covington E, Heit H, et-al. Definitions related to the use of opioids for the treatment of pain: a consensus document from the American Academy of Pain Medicine, the American Pain Society and the American Society of Addiction Medicine. Available at: http://www.ampainsoc.org. Accessed November 17, 2007.

[17] Kaiko R, Wallenstein S, Rogers A, et al. Clinical analgesic studies and sources of variation in analgesic response to morphine. In: Foley K, Inturrisi CE, editors. Opioid analgesics in the management of clinical pain, advanced pain research therapy, vol. 8. New York: Raven Press; 1986.

[18] Fick DM, Cooper JW, Wade WE, et al. Updating the beers criteria for potentially inappropriate medication use in older adults. Arch Intern Med 2003;163:2716–24.

[19] Boureau F, Doubrere JF, Luu M. Study of verbal description in neuropathic pain. Pain 1990; 42:145–52.

[20] Dreiser RL, Le Parc JM, Velicitat P, et al. Oral meloxicam is effective in acute sciatica: two randomized, double-blind trials versus placebo or diclofenac. Inflamm Res 2001;50(Suppl 1): S17–23.

[21] Cohen KL, Harris S. Efficacy and safety of nonsteroidal anti-inflammatory drugs in the therapy of diabetic neuropathy. Arch Intern Med 1987;147:1442–4.

[22] O'Connor AB, Dworkin RH. Neuropathic pain. In: McCarberg B, Passik SD, editors. Expert guide to pain management. Philadelphia: American College of Physicians; 2005. p. 121–44.

[23] Mason L, Moore RA, Derry S, et al. Systematic review of topical capsaicin for the treatment of chronic pain. BMJ 2004;328:991–5.

[24] Kumar D, Marshall HJ. Diabetic peripheral neuropathy: amelioration of pain with transcutaneous electrostimulation. Diabetes Care 1997;20:1702–5.

[25] Carrol EN, Badura AS. Focal intense brief transcutaneous electric nerve stimulation for treatment of radicular and posthoracotomy pain. Arch Phys Med Rehabil 2001;82:262–4.

[26] Eisenberg DM, Kessler RC, Van Rompay MI, et al. Perceptions about complementary therapies relative to conventional therapies among adults who use both: results from a national survey. Ann Intern Med 2001;135:344–51.

[27] The Joint commission Web site. Available at: www.jcaho.org. Accessed November 17, 2007.

THE MEDICAL
CLINICS
OF NORTH AMERICA

Med Clin N Am 92 (2008) 387–406

Acute Hospital Care for the Elderly Patient: Its Impact on Clinical and Hospital Systems of Care

Paula M. Podrazik, MD[a],*, Chad T. Whelan, MD[b]

[a]Section of Geriatrics, Department of Medicine, University of Chicago,
5841 South Maryland Avenue, MC6098, Chicago, IL 60637, USA
[b]Section of General Internal Medicine, Department of Medicine, University of Chicago,
5841 South Maryland Avenue, MC 2007, Chicago, IL 60637, USA

Elderly patients are frequently hospitalized with complex medical issues or issues related to frailty. In many cases, skill and time are required during the course of an acute hospitalization to negotiate patient care decisions with the patient and caregivers through the end of life. Approximately half of the hospital beds in the United States are presently occupied by those over age 65. However, the disproportionate numerical increase of elderly projected in the coming decades—particularly the oldest old (greater than 85 years) [1] who are more likely to be medically complex or frail [2] and have twice the rate of hospitalizations when compared with the youngest old (aged 65–74) [3]—will have a further impact on health care expenditures. Currently, the cost for care of the elderly at the end of life accounts for 10% to 12% of the total United States health care budget and 28% of the Medicare budget [4]. In addition, a greater number of other health care resources will be needed, especially after-hospitalization services [5] that include skilled nursing care, in-patient rehabilitation, visiting nursing services, and long-term care.

Furthermore, if a hospitalization outcome is largely dependent on the impact of the acute illness, the patient's baseline vulnerability, and the hazards of the hospitalization process (including medical error) (Fig. 1), the elderly patient then is at a decided disadvantage in all three aspects. Elderly patients have a high prevalence of acute illness, and when compared with

---

* Corresponding author.
E-mail address: ppodrazi@medicine.bsd.uchicago.edu (P.M. Podrazik).

0025-7125/08/$ - see front matter © 2008 Elsevier Inc. All rights reserved.
doi:10.1016/j.mcna.2007.11.004   *medical.theclinics.com*

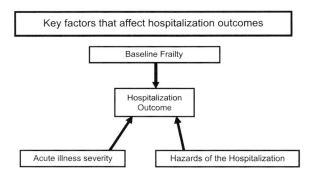

Fig. 1. Key factors that affect hospitalization outcomes.

younger patients, hospitalizations of the elderly are more frequent, severe, and protracted [6]. The older patient's baseline vulnerability and risk of iatrogenic complications with hospitalization [7,8] rate is as high as 29% to 38%. These factors together contribute to a greater frequency of hospitalization, greater length of stay, and higher risk of readmission.

Finally, acute hospitalization for an elderly patient usually represents only one relatively brief health care encounter within a much larger health care framework that covers multiple caregivers, health care professionals, and settings for such care.

Clinical care of the elderly hospitalized patient: areas for improvement

One curricular framework targets four commonly seen, high-impact areas of hospital-based clinical care for the elderly. These areas include: (1) identifying frailty or vulnerability; (2) avoiding hazards of hospitalization, including delirium, falls, indwelling urinary catheter (IUC) use, deconditioning, adverse drug reactions and errors in drug administration, and pressure ulcers; (3) palliating and addressing end-of-life issues; and (4) improving transitions of care (Box 1) [9].

Elderly patients are significantly affected by hospitalization, with rates of iatrogenic complications approaching three to five times those of younger patients [10,11], a 35% risk of functional decline [5], increased incidence of delirium, greater risk of rehospitalization, and higher rates of institutionalization. Labeling the hospital "unsafe" does not provide the solution, given the high prevalence of acute illness in the elderly and need for acute hospitalization. Instead, there exist avenues of education that can bridge demonstrable knowledge gaps in many clinical areas, such as end-of-life care [12,13], delirium and its prevention [14], and frailty [15,16].

There is already heightened awareness regarding some areas of care that are especially relevant to the elderly. These include pain management,

---

Box 1. Curriculum for the hospitalized aging medical patient geriatrics topics

Geriatric topics

Theme #1: Identification of the frail or vulnerable elder
- Identify and assess the vulnerable hospitalized older patient
- Dementia in hospitalized older medical patients: recognizing and screening for dementia, assessing medical decision making capacity, implications for the treatment of nondementia illness, pain assessment, improving the posthospitalization transition of care

Theme #2: Recognize and avoid hazards of hospitalization
- Delirium: diagnosis, treatment, risk stratification, and prevention
- Falls: assessment and prevention
- Foley catheters: scope of the problem, appropriate indications and management
- Deconditioning: scope of the problem, prevention
- Adverse drug reactions and medication errors: principles of drug review
- Pressure ulcers: assessment, treatment, and prevention

Theme #3: Palliate and address end-of-life issues
- Pain control: general principles and use of opiates
- Symptom management in advanced disease: nausea
- Difficult conversations and advanced directives
- Hospice and palliative care and changing goals of care

Theme #4: Improve transitions of care
- The ideal hospital discharge: core components and determining destination
- Destinations of posthospital care: nursing homes for skilled rehabilitation and long-term care

---

end-of-life care, and preventing hazards of hospitalization, including medication error, falls, and delirium [17]. Much of the clinical focus on these issues is fueled by external factors, such as payers, the Joint Commission (TJC) [18], and patient and family advocacy groups. Yet, these areas have to be better defined, standardized, and systematized for the older patient population.

This article addresses and focuses on important patient care issues for older adults, including the issue of frailty, hazards of hospitalization, and transitions of care. In addition to these core clinical areas of knowledge and skills, the authors discuss systems improvements that benefit the hospitalized elderly, and particularly the frail elderly.

Identifying frailty

Definitions and impact on hospital care

When one hears the word "frail" in the context of an elderly patient, a number of words come to mind, including: "advanced age," "nursing home patient," "needs assistance," or "confused." Establishing a specific definition or phenotype of frailty seems to be as elusive as the words used to describe a frail elder. Definitions and measures of frailty in the elderly certainly exist [19]. In the Assessing the Care of the Vulnerable Elder (ACOVE) study, investigators developed one such definition by estimating the risk of frailty via a United States nationally representative sample of community-dwelling elders over 65 years [20]. Employing Medicare Current Beneficiary Survey data, the ACOVE investigators determined that functional status was a more important predictor of functional decline and death than any specific medical condition, and identified approximately 32% of community-dwelling elders as "vulnerable," with a fourfold increased risk of functional decline or death over a 2-year period. This "vulnerability" risk was determined through the Vulnerable Elders Survey (VES)-13 [21], a phone screen tool based on age, self-rated health, and aspects of functional status. Using the ACOVE model, the phenotypic characteristics of vulnerable elder—established as being at advanced age with functional impairments—not only puts into perspective our verbal descriptions of "frail" but adds definition and the link to clinical outcomes.

Surveying patients over 65 with the VES-13 in an urban academic medical center determined a vulnerable elder rate of approximately 25% of adult patients on the general medicine service [22]. The implications of frailty in a hospitalized elder include further functional and cognitive decline [23–25], increased risk of delirium [26], prolonged hospitalization, and increased cost and mortality [27]. For the busy hospitalist, recognizing the frail or vulnerable elder at the point of admission is crucial in determining the need to screen for dementia and functional status, and to help frame patient care and discussions with a better understanding of the medical complexity, prognosis, and risk of adverse outcomes. The hospitalist's identification of the frail elderly patient also serves as an important determinant for preventing delirium, deconditioning, falls, and pressure ulcers, and for instituting comprehensive discharge planning.

Using age criteria alone may help to capture a large number of such potentially frail or vulnerable older patients. For example, the prevalence of dementia increases with age, rising from an incidence of 5% to 10% at age 65, and up to nearly 50% at age 85 [28]. Similarly, the incidence of difficulties with basic life activities increases with age; approximately 26% of the 74- to 84-year-old age group (the "older old") have some difficulty, and this rises to approximately 58% of the 85-plus (the "oldest old") age group [29,30]. Not surprisingly, age and functional status predicted risk of increased morbidity and mortality outcomes in the ACOVE studies [20] for the community-dwelling elder. Although acute care for elders (ACE) hospital units are not widespread (largely because costs per case are not proportionately reduced to the shorter stays documented [31]), they provide another model that typically uses age criterion as one point of entry. While not standardized across the ACE units in operation in the United States, the most common age group is 71 to 80 years of age [31]. Some younger patients with numerous comorbidities may also be at risk for problems seen in an older population. However, using an age criterion of greater than 70 years to screen for cognitive and functional status is a reasonable starting point and is supported by several studies in the literature.

Dementia

While dementia is common in the elderly patient, it is often not diagnosed or fully recognized [32,33]. Screening for dementia in the hospitalized elder is particularly important in the patient who is losing weight, noncompliant with medications, readmitted to the hospital, or admitted from the nursing home. Finding that a patient's insight and judgment are significantly impaired can have a life-altering impact on the patient's ability to make major health care decisions during hospitalization and to live or operate an automobile independently at discharge. Similarly, results of cognitive screening can significantly affect the management of other nondementia-related illness, end-of-life issues (such as feeding tube placement), and signal an increased risk of delirium and readmission. A study of the predisposing factors that affect the risk of delirium in the elderly hospitalized patient showed that a mini-mental status examination (MMSE) of less than 24/30 increased the risk of delirium to 2.82 times that of the nondemented older hospitalized patient [26].

While the clinical diagnosis of dementia is still based on the Diagnostic and Statistical Manual of Mental Disorders, 4th edition, criteria [34], two commonly used screening tools, the MMSE [35] and the mini-cog (Box 2) [36], identify the elderly at high risk for dementia. Both screening tests have similar sensitivities, and although the mini-cog has not been specifically validated for the hospital setting, it is faster to administer at bedside. A limitation of the MMSE and the mini-cog is that they do not directly screen for executive function, such as planning, organizing, or prioritizing, often requiring further investigation by the physician.

Some organizations have specific system initiatives to prevent delirium in patients with underlying dementia. However, even in the absence of these programs, hospitalists can use tools, such as an orientation board, to help to decrease confusion for an in-patient with dementia. An orientation board prominently lists the day, the date, the name of the next meal, the current weather, and other information that helps the patient

---

Box 2. Dementia screening tool: mini-cog

- Step 1: Remember and repeat three unrelated words
- Step 2: Clock-drawing test (CDT)—distracter
- Step 3: Repeat three previously presented words
- Step 4: Scoring: 1 point for each recalled word
  - Score = 0; positive screen for dementia
  - Score = 1–2 with abnormal CDT; positive screen for dementia
  - Score = 1–2 with normal CDT; negative screen for dementia
  - Score = 3; negative screen for dementia

Adapted from Borson S, Scanlan J, Brush M, et al. The mini-cog: a cognitive "vital signs" measure for dementia screening in multi-lingual elderly. Int J Geriatr Psychiatry 2000;15(11):1021–27, with permission.

---

with reality orientation. Use of an orientation board and a program of cognitive stimulation decreased the confusion rate from 26% to 8% in the Hospital Elder Life Program (HELP) [37]. The HELP program was initially reported as a multicomponent intervention in 1999, targeting modifiable risk factors, and was later transformed into a formal program that is commonly known as the HELP program. The program has target risk factors and patient groups, associated interventions, and specific outcomes of interest (Table 1). In addition, having family or caregivers stay with the patient overnight, avoiding physical restraints, removing unnecessary foley catheters, and reducing polypharmacy are other important interventions.

While delirium may be the most common cause of severe behavioral disturbances in hospitalized patients with underlying dementia, many patients with dementia may have baseline behavioral patterns that are problematic in the acute hospital setting. Up to two-thirds of patients with dementia exhibit sleep disturbances, agitation, aggression, hallucinations, and wandering. Preventing delirium is important, but managing these behaviors is also critical to provide a safe hospitalization for these patients. These patients may require pharmacologic therapy. Antipsychotics and benzodiazepines are the most commonly used agents to treat agitation and aggression. However, in the elderly, benzodiazepines should not be a first-line agent. Therefore, antipsychotics should be considered first-line therapy. Typical antipsychotics, such as haloperidol, are felt to be safe and effective, but do not have strong clinical trial data to support their use in the in-patient setting for this purpose. Haloperidol, especially when given intravenously, can cause prolongation of the QT interval, so the intravenous route should be avoided. The atypical antipsychotics, such as olanzapine and risperidone, have clinical trial data that suggest a moderate effect in the chronic treatment of these effects. However, there are published studies that demonstrate an increased mortality effect in elderly patients treated with these atypical antipsychotics when used chronically [38,39]. Therefore, antipsychotics should be used when necessary, but consideration for these side effects needs to be given.

Functional impairment

Activities of daily living (ADLs) and instrumental activities of daily living (IADLs) are commonly employed in research and clinical assessment as measures to determine degree and type of functional impairment. Testing for patient mobility by observing the patient's gait and ability to transfer from bed or chair, and using a more formal screen (such as the "get up and go" test) [40] (Fig. 2) will provide more information into the kinds of physical therapy or occupational therapy needed, and the immediate discharge destination (eg, home physical therapy versus acute rehabilitation).

Functional measures are strong predictors of mortality in the hospitalized older patient, and study evidence suggests these measures contribute more to prognosis than the combined measures of comorbidity, disease severity, and staging or diagnosis [41]. This echoes the findings of the ACOVE investigators [20] in the community-dwelling elder. Many of the interventions in clinical trials for improving the outcomes of the hospitalized older patient target functional decline. While most of these interventions involve interdisciplinary and team care—such as inpatient geriatric evaluation and management units [42], ACE units [43,44], and HELP [37]—the practicing hospitalist can perform baseline screening of ADLs and IADLs, and institute early mobilization with the help of physical or occupational therapy, nursing, and family or caregivers. A set of four simple screening questions can identify older patients at significant risk for functional decline while in the hospital. They are:

1. Does the patient have a decubitus ulcer?
2. Are there baseline cognitive deficits?
3. Is there baseline functional impairment?
4. Is baseline social activity low?

Zero positive responses places the patient at low risk for functional decline during the hospitalization (8%), one to two positive responses results in moderate risk (28%), and three to four positive responses is high risk (63%) [45]. The HELP program has been shown to not only prevent delirium, but to also reduce the risk of functional impairment.

Frailty and systems interventions

In identification of patients at increased risk for hazards of hospitalization, crucial and systematic screening can be implemented for patients through use of a simple age criterion. Physicians working with a multidisciplinary team can develop methods of screening this large segment of hospitalized patients.

Table 1
Risk factors for delirium and intervention protocols

Targeted risk factor and eligible patients	Standardized intervention protocols	Targeted outcome for reassessment
Cognitive impairment[a] All patients, protocol once daily; patients with base-line MMSE score of < 20 or orientation score of < 8, protocol three times daily	Orientation protocol: board with names of care-team members and day's schedule; communication to reorient to surroundings. Therapeutic-activities protocol: cognitively stimulating activities three times daily (eg, discussion of current events, structured reminiscence, or word games). Nonpharmacologic sleep protocol: at bedtime, warm drink (milk or herbal tea), relaxation tapes or music, and back massage. Sleep-enhancement protocol: unit-wide noise-reduction strategies (eg, silent pill crushers, vibrating beepers, and quiet hallways) and schedule adjustments to allow sleep (eg, rescheduling of medications and procedures). Early mobilization protocol: ambulation or active range-of-motion exercises three times daily; minimal use of immobilizing equipment (eg, bladder catheters or physical restraints)	Change in orientation score
Sleep deprivation All patients; need for protocol assessed once daily		Change in rate of use of sedative drug for sleep[b]

Risk factor	Intervention	Outcome measure
Immobility All patients: ambulation whenever possible, and range-of-motion exercises when patients are chronically nonambulatory, bed or wheel-chair bound, immobilized (eg, because of an extremity fracture or deep venous thrombosis), or when prescribed bed rest.		Change in activities of daily living score
Visual impairment Patients with <20/70 visual acuity on binocular near-vision testing	Vision protocol: visual aids (eg, glasses or magnifying lenses) and adaptive equipment (eg, large illuminated telephone key-pads, large-print books, and fluorescent tape on call bell), with daily reinforcement of their use.	Early correction of vision, < 48 hrs after admission
Hearing impairment Patients hearing <6 of 12 whispers on Whisper Test	Hearing protocol: portable amplifying devices, earwax disimpaction, and special communication techniques, with daily reinforcement of these adaptations.	Change in Whisper Test score
Dehydration Patients with ratio of blood urea nitrogen to creatinine >18, screened for protocol by geriatric nurse-specialist	Dehydration protocol: early recognition of dehydration and volume repletion (eg, encouragement of oral intake of fluids)	Change in ratio of blood urea nitrogen to creatinine

[a] The orientation score consisted of results on the first 10 items on the MMSE.

[b] Sedative drugs included standard hypnotic agents, benzodiazepines, and antihistamines, used as needed for sleep.

Reprinted from Inouye S, Bogardus ST, Charpentier PA, et al. A multicomponent intervention to prevent delirium in hospitalized older patients. NEJM 1999;340:669–76, with permission. Copyright © 1999, Massachusetts Medical Society.

Get Up and Go Test

The "Get Up and Go Test" is an assessment that should be conducted as part of a routine evaluation when dealing with older persons. Its purpose is to detect "fallers" and to identify those who need evaluation.

The staff should be trained to perform the "Get Up and Go Test" at check-in and query those with gait or balance problems for falls.

INITIAL CHECK

All older persons who report a single fall should be observed as they:

• From a sitting position, stand without using their arms for support.

• Walk several paces, turn, and return to the chair.

• Sit back in the chair without using their arms for support.

Individuals who have difficulty or demonstrate unsteadiness performing this test require further assessment.

FOLLOW-UP ASSESSMENT

In the follow-up assessment, ask the person to:

• Sit.

• Stand without using their arms for support.

• Close their eyes for a few seconds, while standing in place.

• Stand with eyes closed, while you push gently on his or her sternum.

• Walk a short distance and come to a complete stop.

• Turn around and return to the chair.

• Sit in the chair without using their arms for support.

While conducting the test, pay attention to any abnormal movements. As you observe, answer the questions below. Record your assessment in the Yes or No boxes provided and/or on the "Falls Evaluation: Initial Visit" form.

Follow-Up Assessment Observations

• Is the person steady and balanced when sitting upright?	☼	No ☼	Yes
• Is the person able to stand with the arms folded?	☼	No ☼	Yes
• When standing, is the person steady in narrow stance?	☼	No ☼	Yes
• With eyes closed, does the person remain steady?	☼	No ☼	Yes
• When nudged, does the person recover without difficulty?	☼	No ☼	Yes
• Does with person start walking without hesitancy?	☼	No ☼	Yes
• When walking, does each foot clear the floor well?	☼	No ☼	Yes
• Is there step symmetry, with the steps equal length and regular ?	☼	No ☼	Yes
• Does the person take continuous, regular steps?	☼	No ☼	Yes
• Does the person walk straight without a walking aid?	☼	No ☼	Yes
• Does the person stand with heels close together?	☼	No ☼	Yes
• Is the person able to sit safely and judge distance correctly?	☼	No ☼	Yes

Additional Observations

Fig. 2. The "Get Up and Go Test." (*From* Mathias S, Nayak US, Issacs B. Balance in elderly patients: The "get-up and go" test. Arch Phys Med Rehabil 1986;67:387–9; with permission.)

Screening can be done by physicians or nurses, but can also be done using nonclinical volunteers [46].

Of the multidisciplinary interventions that have been published, the HELP program has a positive impact on the cognitive and functional status of the elderly patient. This program does require a committed team, including physician sponsorship to incorporate into routine practice the types of screening and interventions used in the HELP program. Geriatricians and hospitalists would be ideal leaders in initiating these types of systematic improvements to the way patient-care is provided within their own medical center. An example of incorporation of the HELP program in a community hospital follows in the delirium section.

Avoiding hazards of hospitalization

Hazards of hospitalization, an overview

Some of the hazards of being hospitalized include iatrogenic illness, such as medication errors, nosocomial infection, and errors during diagnostic or therapeutic procedures. In addition to health system issues that may contribute to patient safety, the elderly patient's baseline vulnerability and severity of illness play a large role. For example, the incidence of delirium is greater in an older patient with an MMSE of less than 24, a severe illness, or an iatrogenic event [26]. High-risk areas related to hospitalization are important to target in daily medical practice and as areas for system redesign and standardization. Some important clinical issues include the development of pressure ulcers or delirium, preventing deconditioning and further functional decline, and addressing the risk of adverse drug reactions and errors of medication administration in the elderly hospitalized patient. This article's discussion of hazards of hospitalization will focus on delirium identification and strategies for its prevention, adverse drug events and medication review, and reducing the number of unnecessary urinary catheters.

Delirium identification and strategies for prevention

The incidence of delirium in the hospitalized older patient is as high as 50%, including increased mortality, length of hospital stay, and placement in long-term care [11,47,48]. However, it typically goes unrecognized by both nurses and physicians [49,50]. Important steps in improving rates of delirium are developing a strategy for identifying delirium and understanding predisposing and precipitating risk factors. Only with this understanding in place can a successful strategy for delirium preventing be developed and implemented.

The Confusion Assessment Method (CAM) (Fig. 3) [51], a standardized screening tool for making the diagnosis of delirium, has been validated for use in a variety of hospital settings, including the emergency department, inpatient unit, and intensive care unit. Based on work by Inouye and others,

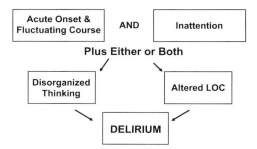

Fig. 3. Confusion assessment method. LOC, level of consciousness. (*Data from* Inouye SK, van Dyck CH, Alessi CA, et al. Clarifying confusion: the confusion assessment method. A new method for detection of delirium. Ann Intern Med 1990;113:941–8.)

in a study group comprised of patients older than 70 years old, increased risk of developing delirium included vision impairment, severe illness (a composite variable based on the acute physiology and chronic health evaluation or APACHE score greater than 16 or a nurse rating of "severe"), cognitive impairment (MMSE less than 24), and blood urea nitrogen/creatinine ratio greater than or equal to 18 [26]. Precipitating factors for delirium in the elderly patient during the acute hospitalization process included use of physical restraints or a bladder catheter, three or more medications added, an iatrogenic event, or malnutrition [52].

The Yale Delirium Prevention Trial studied the impact of a set of delirium prevention interventions. These included interventions to prevent cognitive impairment, sleep deprivation, immobility, dehydration, and vision or hearing impairment [14,37]. These interventions were low-tech but labor intensive, reduced the incidence of delirium significantly from 15% to 10% in the intervention group, and decreased the total number of days with delirium and number of episodes. There was no significant effect on severity or recurrence rate of those once delirious. Additionally, there was an 8% decline in MMSE by two or more points (control 26%) and a 14% decline by two or more ADLs (control 33%) in those enrolled in this study.

While HELP-funded programs may be difficult to replicate in other settings, the cost-savings associated with this program have made it appealing to many institutions. A Pittsburgh community hospital without research funding or infrastructure established a modified HELP program, demonstrating clinical effectiveness and cost-saving. With the HELP intervention, delirium rates dropped by 14.4% and total cost decreased $626,261 for a 40-bed unit over a 6-month survey period. Nursing and family satisfaction ratings were very favorable. Furthermore, these benefits were sustained. This community hospital project did eliminate some of the components of the original HELP program—the exercise and fluid repletion portions— because of resource limitations [46].

While efforts to prevent delirium in at-risk patients are essential, delirium will still occur. Two key steps are essential in managing patients with delirium, as identified when using a tool such as the CAM. The first is to identify an underlying cause, particularly those that have reversible medical causes. These include fluid and electrolyte imbalances, metabolic derangements, infections, adverse drug reactions, hypoperfusion, and withdrawl effects. Treatment of the underlying medical cause is essential and should be initiated immediately. However, patients with significant behavioral disorders secondary to delirium may require interventions to control those behaviors. Restraints should be avoided if at all possible. If used, they should be of the least restrictive and for the shortest period of time possible. More commonly, pharmacologic management is required. Like the treatment of behavioral disturbances in patients with dementia, antipsychotics, particularly the typical antipsychotics, are the first-line pharmacologic treatment option for these patients. These medications should be discontinued as soon as safely possible.

Adverse drug events, polypharmacy, and medication review

An adverse drug reaction (ADR) is usually defined as any noxious drug effect occurring at standard drug treatment doses. ADRs account for hospital admission rates of 3% to 10%. The in-hospital ADR rate is approximately 2%, with the fatal in-hospital ADR rate at 0.19% [53]. ADRs in hospitalized patients also result in excess length of stay and cost [54].

Bates and colleagues [55] looked at "preventable" in-hospital drug errors and found that one-third of the errors were preventable but accounted for 50% of the cost. Analgesics, sedatives, and psychoactive drugs were the most common of the "culprit" drugs and delirium was a common presentation in the "preventable" in-hospital ADR group.

The elderly patient is already at increased risk of ADRs, largely because of the greater number of medications he or she may be on and the additional number of comorbidities seen with aging. However, age is not an independent risk factor for developing ADRs [56].

The term "polypharmacy" is frequently defined as taking five or more medications. As defined, polypharmacy emphasizes the greater risk of drug interactions with increasing numbers of medications and the resulting potential for accompanying adverse drug effects. However, defining polypharmacy without a measure of appropriateness may not be as clinically useful in the elderly, who often require five or more medications.

Medication oversight is a time-consuming endeavor involving a systematic and rigorous review of each medication for appropriateness in conjunction with comorbidities and the other medications the patient may be taking. These systematic reviews may be beneficial when conducted by pharmacists [57]. However, there are components of medication review that certainly lend themselves to the use of integrated technologies, such as the review of medications upon admission and reconciliation of medications upon discharge. Another approach to medication review is use of explicit criteria for inclusion or exclusion of medications noted on an elderly patient's medication list.

The Beers list of medications [58] is a list of potentially hazardous medications for older adults. It was developed as a guide for prescribing based on expert consensus after rigorous literature review. It states that older patients are more prone to ADRs, with specific medications or classes of medications that cause a high likelihood of adverse effects with little proven therapeutic benefit. The Beers recommendation is that the medications or classes of medications with a high severity rating should be avoided, and that often a safer alternative exists. Using the Beers recommendations as the only tool for medication review is inadequate, but is a good starting point to identify medications with significant side effects in the older adult.

For the hospitalist, the elderly patient's entry to the hospital is an important juncture for medication review, especially at admission and discharge. This situation presents an opportunity to reduce polypharmacy at admission, as approximately 50% of older community-dwelling patients take one or more unnecessary medication [59]. This is all the more important because at discharge more medications are usually added to the elderly patient's medication list [60].

The Joint Commission's requirement for a medication reconciliation process mandates a need to develop systems to review medication lists at points-of-care transition. Hospitalists involved in the care of the elderly can take the lead in developing such systematic safety nets intended to improve care. This process can be automated for those hospitals with a computerized order entry and embedded clinical decision-making support. These integrated electronic systems substantially reduce medical error rates [61]. When medication reconciliation processes are instituted electronically, the physician is able to capture and convey the crucially important clinical information needed to target unnecessary or harmful medication. Even in hospitals without these integrated technologic systems, a TJC mandated medication reconciliation process must be established using a manual process.

Incorporating pharmacists into the review of medications at discharge may prove effective at improving the appropriateness of discharge medications. In a single site study, hospitalized older patients who were being discharged to a long-term care facility had a pharmacist-based medication review which resulted in a lower rate of inappropriate medications [62]. While this study showed favorable trends in clinical outcomes, the clinically relevant decrease in hospital usage and adverse drug events did not reach statistical significance. With such promising clinical outcomes, hospitals that already use pharmacists in the discharge process could incorporate pharmacist-driven medication review of frail patients using the Medication Appropriateness Index [57].

Urinary catheters

Indwelling urinary catheters are used in approximately 25% of hospitalized elderly, account for 40% of nosocomial infections [63,64], and are a risk factor for precipitating delirium [52] and falls [65]. The widely accepted indications for IUCs include inability to void, brief after anesthesia use, monitoring of urine output in a patient unable to comply, protection of an open wound in patients with urinary incontinence, or as part of a palliative care plan. Unfortunately, up to one-third of physicians are not even aware that an IUC has been placed [66]. Many of these catheters are placed at other patient-care sites, such as the emergency department or intensive care unit. Often the original need for the catheter has resolved and the catheter now becomes a "forgotten" focus of potential infection and other hazards in the elderly patient.

IUC use in the hospitalized elderly patient is an example of a hospital-care issue that lends itself to a number of simple systems interventions. For those institutions with a computerized order entry, embedded clinical decision support can be effective in reducing the number of IUCs employed without appropriate indication. In a Veterans Administration study, a combination of an electronic medical reminder and an automated 72-hour default stop date reduced the average use duration of IUCs by 3 days [67]. For those institutions without this level of electronic medical record, similar paper reminders can be effective [68]. Finally, for male patients who require a catheter for reasons other than urinary retention, condom catheters may be an alternative. In addition to being rated as more comfortable, condom catheters have been shown to reduce the risk of bacteriuria, symptomatic urinary tract infections, and death [69]. Hospitalists can advocate reducing the number of IUCs by assisting their institutions in developing electronic or paper reminder systems and incorporating condom catheters into a hospital IUC protocol.

Improve transitions of care

Coordination of after hospitalization health care—particularly of the medically complex, frail, or functionally debilitated elderly patient—requires anticipatory discharge planning, starting typically at the patient's point of entry into the hospital. Advanced and integrated systems of communication and coordination are needed to support such expanded and integrated patient-care and follow-up at discharge. Such discharge planning often incorporates family, caregivers, nursing, social work, primary care physicians and specialists, pharmacists, and nurse practitioners. To further add to the complexity of the communication and systems coordination needed in the elderly patient population, the after hospitalization follow-up care is often given in a variety of settings, including the patient's or caregiver's home, physician's office, skilled nursing or acute rehabilitaton, and long-term care facilities.

While patient discharge processes vary among hospitals, there are key components to any successful discharge that can be generalized across institutions. The Society of Hospital Medicine's Hospital Quality and Patient Safety Committee developed such components in a discharge check sheet (Table 2) [70], derived by the consensus of experts and rigorous review of

Table 2
Ideal discharge of the elderly patient: a hospitalist checklist

Data elements	Process		
	Disharge summary	Patient instructions	Communication to follow-up clinician on day of discharge
Presenting problem that precipitated hospitalization	x	x	x
Key findings and test results	x		
Final primary and secondary diagnoses	x	x	x
Brief hospital course	x		x
Condition at discharge, including functional status and cognitive status, if relevant	x – Functional status o – Cognitive status		
Discharge destination (and rationale, if not obvious)	x		x
Discharge medications:			
Written schedule	x	x	x
Include purpose and cautious (if appropriate) for each	o	x	o
Comparison with preadmission medications, (new, changes in dose/ frequency unchanged, "medications should no longer take")	x	x	x
Follow-up appointments with name of provider, date, address, phone number, visit purpose, suggested management plan	x	x	x
All pending labs or tests, responsible person to whom results will be sent	x		x
Recommendations of and subspecialty consultants	x		o
Documentation of patient education and understanding	x		
Any anticipated problems and suggested interventions	x	x	x
24/7 call-back number	x	x	
Identify referring and receiving providers	x	x	
Resuscitation status and any other pertinent end-of-life issues	o		

x, required element; o, optional element

Reprinted from Halasyamani L, Kripilani S, Coleman E, et al. Transition of care for hospitalized elderly patients—development of a discharge checklist for hospitalists. J Hosp Med 2006;1:354–60, with permission. Copyright © 2006, John Wiley & Sons, Inc.

the literature and existing products. This peer reviewed tool, although not yet formally evaluated, provides the key clinical care elements in the discharge summary section and sections on patient instructions, along with communication to the patient's physicians in other institutions or in the outpatient setting. This discharge checklist can be used by the individual hospitalist or hospital-wide in the discharge process.

Summary

A significant portion of hospital care involves elderly patients who have frequent and severe disease presentations, higher risk of iatrogenic injury during hospitalization, and greater baseline vulnerability. These risks frequently result in longer and more frequent hospitalizations.

The frailty and complication rates of the elderly population underscore the importance of hospital-based programs of education, and screening for cognitive and functional impairments, to determine risk and needed additional care and services during hospitalization and at discharge. In addition, physicians are needed to take the lead in instituting programs of prevention (eg, delirium, ADRs, unnecessary IUC use) and improving the systems of care with integrated technologies (eg, aspects of discharge planning, medication reconciliation, and reduction of medication error). As such, it is a multitiered approach, with interventions in the areas of education, screening, prevention, and systems of care improvements, that is needed to improve the clinical care and outcomes of the hospitalized elderly patient.

References

[1] Defrancis CJ, Hall MJ. 2002 National Hospital Discharge survey. Advance data from vital and health statistics. No.342. Hyattsville (MD): National Center for Health Statistics; 2002.

[2] Naylor M, Brooten D, Campbell R, et al. Comprehensive discharge planning and home follow-up of hospitalized elders: a randomized controlled trial. JAMA 1999;281:613–20.

[3] Kozak LJ, Hall MJ, Owings MF. 2000 National Hospital Discharge survey: annual summary with detailed diagnosis and procedure data. Vital health statistics No. 13(153). Hyattsville (MD): National Center for Health Statistics; 2002.

[4] Lubitz JD, Riley GF. Trends in Medicare payments in the last year of life. N Engl J Med 1993;328:1092–6.

[5] Covinsky KE, Palmer RM, Fortinsky RH, et al. Loss of independence in activities of daily living in older adults hospitalized with medical illnesses: increased vulnerability with age. J Am Geriatr Soc 2003;51:451–8.

[6] Burns R, Nichols L. Factors predicting readmission of older general medicine patients. J Gen Intern Med 1991;6:389–93.

[7] Steel K, Gertman PM, Crescenzi C, et al. Iatrogenic illness on a general medicine service at a university hospital. N Engl J Med 1981;304:638–42.

[8] Becker PM, McVey LJ, Saltz CC, et al. Hospital acquired complications in a randomized controlled clinical trial of a geriatric consultation team. JAMA 1987;257:2313–7.

[9] Curriculum for the hospitalized aging medical patient (CHAMP). Available on the Portal of Online Geriatics Education. http://www.pogoe.org. Supported by the Donald W. Reynolds Foundation.

[10] Brennan TA, Leape LL, Laird NM, et al. Incidence of adverse events and negligence in hospitalized patients. N Engl J Med 1991;324:370–6.

[11] Gillick MR, Serrell NA, Gillick LS. Adverse consequences of hospitalization in the elderly. Soc Sci Med 1982;16:1033–8.

[12] The Support Principal investigators. A controlled trial to improve care for seriously ill hospitalized patients: the study to understand prognosis and preferences for outcomes and risks of treatments (Support). JAMA 1995;274:1591–8.

[13] Cassel CK. Overview on attitudes of physicians toward caring for the dying patient. In: Caring for the Dying: Identification and Promotion of Physician Competency. Philadelphia: American Board of Internal Medicine; 1996. p. 1–4.

[14] Inouye SK, Wagner DR, Acampora D, et al. A controlled trial of a nursing-centered intervention in the hospitalized elderly medical patients: The Yale Geriatric Care Program. J Am Geriatr Soc 1993;41:1353–60.

[15] Hirch CH, Sommers L, Olsen A, et al. The natural history of functional morbidity in hospitalized older patients. J Am Geriatr Soc 1990;38:1296–303.

[16] Counsell SR, Kennedy RD, Szwabo P, et al. Curriculum recommendations for resident training in geriatrics interdisciplinary team care. J Am Geriart Soc 1999;47:1145–8.

[17] Dressler DD, Pistoria MJ, Budnitz TL, et al. Core competencies in hospital medicine: Development and methodology. J Hosp Med 2006;1:48–56.

[18] The Joint Commission. Available at: http://www.jointcommission.org. Accessed January 29, 2008.

[19] Fried L, Tangen CM, Walston J, et al. Frailty in older adults: evidence for a phenotype. J Gerontol A Biol Sci Med Sci 2001;56A(3):M146–56.

[20] Wenger NS, Shekelle PG, the ACOVE Investigators. Assessing care of vulnerable elders: ACOVE project overview. Ann Intern Med 2001;135:642–6.

[21] Saliba D, Elliott M, Rubenstein L, et al. The Vulnerable Elders Survey: a tool for identifying vulnerable older people in the community. J Am Geriatr Soc 2001;49:1691–9.

[22] Arora VM, Johnson M, Olson J, et al. Using Assessing Care of Vulnerable Elders Quality Indicators to Measure Quality of Hospital Care for Vulnerable Elders. J Am Geriatr Soc 2007;55:1705–11.

[23] Sager M, Franke T, Inouye SK, et al. Functional outcomes of acute medical illness and hospitalizations in older persons. Arch Intern Med 1996;156:645–52.

[24] Sands L, Yaffe K, Covinski K, et al. Cognitive screening predicts magnitude of functional recovery from admission to 3 months after discharge in hospitalized elderly. J Gerontol A Biol Sci Med Sci 2003;58:37–45.

[25] Albert SM, Costa R, Merchant C, et al. Hospitalization and Alzheimer's disease: results from a community-based study. J Gerontol A Biol Sci Med Sci 1999;54:M267–71.

[26] Inouye SK, Viscoli CM, Horwitz RI, et al. A predictive model for delirium in hospitalized elderly medical patients based on admission characteristics. Ann Intern Med 1993;119: 474–81.

[27] Walter LC, Brand RJ, Counsell SR, et al. Prognostic Index for 1-year mortality on older hospitalized adults. JAMA 2001;285:2987–94.

[28] Brookmeyer R, Gray S, Kawas C. Projections of Alzheimer's disease in the United States and the public health impact of delaying disease onset. Am J Public Health 1998; 88:1337–42.

[29] Katz S, Ford A, Moskowitz R, et al. Studies of illness in the aged. The index of ADL: a standardized measure of biological and psychosocial function. JAMA 1963;185:914–9.

[30] Lawton M, Brody E. Assessment of older people: self-maintaining and instrumental activities of daily living. Gerontologist 1969;9(3):179–86.

[31] Jayadevappa R, Bloom BS, Raziano DB, et al. Dissemination of characteristics of acute care for elders (ACE) units in the United States. Int J Technol Assess Health Care 2003; 19:220–7.

[32] Sternberg SA, Wolfson C, Baumgarten M. Undetected dementia in community-dwelling older people: the Canadian study of health and aging. J Am Geriatr Soc 2000;48:1430–4.

[33] Boustani M, Callahan CM, Unverzagt FW, et al. Implementing a screening and diagnosis program for dementia in primary care. J Gen Intern Med 2005;20:572–7.

[34] American Psychiatric Association. Diagnostic and statistical manual of mental disorders; DSM IV. 4th edition. Washington, DC: American Psychiatric Association; 1994, p. 123–130.

[35] Folstein M, Folstein S, McHugh P. Mini-mental state: a practical method for grading the cognitive state of patients for the clinician. J Psychiatr Res 1975;12:189–98.

[36] Borson S, Scanlan J, Brush M, et al. The mini-cog: a cognitive:"vital signs"measure for dementia screening in multi-lingual elderly. Int J Geriatr Psychiatry 2000;15(11):1021–7.

[37] Inouye SK, Bogardus ST, Baker DI, et al. The Hospital Elder Life Program: a model of care to prevent cognitive and functional decline in older hospitalized patients. J Am Geriatr Soc 2000;48:1679–706.

[38] Schneider LS, Dagerman KS, Insel P. Risk of death with atypical antipsychotic drug treatment for dementia: meta-analysis of randomized placebo-controlled trials. JAMA 2005; 294(15):1934–43.

[39] Atypical antipsychotics in the elderly. Medical Letter on Drugs & Therapeutics 2005;47: 61–2.

[40] Mathias S, Navak US, Isaacs B. Balance in elderly patients: the "get-up and go" test. Arch Phys Med Rehabil 1986;67(6):387–9.

[41] Inouye SK, Peduzzi PN, Robinson JT, et al. Importance of functional measures in predicting mortality among older hospitalized patients. JAMA 1998;279:1187–93.

[42] Cohn HJ, Feussner JR, Weinberger M, et al. A controlled trial of inpatient and outpatient geriatric evaluation and management. N Engl J Med 2002;346:905–12.

[43] Landefeld CS, Palmer RM, Kresevic D, et al. A randomized trial of care in a hospital medical unit especially designed to improve the functional outcomes of acutely ill older patients. N Engl J Med 1995;332:1338–44.

[44] Counsell SR, Holder CM, Liebenauer LL, et al. Effects of a multicomponent intervention on functional outcomes and process of care in hospitalized older patients: a randomized controlled trial of acute care for elders (ACE) in a community hospital. J Am Geriatr Soc 2000;48:1572–81.

[45] Inouye SK, Wagner DR, Acampora D, et al. A predictive index for functional decline in hospitalized elderly patients. J Gen Intern Med 1993;8(12):645–52.

[46] Rubin FH, Williams JT, Lescisin DA, et al. Replicating the Hospital Elder Life Program in a community hospital and demonstrating effectiveness using quality improvement methodology. J Am Geriatr Soc 2006;54:969–74.

[47] Chisholm SE, Deniston OL, Ingrisan RM, et al. Prevalence of confusion in elderly hospitalized patients. J Gerentol Nurs 1982;8:87–96.

[48] Inouye SK, Schlesinger MJ, Lydon TJ. Delirium: a symptom of how hospital care is failing older persons and a window to improve quality of hospital care. Am J Med 1999;106: 563–73.

[49] Meagher DJ, Trzepacz PT. Motoric subtypes of delirium. Semin Clin Neuropsychiatry 2000; 5:75–85.

[50] O'Keeffe ST, Lavan JN. Clinical significance of delirium subtypes in older people. Age Ageing 1999;28:115–9.

[51] Inouye SK, van Dyck CH, Alessi CA, et al. Clarifying confusion: the confusion assessment method. A new method for detecting delirium. Ann Intern Med 1990;113:941–8.

[52] Inouye SK, Charpentier PA. Precipitating factors for delirium in hospitalized elderly persons: predictive model and interrelationship with baseline vulnerability. JAMA 1996;275: 852–7.

[53] Lazarou J, Pomeranz BH, Corey PN. Incidence of adverse drug reactions in hospitalized patients: a meta-analysis of prospective studies. JAMA 1998;279:1200–5.

[54] Classen DC, Pestotnik SL, Evans RS, et al. Adverse drug events in hospitalized patients. Excess length of stay, extra costs, and attributable mortality. JAMA 1997;277:301–6.

[55] Bates DW, Spell N, Cullen DJ, et al. The costs of adverse drug events in hospitalized patients. JAMA 1997;277:307–11.

[56] Carbonin P, Pahor M, Bernabei R, et al. Is age an independent risk factor for adverse drug reactions in hospitalized medical patients? J Am Geriatr Soc 1991;39:1093–9.

[57] Hanlon JT, Schmader KE, Samsa GP, et al. A method for assessing drug therapy appropriateness. J Clin Epidemiol 1992;45:1045–51.

[58] Fick DM, Cooper JW, Wade WE, et al. Updating the Beers criteria for potentially inappropriate medication use in older adults. Arch Intern Med 2003;163:2716–24.

[59] Schmader K, Hanlon JT, Weinberger M, et al. Appropriateness of medication prescribing in ambulatory elderly patients. J Am Geriatr Soc 1994;42:1241–7.

[60] Beers M, Dang J, Hasegawa J, et al. Influence of hospitalization on drug therapy in the elderly. J Am Geriatr Soc 1989;37:679–83.

[61] Kaushal R, Shojania KG, Bates DW. Effects of computerized physician order entry and clinical decision support systems on medication safety: a systematic review. Arch Intern Med 2003;163:1409–16.

[62] Crotty M, Rowett D, Spurling L, et al. Does the addition of a pharmacist transition coordinatory improve evidence-based medication management and health outcomes in older adults moving from the hospital to a long-term care facility? Results of a randomized, controlled trial. Am J Geriatr Pharmacother 2004;2:257–64.

[63] Holroyd-Leduc JM, Mehta KM, Covinsky KE. Urinary incontinence and its association with death, nursing home admission, and functional decline. J Am Geriatr Soc 2004;52:712–8.

[64] Ouslander JG, Greengold B, Chen S. Complications of chronic urethral indwelling catheters among male nursing home patients: a prospective study. J Urol 1987;138:1191–5.

[65] Cesari M, Landi F, Torre S, et al. Prevalence and risk factors for falls in an older community-dwelling population. J Gerontol A Biol Sci Med Sci 2002;57:M722–6.

[66] Jain P, Parada JP, David A, et al. Overuse of the indwelling urinary tract catheter in hospitalized medical patients. Arch Intern Med 1995;155:1425–9.

[67] Cornia PB, Amory JK, Fraser S, et al. Computer-based order entry decreases duration of indwelling urinary catheterization in hospitalized patients. Am J Med 2003;114:404–7.

[68] Saint S, Kaufman SR, Thompson M, et al. A reminder reduces urinary catheterization in hospitalized patients. Jt Comm J Qual Patient Saf 2005;31:455–62.

[69] Saint S, Kaufman SR, Rogers MA, et al. Condom versus indwelling urinary catheters: a randomized trial. J Am Geriatr Soc 2006;54:1055–61.

[70] Halasyamani L, Kripilani S, Coleman E, et al. Transition of care for hospitalized elderly patients—development of a discharge checklist for hospitalists. J Hosp Med 2006;1:354–60.

THE MEDICAL
CLINICS
OF NORTH AMERICA

Med Clin N Am 92 (2008) 407–425

Diabetes Management in the Hospital

Thomas W. Donner, MD[a,b,*],
Kristin M. Flammer, MD[a]

[a]*Division of Endocrinology, Diabetes and Nutrition, University of Maryland School of Medicine, 22 S. Greene Street, Room N3W130, Baltimore, MD 21201, USA*
[b]*Joslin Diabetes Center Affiliate, University of Maryland School of Medicine, 22 South Greene Street, Room N6W100, Baltimore, MD 21201, USA*

Diabetes is an increasingly prevalent disease, with 9.3% of adults 20 years or older in the United States now afflicted [1]. Patients with diabetes make up a disproportionate percentage of those admitted to the hospital, because of more frequent hospitalizations for cardiovascular, cerebrovascular, and peripheral vascular disease; renal failure; infections; and lower extremity amputations. While landmark studies in the 1990s demonstrated reduced micro- and macrovascular events with aggressive diabetes control in outpatients [2–5], only recently has evidence supported aggressive inpatient diabetes control. Historically, inpatient hyperglycemia has been viewed as an expected outcome of a stressful illness among glucose-intolerant individuals. Physicians have traditionally delegated inpatient diabetes management as secondary in importance to the acute illness, often instituting sliding scale insulin as the only means to address hyperglycemia [6]. However, diabetes has now been identified as an independent risk factor for adverse inpatient outcomes [7,8]. Randomized studies have also shown that aggressive treatment of hyperglycemia in the intensive care unit setting leads to reduced morbidity and mortality [9–11]. This article will review the adverse effects of hyperglycemia among hospitalized patients, and provide treatment recommendations.

Prevalence of diabetes and hyperglycemia

Patients with diabetes are two to five times more likely to be hospitalized than patients without diabetes and many patients are undiagnosed before

---

* Corresponding author. Division of Endocrinology, Diabetes and Nutrition, University of Maryland School of Medicine, 22 S. Greene Street, Room N3W130, Baltimore, MD 21201.
E-mail address: tdonner@medicine.umaryland.edu (T.W. Donner).

hospitalization. Among patients admitted to an inner city teaching hospital, 13% of patients had one or more plasma glucose levels higher than 200 mg/dL [12]. Of these, 68% carried a diagnosis of diabetes while 32% were newly diagnosed. Among patients admitted to general medical and surgical wards in a community hospital, 38% were found to have one or more fasting glucose levels 126 mg/dL or higher or random glucose levels 200 mg/dL or higher [13]. Of these, 67% had a known history of diabetes, and 33% had no prior diabetes diagnosis. Hyperglycemia is also associated with increased resource use and worse clinical outcomes. Hyperglycemic patients were more likely to be admitted to the intensive care unit ($P < .01$), or discharged to a transitional care unit or nursing home ($P < .01$). Those with new hyperglycemia had a significantly longer inpatient length of stay when compared with euglycemic patients (9.0 ± 0.7 versus 4.5 ± 0.1 days, $P < .01$). In 2002, the financial burden of inpatient diabetes care in the United States was $42 billion, representing 41% of the total health care expenditures for patients with diabetes [14]. These patients also had an annual per capita inpatient health care expenditure nearly five times that of patients without diabetes.

Hyperglycemia is common among patients with diabetes admitted to the hospital because of illness-related elevations in counter-regulatory hormones, glucocorticoid therapy, dextrose-containing IV solutions, and parenteral nutrition. Despite being alerted to uncontrolled hyperglycemia by elevated bedside and laboratory glucose readings, clinicians tend to poorly manage inpatient diabetes. A survey of 44 US hospitals identified 999 adult general medical and surgical patients with primary or secondary discharge diagnoses of diabetes. Of these, 60% were found to have at least one glucose level greater than 250 mg/dL. Persistent hyperglycemia, defined as glucose levels greater than 200 mg/dL for 3 consecutive days, was found in between 18% and 38% of patients. Basal insulins were often held in patients known to be insulin deficient: 16% of patients with type 1 diabetes and 35% of patients with type 2 diabetes on insulin as outpatients were treated with sliding scale insulin therapy alone [15]. Even though the diabetes appeared to be undertreated in these patients, glucose levels of less than 60 mg/dL were also common, seen in 12% to 18% of those studied.

Pathogenesis of adverse outcomes

The etiology of adverse outcomes among patients with hyperglycemia is multifactorial, with a number of organ systems being impaired. Studies have found that most of these abnormalities are reversible when glucose levels are normalized. Hyperglycemia has detrimental effects on phagocyte function and cellular immunity, placing patients at increased risk of infectious complications. Elevated glucose levels cause abnormalities in polymorphonuclear leukocyte mobilization, chemotaxis, adherence, phagocytosis, and intracellular killing [16–19]. Even transient hyperglycemia in nondiabetic individuals reduces the number of circulating lymphocytes [20]. Reductions in CD-4 and CD-8 cells in hyperglycemic patients with diabetes normalized after euglycemia was achieved [21].

Hyperglycemia is known to be a proinflammatory state with elevations in C-reactive protein, interleukin (IL)-6, IL-18, and tumor necrosis factor-α. Acute hyperglycemia has also been shown to be a prothrombotic state with elevated levels of plasminogen activator inhibitor-1 and fibrinogen, decreased tissue plasminogen activator levels, and increased platelet aggregation and adhesion [22–24]. Acute hyperglycemia is associated with endothelial dysfunction associated with reduced nitric oxide levels [25]. Such changes are felt to directly lead to impaired cellular immunity, increased oxidative stress, inflammation, increased cellular apoptosis, impaired wound healing, ischemia, and acidosis, resulting in increased morbidity, prolonged hospital length of stay, and increased death rates [7]. These deleterious effects have been associated with prolonged hospital length of stay and increased costs. In post–coronary bypass surgery patients, each 50 mg/dL increase in mean glucose levels increased length of stay by 0.76 days and hospital costs by $2840 [26]. Another study in CABG patients found that each 30 mg/dL increase in 3-day mean postoperative glucose added 1 day to hospital length of stay and $1150 in hospital costs [27].

Hyperglycemia and adverse outcomes

Studies have demonstrated a correlation between adverse outcomes and inpatient hyperglycemia in a variety of clinical settings. In a retrospective data review of 1826 consecutive patients admitted to an intensive care unit, there was a direct and positive correlation between glucose levels and mortality [28]. When compared with patients whose mean glucose ranged between 88 and 99 mg/dL, there was a threefold increase in mortality among patients whose mean glucose level ranged from 160 to 179 mg/dL [28]. The highest hospital mortality rate (42.5%) was seen among patients whose mean glucose values exceeded 300 mg/dL. A similar, progressive increase in hospital mortality was seen in 3554 patients with diabetes undergoing coronary artery bypass grafting. Patients whose mean postoperative glucose was less than 150 mg/dL had a 0.9% mortality compared with 14.5% mortality in patients whose mean postoperative glucose was 250 mg/dL [29]. Postoperative infections have been shown to be directly related to glycemic control. Deep sternal wound infection rates were 13% in patients whose glucose ranged between 100 and 150 mg/dL compared with 67% in those whose 1-day postoperative glucose ranged from 250 to 300 mg/dL [30]. In a prospective study of 336 patients admitted to the hospital with an acute myocardial infarction, 1-year mortality rates were found to be highest among those with diabetes (44%), followed by those with severe impaired glucose tolerance (30%), mild impaired glucose tolerance (13%), and normoglycemia (9%) [31]. In this study, admission glucose and diabetes were independent predictors of mortality. Similarly, among 63 acute stroke patients, a 90-mg/dL increase in admission glucose was associated with a 5.6-cm^3 increase in final infarct size [32].

The rationale for tight glycemic control in the hospital

Recent studies have demonstrated improved clinical outcomes in the acute care setting associated with aggressive glycemic control. To assess the impact of intensified diabetes control following coronary bypass surgery, Furnary and colleagues [27] studied the effect of changing from subcutaneous sliding-scale insulin to a continuous insulin infusion. Hyperglycemia in the first 3 postoperative days was found to be independently predictive of mortality ($P < .0001$) and deep sternal wound infections ($P = .0001$). Continuous insulin infusion with a target glucose levels of <150 mg/dL independently led to a 60% reduction in mortality and a 77% reduction in deep sternal wound infections. Because the majority of excess mortality associated with hyperglycemia was cardiac related, the authors speculated that the clinical improvement seen may have been because of improved myocardial adenosine triphosphate production.

The Diabetes Insulin-Glucose Infusion in Acute Myocardial Infarction (DIGAMI) study investigated patients presenting with an acute myocardial infarction and glucose levels greater than 200 mg/dL [10]. Subjects who were randomized to intensive insulin therapy received intravenous (IV) insulin for 24 hours or more followed by multiple daily insulin injections, resulting in a 24-hour mean glucose of 173 mg/dL. Conventionally treated patients received subcutaneous insulin for glucose levels over 200, leading to a mean glucose of 211 mg/dL. Intensive insulin therapy led to a 28% reduction in mortality ($P = .011$).

In a Belgian surgical intensive care unit, 1548 patients were randomized to IV insulin therapy and a target glucose of 80 to 110 mg/dL, or conventional therapy with a target glucose between 180 and 200 mg/dL and IV insulin only when the blood glucose rose to greater than 250 mg/dL [9]. Intensive insulin therapy resulted in a mean AM glucose of 103 mg/dL in the intensively treated patients and 153 mg/dL in conventionally treated patients. Patients randomized to intensive insulin therapy had a 40% reduction in ICU mortality ($P < .04$). Each 20-mg/dL blood glucose elevation was associated with a 30% increased mortality risk. Intensive insulin therapy also led to reductions in overall hospital mortality (34%), sepsis (46%), need for dialysis (41%), transfusion rates (50%), and cardioneuropathy (44%). The lower mortality rate was attributed mainly to patients whose ICU stay was longer than 5 days. A subsequent study using the same protocol was performed in their medical ICU [33]. While mortality was not improved by intensive insulin therapy among all patients, those in the ICU for 3 days or more had lower in-hospital mortality rates (43.0% versus 52.5%, $P < .009$). More deaths occurred in the intensive insulin treatment group among patients whose ICU stay was less than 3 days. The significance of this finding is unclear, since higher numbers of patients in the intensive insulin therapy group had their care limited or withdrawn because of medical futility. Intensive insulin therapy also led to lower rates of kidney injury, need for mechanical ventilation, and duration of ICU stay. Three ICU studies suggest that 3 to 5 days of intensified diabetes management are required to reduce mortality [27,29,33]. Hypoglycemia was considerably more common among intensively controlled patients than among conventionally controlled patients in the surgical ICU (5.2% versus 0.7%) [9] and medical ICU (18.7% versus 3.1%), [33]. Hypoglycemia independently predicted a higher risk of death in medical ICU patients. It remains to be determined whether intensive insulin therapy should be avoided in patients with conditions predisposing to hypoglycemia, such as sepsis, hepatic and renal failure, and glucocorticoid deficiency [34]. Studies showing mortality benefits from tight diabetes control have been limited to surgical and medical ICU settings. Given the potential for hypoglycemia, aggressive insulin protocols should be employed only in settings where hypoglycemia can be adequately prevented, recognized, and treated.

Inpatient diabetes management

The goal of hyperglycemia management in the hospital is to normalize glucose levels while avoiding hypoglycemia. Treatment of hyperglycemia helps correct a catabolic metabolic state, improves white cell function and wound healing, and prevents an osmotic diuresis and the progression of hyperglycemia to ketoacidosis or a hyperglycemic, hyperosmolar state. The American College of Endocrinology (ACE) [8], and American Diabetes Association (ADA) [35] have identified targets of glycemic control based on the findings of randomized clinical trials and observational studies (Table 1). The glucose target for patients in the critical care setting is 110 mg/dL. Those in noncritical inpatient settings should have preprandial glucose levels of less than 110 mg/dL (ACE) or 90 to 130 mg/dL (ADA) and postprandial glucose of less than 180 mg/dL. Pregnant patients should be targeted to a premeal glucose of less than 100 mg/dL and 1-hour postprandial glucose of less than 120 mg/dL (ACE). Pregnant patients in labor and delivery should strive for a glucose target of 100 mg/dL (ACE).

Clinicians face a number of obstacles to attaining good inpatient glycemic control. Patients with diabetes are typically admitted for diagnoses other than uncontrolled hyperglycemia. For this reason, diabetes management often is of secondary importance to the disorder causing hospitalization. The stress of the underlying illness often leads to the secretion of counter-regulatory hormones including cortisol, catecholamines, and glucagon, which worsen insulin resistance. The administration of hypoglycemic agents to control diabetes is often complicated by irregular and

Table 1
Inpatient glycemic targets

Clinical setting	American College of Endocrinology [8]	2007 American Diabetes Association Guidelines [35]
• ICU Patients	80–110 mg/dL	As close to 110 mg/dL as possible, generally <180 mg/dL
• Medical/Surgical Floor		
Preprandial	80–110 mg/dL	90–130 mg/dL
Postprandial	<180 mg/dL	<180 mg/dL
• Pregnant patients		
Preprandial	< 100 mg/dL	
Postprandial	< 120 mg/dL	
Labor and delivery	< 100 mg/dL	

unpredictable eating patterns because of anorexia, nausea, or fasting for diagnostic tests or procedures. Therapeutic medications including glucocorticoids frequently exacerbate underlying hyperglycemia or lead to development of new hyperglycemia. These factors contribute to many clinicians resorting to sliding scale insulin therapy to peripherally address the hyperglycemia on general medical and surgical wards. This practice persists despite a growing body of literature demonstrating that the sliding scale is ineffective and potentially dangerous [6,36–38]. Sliding scales replace insulin in a nonphysiologic manner, do not take into account individual differences in insulin requirements, and focus attention on isolated reactions to hyperglycemia rather than maintenance of normoglycemia. When used alone, sliding scale insulin leads to more widely fluctuating glucose levels and an up to threefold increased risk of hyperglycemia (glucose greater than 200 mg/dL) when compared with treatment with an oral agent with or without a standing order for a long-acting insulin, and no sliding scale insulin [36]. The use of sliding scale insulin places patients with type 1 diabetes at high risk for ketoacidosis if a basal insulin is not added. For these reasons, the use of sliding scale insulin alone is discouraged.

Oral hypoglycemic therapy

Oral hypoglycemic agents are frequently contraindicated in the inpatient setting [7]. Furthermore, most of these agents have a relatively slow onset of action. Sulfonylureas increase the risk of hypoglycemia because of their long duration of action in a patient population with inconsistent meal intake and timing [39]. Metformin carries a risk of lactic acidosis, and should therefore be restricted among inpatients with conditions predisposing them to lactic acidosis. These include infections, renal or hepatic insufficiency, congestive heart failure, hypoxia, or iodinated contrast studies. Metformin may also worsen underlying nausea and diarrhea, and suppress appetite. Thiazolidinediones can be safely continued in most patients. Because they can cause salt and water retention, these agents are best withheld in edematous patients, or in those with advanced or uncompensated heart failure. Experience with exenatide, a glucagon-like peptide-1 (GLP-1) mimetic, and the dipeptidyl peptidase-4 inhibitor sitagliptin, is limited in the inpatient setting. Because exenatide can lead to nausea and vomiting, this agent should typically be withheld in patients with gastrointestinal symptoms. Sitagliptin should be safe to continue in the inpatient setting because of its favorable side-effect profile and low hypoglycemia risk due to glucose-dependent insulin secretion [40]. Both these agents need additional study in the inpatient setting. The alpha glucosidase inhibitors, acarbose and miglitol, are only modestly potent agents that have frequent gastrointestinal adverse effects including bloating, flatulence, and diarrhea. For this reason, these agents should also be discontinued upon admission to the hospital in most patients.

Insulin therapy

Insulin therapy has been shown to effectively control hyperglycemia in a number of inpatient settings and is the most effective treatment for inpatient diabetes control. Increasing attention is now being paid to the importance of physiologic, individualized insulin regimens in the inpatient setting. Current practice guidelines argue for the use of subcutaneous insulin regimens that take into consideration the same basal, mealtime, and supplemental needs that have become the mainstay of intensive outpatient insulin therapy [7,34,35,38,41–43]. Suggested inpatient insulin regimens based on these guidelines are summarized in Table 2. Long-acting "basal" insulin can effectively prevent excess gluconeogenesis and ketogenesis in both type 1 and type 2 diabetes patients. Prandial or "bolus" insulin can be adapted to the patient's nutritional status whether they receive IV dextrose, enteral feeds, total parenteral nutrition, or oral nutritional supplements. Insulin formulations available for basal and prandial use are reviewed in Table 3. In patients with variable oral intake, the bolus insulin can also be administered after the meal, based on the portion of the meal eaten. Because of their rapid absorption, the insulin analogs lispro, aspart, and glulisine are the preferred prandial insulins. They can effectively control postprandial hyperglycemia when dosed either immediately before or after a meal. In selected inpatient settings, the patient's bolus insulin schedule may also be titrated based on the amount of carbohydrate eaten at meals. In patients with Type 1 diabetes or in lean type 2 patients, 1 unit of rapid-acting insulin may be administered per 15 g of carbohydrate at meals, or alternatively one may use 1 unit per 10 g of carbohydrate in more insulin-resistant patients. "Hold" orders should be written for prandial insulins

Table 2
Suggested inpatient insulin regimens

Patient NPO or Limited PO	
• On home insulin, controlled	• Continue 80%–100% glargine or detemir dose
	Continue 50%–80% NPH doses or convert to glargine or detemir
• New to insulin	• Basal insulin 0.2 U/kg/day
	Correctional rapid-acting insulin every 4–6 hours
Patient eating	
• On home insulin, controlled	• Continue home regimen
• New to insulin	• Total insulin daily dose 0.4–1.0 U/kg/day
Consider less-aggressive dosing ranges in:	Divide basal/prandial doses 50%/50%
• Increased insulin sensitivity	• Type 1 diabetic patients, elderly
• Decreased insulin clearance	• Renal, cardiac failure
• Diminished glycogen stores	• Severe liver disease, marked malnutrition
Consider more aggressive dosing in:	
• Increased insulin resistance	• Infections or surgical wounds may require higher basal/prandial ratio
	• Metabolic syndrome/obesity
	• Patients markedly hyperglycemic on admission

when the patient is made NPO (nothing by mouth), or misses a meal because of a test or procedure.

Subcutaneous insulin should be continued in all type 1 and most type 2 diabetes patients who are on insulin as outpatients. For patients admitted on a nonpeaking basal insulin such as insulin glargine or insulin detemir, the outpatient dose of these insulins should be continued on admission to prevent ketoacidosis and suppress hepatic gluconeogenesis. For patients with type 2 diabetes on these insulins whose insulin requirements often decrease when NPO, one should decrease the glargine or detemir dose to 80% of the outpatient dosage. The use of neutral protamine Hagadorn (NPH)

Table 3
Properties of subcutaneous insulin preparations

Insulin	Onset	Peak effect	Duration of action
Basal			
• NPH	2–4 hours	4–8 hours	12–16 hours
• Glargine	2–4 hours	None	20–24 hours
• Detemir	2–4 hours	None	12–24 hours
Prandial/Supplemental			
• Regular (short-acting)	30–60 minutes	2–3 hours	6–10 hours
• Insulin analogs (rapid-acting)	5–15 minutes	30–90 minutes	4–6 hours
Lispro			
Aspart			
Gulisine			

insulin in the hospital is associated with higher rates of hypoglycemia, and its use is therefore discouraged. Should NPH be continued during hospitalization, the dose should be reduced by 50% to reduce the risk of hypoglycemia. For type 2 diabetes patients in whom oral hyperglycemic agents are discontinued on admission or in patients controlled with diet and exercise alone, insulin glargine may be safely started at a dose of 0.2 to 0.5 units/ kg daily [7,41,44], if more than one glucose fingerstick glucose measurement rises to over 180 mg/dL in a 24-hour period.

It is recommended that bedside fingerstick glucose measurements be obtained before each meal and at bedtime among patients who are eating, and every 6 hours in patients who are fasting or receiving continuous enteral or parenteral nutritional support. A 3 AM fingerstick glucose measurement is recommended in patients in whom the basal insulin dose is increased so as to capture any nocturnal hypoglycemia. In patients with type 2 diabetes, should there be excessive daytime hyperglycemia on a basal insulin alone, a premeal rapid-acting insulin should be added before meals. The dosage of prandial insulin can also be started at 0.2 to 0.5 units/kg divided among the three meals. The selection of initial basal and prandial insulin doses should factor in the severity and type of medical illnesses, diabetes classification, and weight (as a measure of insulin resistance).

Supplemental doses of rapid-acting insulin are used to correct hyperglycemia while basal and prandial insulin regimens are being optimized. These orders differ from sliding scale insulin since they are not used to replace basal/prandial regimens. The dose of supplemental insulin should be tailored to a patient's insulin sensitivity to avoid provoking hypoglycemia while still achieving an effective glucose reduction. Lean patients with type 1 diabetes generally require more conservative correctional dosages, on the order of 1 unit to reduce glucose 50 to 70 mg/dL, while more insulin-resistant patients commonly require higher doses, on the order of 1 unit to reduce glucose 10 to 40 mg/dL. In patients on insulin, the "rule of 1800" can be used to estimate the amount of supplemental insulin to order [45]. The patient's total daily insulin dose divided into 1800 provides the estimated mg/dL fall in glucose with 1 unit of insulin. For example, if a patient is receiving 60 units of insulin daily, 1 unit of insulin would be estimated to lower blood glucose (1800/60) 30 mg/dL. Supplemental insulin is given at mealtime, in addition to standing prandial insulin doses. To help prevent nocturnal hypoglycemia, supplemental insulin should be administered at a reduced dose at bedtime. Glucose goals of 100 mg/dL premeal and 140 mg/dL at bedtime should be targeted when correcting hyperglycemia in the hospital. Rapid-acting insulin analogs are generally preferred to regular insulin, given their lower risk for insulin stacking and hypoglycemia [35].

The use of a multifaceted subcutaneous insulin protocol has been shown to improve inpatient glycemic control. Desantis and colleagues [44] used an insulin protocol with basal, bolus, and supplemental insulins in patients with diabetes on surgical wards. When compared with historical glycemic control on the same surgical services, mean blood glucose was reduced from 163 ± 68 mg/dL to 146 ± 56 mg/dL, with glucose levels of less than 60 mg/dL in only 1.3% versus 1.4% of glucose measurements.

As inpatient insulin orders become more complex, the potential for medication errors increases. Intensive insulin therapy requires both ongoing staff education, and precise written orders. Preprinted order sets prompting physicians to consider basal, bolus, or correctional insulin have been published by a number of centers [38,42,46–48]. Order sets generally include low-, medium-, and high-dose correctional insulin options. Studies suggest that standardized order forms significantly reduce medication errors, and prompt providers to consider insulin choices more carefully. The University of Maryland inpatient order form has been well received by the physician and nursing staff (Fig. 1).

Standardized protocols for the treatment and prevention of hypoglycemia have also been published [42,49,50]. Their routine use is recommended by both the ADA and ACE [6]. It should be noted that many inpatient hypoglycemic episodes are preceded by events such as nausea/vomiting, steroid dose reduction, change in diet, change or interruption of tube feed administration, sepsis, worsening renal function, and altered levels of consciousness [35]. Providers should be proactive in adjusting insulin downwards in such settings.

Intravenous insulin therapy

Intravenous insulin therapy is recommended in a number of acute clinical settings to achieve rapid glycemic control. Such conditions include hyperglycemic emergencies such as diabetic ketoacidosis (DKA) and hyperglycemic hyperosmolic syndrome, myocardial infarction, stroke, intensive care units, type 1 diabetes patients having surgery, prolonged fasting in an insulin-deficient patient, labor and delivery, and when marked hyperglycemia accompanies glucocorticoid therapy [7,51]. In these settings it is recommended that clinicians use an IV insulin protocol that is effective at keeping glucose levels in the target range and allows for easy titration of insulin dosages [7,47]. A number of IV insulin algorithms have now been published with documentation of successful clinical outcomes. Several of these, however, including the ICU protocol of Catholic University of Leuvin, Belgium, are fairly complex and associated with higher rates of hypoglycemia [9,33]. The Portland protocol has been shown to be effective and safe in the perioperative period in thoracic surgery patients [27]. The Stanford Hospital protocol was used successfully in a mixed medical/surgical intensive care unit [28]. The Northwestern University IV insulin protocol used a target glucose range of 80 to 110 mg/dL, and led to rapid achievement of the glycemic target (10.6 ± 5.2 hours on average), successful glycemic control (mean capillary glucose of 135 ± 50 mg/dL), and low rates of hypoglycemia (blood glucose levels of ≤ 60 mg/dL in 1.5% of glucose readings) [44].

University of Maryland Medical Center

Diabetes Preprinted Orders

PLEASE NOTE: It is required that the Prescriber's signature is provided on **each** Order. For multiple Orders in one Order session. it is required that the Prescriber's printed name, pager number, and ID # are provided on the first Order of each page of multiple Orders At end of Ordering session, "X-out" Rx boxes not used.

WEIGHT		HEIGHT		ALLERGY		

IMPRINT ORDER SHEET WITH PATIENT S ID PLATE BEFORE USING

MEDICATION AND I.V. FLUID ORDERS

Rx1   Check if ☐ TRANSFER ☐ ADMIT ☐ POST OP | ☐ VERBAL ORDER/Read Back Complete

NURSE'S SIGNATURE

MEDICATION OR FLUID (Generic Name)	DOSE OR AMT	ROUTE	FREQUENCY	INDICATION (Required for PRN or Range Order)
Basal Insulin				Hyperglycemia/Diabetes
☐ Glargine (Lantus)	_____ units	subcut	☐ before breakfast	
☐ NPH	_____ units		☐ before dinner	
	_____ units		☐ before bedtime	

DATE	TIME	PRESCRIBER'S PRINTED NAME	PRESCRIBER'S SIGNATURE	PRESCRIBER'S ID#	PRESCRIBER'S PAGER#

Rx2   Check if ☐ TRANSFER ☐ ADMIT ☐ POST OP | ☐ VERBAL ORDER/Read Back Complete

NURSE'S SIGNATURE

MEDICATION OR FLUID (Generic Name)	DOSE OR AMT	ROUTE	FREQUENCY	INDICATION (Required for PRN or Range Order)
Prandial Insulin				Hyperglycemia/Diabetes
☐ Aspart (Novolog)	_____ units	subcut	☐ before breakfast	
	_____ units		☐ before lunch	
☐ Regular	_____ units		☐ before dinner	

☐ Give Aspart (Novolog) insulin when meal tray is delivered to patient

☐ Give Regular insulin 30 minutes prior to meal tray being delivered to patient.

DATE	TIME	PRESCRIBER'S PRINTED NAME	PRESCRIBER'S SIGNATURE	PRESCRIBER'S ID#	PRESCRIBER'S PAGER#

Rx3   Check if ☐ TRANSFER ☐ ADMIT ☐ POST OP | ☐ VERBAL ORDER/Read Back Complete

NURSE'S SIGNATURE

MEDICATION OR FLUID (Generic Name)	DOSE OR AMT	ROUTE	FREQUENCY	INDICATION (Required for PRN or Range Order)
Correction Insulin				Hyperglycemia/Diabetes
☐ Aspart (Novolog)		subcut	☐ before breakfast	
☐ Regular			☐ before lunch	
Blood sugar			☐ before dinner	
☐ Low dose				
150-199	1 unit			
200-249	2 units			
250-299	3 units			
300-349	4 units			
>350	5 units			
☐ Medium dose				
150-199	1 unit			
200-249	3 units			
250-299	5 units			
300-349	7 units			
>350	8 units			
☐ High dose				
150-199	2 units			
200-249	4 units			
250-299	7 units			
300-349	10 units			
>350	12 units			
☐ Individual				
150-199	_____ units			
200-249	_____ units			
250-299	_____ units			
300-349	_____ units			
>350	_____ units			

☐ When patient is NPO for a procedure, hold Prandial and Correction Insulin, and:
♦ Give 80% of dose of Glargine.
♦ Give half of morning NPH dose

☐ BS<70 mg/dL
♦ If patient awake and able to take P.O., give 15 gms of carbohydrate (3 glucose tablets OR 4 oz. (1/2 cup) fruit juice OR 6 oz regular soda OR 1 cup low fat milk).
♦ If patient not alert or cannot take P O , give 25 ml D50W, IV Push
♦ Recheck glucose q 15 min until BG>80 mg/dL
♦ Repeat 15 gms of carbohydrate P O. or 25 ml D50 IV Push q 15 min until glucose level is >70 mg/dL

Call House Officer for BS<70 mg/dL or BS>350 mg/dL

DATE	TIME	PRESCRIBER'S PRINTED NAME	PRESCRIBER'S SIGNATURE	PRESCRIBER'S ID#	PRESCRIBER S PAGER#

NON-MEDICATION ORDERS

For ordering physician consults and for procedure/tests not yet available through PowerChart. For all other Orders, please use PowerChart.

DATE	TIME	Non-Medication Orders	Prescriber's Signature	Prescriber's Pager #	Prescriber's ID #	Nurse's Signature

Go to diabetes order form in PowerChart to complete non-medication diabetes orders.

PO9B (rev. 01/06)

Fig. 1. University of Maryland diabetes order form. (*Courtesy of* University of Maryland Medical Center, Baltimore, MD; with permission.)

It is recommended that IV insulin be continued until patients are medically stable and tolerating oral nutrition. A bolus dose of insulin should be given when patients are started back on meals while still on IV insulin therapy to avoid increases in insulin drip rates in response to post prandial glucose elevations. When patients are stable for the transition to subcutaneous insulin, the insulin regimen should meet both basal and prandial insulin needs. The 24-hour basal insulin requirements in patients not requiring IV dextrose can be estimated by calculating the amount of IV insulin infused for a 6- to 8-hour period when the patient was not eating, typically overnight. Insulin glargine can be administered at 80% of that 24-hour total as a daily injection [51]. Rapid-acting prandial insulin can then be added as needed to control postprandial hyperglycemia. There is little data available to guide the conversion of patients receiving both IV insulin and IV dextrose to subcutaneous insulin. At the University of Maryland, when both IV insulin and dextrose are to be discontinued, we have successfully used 60% of the calculated 24-hour basal insulin requirement as the daily insulin glargine dose. Because IV insulin has a half-life of only several minutes, it should not be discontinued until subcutaneous insulin has been initiated to prevent recurrent hyperglycemia, or ketoacidosis in type 1 diabetes patients. Intravenous insulin can be safely discontinued 1 hour after the administration of short- or rapid-acting insulins, and 2 hours after the administration of intermediate- or long-acting insulins (Box 1).

Glucocorticoid therapy

Glucocorticoids are commonly used in the inpatient setting, and are well known to complicate diabetes management. While there are no randomized trials comparing treatment strategies for steroid-induced hyperglycemia, insulin is recommended in the acute setting [7,41]. Steroids induce hyperglycemia by stimulating hepatic gluconeogenesis, and by inducing peripheral insulin resistance and diminished insulin secretion [52]. The degree of steroid-induced hyperglycemia varies significantly among individual patients, making insulin requirements difficult to predict. Because they can be rapidly titrated, intravenous insulin infusions are ideal for patients receiving pulse steroid therapy, or as an initial dose-finding strategy in patients who develop marked hyperglycemia [7,53]. In milder cases of steroid-induced hyperglycemia, subcutaneous therapy may first be targeted at preventing postprandial hyperglycemia, which is the dominant glucocorticoid effect [52]. Premeal rapid-acting insulin will effectively control hyperglycemia in these patients. Basal insulin may be required in patients with diabetes before the initiation of glucocorticoids, or in those requiring multiple high doses of rapid-acting insulin. A basal/prandial insulin ratio of 30/70% of the total daily dose has been recommended in these patients [53]. Patients receiving a single daily dose of prednisone may respond best to once-daily NPH (with supplemental

---

Box 1. Transitioning patients from IV to SQ insulin

Example 1

A 76-kg type 2 diabetic man was placed on an insulin drip during a medical ICU admission for sepsis. He is now ready for transfer to the floor. A 5% dextrose in normal saline solution (D5NS) was stopped after he tolerated eating well the night before. Insulin drip requirements were initially variable, but became stable at 2 units/hour overnight while fasting.

Question: How should he be transitioned to subcutaneous insulin?

Answer: The patient's fasting drip rate is stable at 2 units per hour. Over 24 hours, this is a 48-unit basal insulin requirement. To limit hypoglycemia, 80% (38 units) of this dose can be given as subcutaneous insulin glargine. The insulin drip needs to be continued for 2 hours following injection of the long-acting insulin. Rapid-acting insulins can be added premeal as needed to control postprandial hyperglycemia.

Example 2

An insulin-requiring 82-kg type 2 diabetic woman was started on IV insulin and D5 1/2NS after an appendectomy. Her blood sugars were well controlled overnight on an insulin drip at 2 units/hour and she has been cleared to begin eating. Her IV insulin and IV fluids will be discontinued today.

Question: How should she be transitioned to subcutaneous insulin?

Answer: As her IV fluids contain 50 g of glucose/liter, her insulin requirements will be less after fluids are stopped. Her calculated basal insulin requirement is 48 units. To limit hypoglycemia after the IV glucose infusion is discontinued, 60% (29 units) of this dose can be given as insulin glargine 2 hours before stopping the insulin drip. Rapid-acting insulins can be added premeal as needed to control postprandial hyperglycemia.

---

mealtime coverage as needed). When given at the same time, NPH and prednisone have opposing peak and trough effects on blood glucose levels [41]. After choosing any insulin regimen it is important to follow frequent finger stick glucose levels and reevaluate regimens regularly. The need for proactive dose reductions must be anticipated in patients on steroid tapers. Thiazolidinediones may be a helpful adjunct for patients who will require longer-term steroid therapy after discharge [54,55]. Their use in the acute setting is limited by their delayed onset of action (2 to 3 weeks).

Enteral feeding

Tube feeds are well known to induce hyperglycemia and complicate its management in the inpatient setting. Carbohydrate contents are high in most formulas, and enteral feedings are given according to a variety of schedules. Bolus, nocturnal, and continuous feeding regimens are all used, but unscheduled interruptions are common in the inpatient setting. There are no available outcome data comparing different insulin strategies in enterally fed patients. However, a number of centers have published recommendations based on expert opinion. Subcutaneous insulin requirements can be estimated from the number of units of IV insulin needed over a 24-hour period. Basal insulin can also be initiated and dosages adjusted based on supplemental insulin requirements. Patients receiving bolus feeds can usually be managed using a modified basal/prandial protocol, with the prandial insulin dosage starting at 1 unit of rapid-acting insulin for each 10 g carbohydrate. Dosage adjustments are made based on the 2-hour post-bolus glucose level [7]. Nocturnal tube feedings can be covered by NPH insulin. Because of the delayed onset of action of NPH, many patients need to have a short-acting insulin added to control sugars during the first several hours of a nocturnal feeding. For patients receiving continuous tube feeds, 70/30 (NPH/Reg) or NPH insulin preparations administered every 8 hours have been advocated [7,41]. These regimens provide fairly stable insulin levels over a 24-hour period, and allow for doses to be adjusted, or held at several points during the day if feedings are interrupted. Twice-daily glargine doses have also been used in this setting [7,38,56]. To avoid prolonged hypoglycemia when enteral feedings are interrupted on high-dose glargine monotherapy, a reduced glargine dose can be used in conjunction with every 4- to 6-hour short-acting insulins. Finger stick glucose levels should be monitored more frequently in patients who have had enteral feedings interrupted, and intravenous dextrose containing solutions should be infused until the last insulin dose has cleared.

Total parenteral nutrition

The use of total parenteral nutrition (TPN) may double a patient's insulin requirement. This is because of both its high carbohydrate content, and because IV nutrition bypasses intestinal regulators of glucose metabolism such as glucose-dependent insulinotropic polypeptide (GIP) and GLP-1. Among patients with diabetes not previously on insulin, 77% required insulin therapy to maintain glycemic control at a mean dose of 100 units/day [57]. No randomized trials have compared insulin therapies in patients receiving TPN. One commonly used strategy is to add regular insulin to the TPN bag, typically at 1 unit/10 g of infused carbohydrate [41]. This ensures that insulin is held when TPN is stopped, but only allows for insulin dosage adjustments on a daily basis. A more rapid dosage-finding strategy calls for the use of intravenous insulin for the first 24 hours, especially in very poorly controlled patients [7]. Alternatively, subcutaneous basal or 70/30 insulin may be used to supplement the insulin in the TPN bag to more rapidly titrate the insulin dose [38,41].

Patient self-management

Inpatient diabetes management can be especially frustrating for knowledgeable patients who successfully practice intensive diabetes self-management in the outpatient setting. This group largely consists of motivated, type 1 diabetes patients, many of whom employ carbohydrate counting to determine prandial insulin doses. Handing over insulin-dosage decisions to an often less well-educated hospital staff can be worrisome, and occasionally dangerous for such patients. Allowing competent adult patients to practice diabetes self-management in the inpatient setting may be appropriate in stable settings. Clement and colleagues [7] and the ADA [35] have published guidelines for these situations. Patients should be alert, physically able to inject insulin or alter pump settings, and able to demonstrate proficiency in carbohydrate counting, meal dosing, and trouble-shooting skills. The patient, physician, and nursing staff should agree that self-management is appropriate, and physicians should be available to provide assistance when needed. All glucose-monitoring results and insulin dosages given by the patient should be documented in the medical record. Orders to allow patient self-management should be written by a physician, and all members of the team should recognize that provider-directed care may need to be implemented if the patient's clinical condition changes.

Discharge planning

Diabetes treatment regimens and patient education goals should be reviewed as a part of routine discharge planning. If no results over the preceding 2 to 3 months are readily available, hemoglobin A1c (HbA1c) values should be obtained before discharge. These values can help determine whether elevated glucose levels seen in the inpatient setting are a result of longstanding, uncontrolled diabetes, or to the acute stress of the hospitalization. An HbA1c higher than 6% on admission was found to be 100% specific and 57% sensitive in the diagnosis of diabetes [58]. An HbA1c of less than 5.2% excluded diabetes in the same study. However, since an HbA1c level cannot diagnose diabetes, a diagnostic outpatient oral glucose tolerance test is recommended for patients with hyperglycemia during their hospitalization if their inpatient HbA1c is 5.2% or higher. Patients with preexisting diabetes and HbA1c values significantly higher than 7.0% should have their outpatient treatment regimens reevaluated. Patients requiring high doses of insulin (>20 units) before discharge should be discharged on insulin. Thereafter, home glucose monitoring and close outpatient follow-up are needed to facilitate insulin dosage titration as the acute illness resolves. When determining an outpatient diabetes regimen, a patient's resources, social supports, disease insight, and self-management skills need to be considered [6]. Patients should receive specific "survival skill" education regarding medication use, glucose monitoring, and hypoglycemia management. Plans for outpatient follow-up should be confirmed, with referral to a certified diabetes educator for newly diagnosed or poorly controlled patients, to supplement the inpatient education received.

Summary

Hyperglycemia is an increasingly common and often complex condition to manage in the inpatient setting. Numerous clinical trials have demonstrated associations between uncontrolled diabetes and poor clinical outcomes in a number of inpatient settings. It is no longer acceptable for clinicians to fall back on the highly flawed sliding insulin scale as sole therapy for hyperglycemic inpatients. Oral hypoglycemic agents are often contraindicated in the acute care setting. Insulin remains the treatment of choice for most hyperglycemic hospitalized patients and should be prescribed in a physiologic manner, employing basal and bolus insulin as dictated by the clinical setting. Similarly, insulin dosages should be chosen that account for individual patient characteristics that affect insulin sensitivity such as body weight, severity of underlying illness, feeding status, and organ dysfunction. Clinicians need to review bedside glucose readings on a daily basis and respond with insulin dose adjustments, to safely achieve targeted glucose levels. Intravenous insulin should be used liberally in the ICU setting where randomized studies have demonstrated improved outcomes, and as a dose-finding strategy when therapies such as high-dose glucocorticoids, enteral feeds, and TPN complicate glycemic control. Ongoing staff education is needed to ensure intensive inpatient insulin therapy is performed both safely and effectively. Additionally, a patient's diabetes regimen and education goals should be carefully reviewed at the time of discharge. Future studies are required to help better define optimal inpatient glycemic targets and treatment protocols, especially outside of the ICU setting.

References

[1] Cowie CC, Rust KF, Byrd-Holt DD, et al. Prevalence of diabetes and impaired fasting glucose in adults in the U.S. population: National Health and Nutrition Examination Survey 1999–2002. Diabetes Care 2006;29:1263–8.
[2] The Diabetes Control and Complications Trial Research Group. The effect of intensive treatment of diabetes on the development and progression of long-term complications in insulin-dependent diabetes mellitus. N Engl J Med 1993;329:977–86.

[3] Shichiri M, Kishikawa H, Ohkubo Y, et al. Long-term results of the Kumamoto Study on optimal diabetes control in type 2 diabetic patients. Diabetes Care 2000;23(Suppl 2): B21–9.

[4] U.K. Prospective Diabetes Study Group: intensive blood-glucose control with sulfonylureas or insulin compared with conventional treatment and risk of complications in patients with type 2 diabetes. Lancet 1998;352:837–53.

[5] The DCCT/EDIC Study Research Group. Intensive diabetes treatment and cardiovascular disease in patients with type 1 diabetes. N Engl J Med 2005;353:2643–53.

[6] ACE/ADA Task Force on Inpatient Diabetes. American College of Endocrinology and American Diabetes Association consensus statement on inpatient diabetes and glycemic control. Diabetes Care 2006;29:1955–62.

[7] Clement S, Braithwaite SS, Magee MF, et al. The American Diabetes Association Diabetes in Hospitals Writing Committee: management of diabetes and hyperglycemia in hospitals. Diabetes Care 2004;27:553–91.

[8] Garber AJ, Moghissi ES, Bransome ED Jr, et al. The American College of Endocrinology Task Force on Inpatient Diabetes Metabolic Control: American College of Endocrinology position statement on inpatient diabetes and metabolic control. Endocr Pract 2004;10(Suppl 2):4–9.

[9] Van den Berghe G, Wouters P, Weekers F, et al. Intensive insulin therapy in the critically ill patients. N Engl J Med 2001;345:1359–67.

[10] Malmberg K. Prospective randomized study of intensive insulin treatment on long-term survival after acute myocardial infarction in patients with diabetes mellitus. DIGAMI (Diabetes Mellitus, Insulin Glucose Infusion in Acute Myocardial Infarction) Study Group. BMJ 1997;314:1512–5.

[11] Furnary AP, Gao G, Grunkemeier GL, et al. Continuous insulin infusion reduces mortality in patients with diabetes undergoing coronary artery bypass grafting. J Thorac Cardiovasc Surg 2003;125:1007–21.

[12] Levetan CS, Passaro M, Jablonski K, et al. Unrecognized diabetes among hospitalized patients. Diabetes Care 1998;21:246–9.

[13] Umpierrez GE, Isaacs SD, Bazargan N, et al. Hyperglycemia: an independent marker of in-hospital mortality in patients with undiagnosed diabetes. J Clin Endocrinol Metab 2002;87:978–82.

[14] Hogan P, Dall T, Nikolov P, et al. Economic costs of diabetes in the US in 2002. Diabetes Care 2003;26:917–32.

[15] Wexler DJ, Meigs JB, Cagliero E, et al. Prevalence of hyper- and hypoglycemia among inpatients with diabetes. Diabetes Care 2007;30(2):367–8.

[16] Bagdade JD, Steward M, Walters E. Impaired leukocyte function in patients with poorly controlled diabetes. Diabetes 1978;27:677–81.

[17] Alexiewicz J, Kumar D, Smogorzewski M, et al. Polymorphonuclear leukocytes in non-insulin dependent diabetes mellitus: abnormalities in metabolism and function. Ann Intern Med 1995;123:919–24.

[18] Repine JE, Clawson CC, Goetz FC. Bactericidal function of neutrophils from patients with acute bacterial infections and from diabetics. J Infect Dis 1980;142:869.

[19] Ortmeyer J, Mohsenin V. Inhibition of phospholipase D and superoxide generation by glucose in diabetic neutrophils. Life Sci 1996;59:255–62.

[20] Von Kanel R, Mills P, Dimsdale J. Short-term hyperglycemia induces lymphopenia and lymphocyte subset redistribution. Life Sci 2001;69:225–62.

[21] Bouter KP, Meyling FH, Hoekstra JB, et al. Influence of blood glucose levels on peripheral lymphocytes in patients with diabetes mellitus. Diabetes Res Clin Pract 1992;19:77–80.

[22] Morohoshi M, Fujisawa K, Uchimura I, et al. Glucose-dependent interleukin 6 and tumor necrosis factor production by human peripheral blood monocytes in vitro. Diabetes 1996;45: 954–9.

[23] Pandolfi A, Giaccari A, Cilli C, et al. Acute hyperglycemia and acute hyperinsulinemia decrease plasma fibrinolytic activity and increase plaminogen activator inhibitor type 1 in the rat. Acta Diabetol 2001;38:71–7.

[24] Knobler H, Savion N, Shenkman B, et al. Shear-induced platelet adhesion and aggregation on subendothelium are increased in diabetic patients. Thromb Res 1998;90:181–90.

[25] Giugliano D, Marfella R, Coppola L, et al. Vascular effects of acute hyperglycemia in humans are reversed by L-arginine: evidence for reduced availability of nitric oxide during hyperglycemia. Circulation 1997;95:1783–90.

[26] Estrada CA, Young JA, Nifong LW, et al. Outcomes and perioperative hyperglycemia in patients with or without diabetes mellitus undergoing coronary artery bypass grafting. Ann Thorac Surg 2003;75:1392–9.

[27] Furnary AP, Wu Y, Bookin SO. Effect of hyperglycemia and continuous intravenous insulin infusions on outcomes of cardiac surgical procedures: the Portland Diabetic Project. Endocr Pract 2004;10(Suppl 2):21–33.

[28] Krinsley JS. Effect of intensive glucose management protocol on the mortality of critically ill adult patients. Mayo Clin Proc 2004;79:992–1000.

[29] Van den Berghe G, Wouters PJ, Bouillon R, et al. Outcome benefit of intensive insulin therapy in the critically ill: insulin dose versus glycemic control. Crit Care Med 2003;31:359–66.

[30] Zerr KJ, Furnary AP, Grunkemeier GL, et al. Glucose control lowers the risk of wound infection in diabetics after open heart operations. Ann Thorac Surg 1997;63:356–61.

[31] Bolk J, van der Ploeg T, Cornel JH, et al. Impaired glucose metabolism predicts mortality after a myocardial infarction. Int J Cardiol 2001;79:207–14.

[32] Parsons MW, Barber A, Desmond PM, et al. Acute hyperglycemia adversely affects stroke outcome: A magnetic resonance imaging and spectroscopy study. Ann Neurol 2002;52(1):20–8.

[33] Van den Berghe G, Wilmer A, Hermans G, et al. Intensive insulin therapy in the medical ICU. N Engl J Med 2006;354:449–61.

[34] Inzucchi SE. Management of hyperglycemia in the hospital setting. N Engl J Med 2006;355:1903–11.

[35] American Diabetes Association. Standards of medical care in diabetes. Diabetes Care 2007;30(Suppl 1):S27–31.

[36] Queale WS, Siedler AJ, Brancati FL. Glycemic control and sliding scan insulin use in medical inpatients with diabetes mellitus. Arch Intern Med 1997;157:545–52.

[37] Gearhart JG, Duncan JL 3rd, Replogle WH, et al. Efficacy of sliding-scale insulin therapy: a comparison with prospective regimens. Fam Pract Res J 1994;14:313–22.

[38] Hirsch IB, Braithwaite SS, Verderese CA. Practical management of inpatient hyperglycemia. Lakeville (CT): Hilliard Publishing LLC; 2005.

[39] Miller C, Phillips L, Ziemer D, et al. Hypoglycemia in patients with type 2 diabetes. Arch Intern Med 2001;161:1653–9.

[40] Drucker DJ. Enhancing incretin action for the treatment of type 2 diabetes. Diabetes Care 2003;26:2929–40.

[41] Leahy JL. Insulin management of diabetic patients on general medical and surgical floors. Endocr Pract 2006;12(Suppl 3):86–90.

[42] Moghissi ES, Hirsch IB. Hospital management of diabetes. Endocrinol Metab Clin North Am 2005;34:99–116.

[43] Abourizk N, Vora C, Verma P. Inpatient diabetology: the new frontier. J Gen Intern Med 2004;19:466–71.

[44] DeSantis AJ, Schmeltz LR, Schmidt K, et al. Inpatient management of hyperglycemia: the Northwestern experience. Endocr Pract 2006;12:491–505.

[45] Walsh J, Roberts R, Bailey T, et al. Using insulin: everything you need to know for success with insulin. San Diego (CA): Torrey Pines press; 2003.

[46] Markovitz L, Wiechmann R, Harris N, et al. Description and evaluation of a glycemic management protocol for diabetic patients undergoing heart surgery. Endocr Pract 2002;8:10–8.

[47] Moghissi E. Inpatient diabetes. Cleve Clin J Med 2004;71:801–8.

[48] Quevedo SF, Sullivan E, Kington R, et al. Improving diabetes care in the hospital using guideline-directed orders. Diabetes Spectrum 2001;14:226–33.

[49] Donaldson S, Villanuueva G, Rondinelli L, et al. Rush University guidelines and protocols for the management of hyperglycemia in hospitalized patients. Elimination of the sliding scale and improvement of glycemic control throughout the hospital. Diabetes Educ 2006; 32(6):954–62.

[50] Tomky D. Detection, prevention, and treatment of hypoglycemia in the hospital. Diabetes Spectrum 2005;18:39–44.

[51] Bode BW, Braithwaite SS, Steed RD, et al. Intravenous insulin infusion therapy: indications, methods, and transition to subcutaneous insulin. Endocr Pract 2004;10(Suppl 2):71–80.

[52] Trence D. Management of patients on chronic glucocorticoid therapy: an endocrine perspective. Primary Care: Clinics in Office Practice 2003;30:593–605.

[53] Hirsch IB, Paauw DS. Diabetes management in special situations. Endocrinol Metab Clin North Am 1997;26(3):631–45.

[54] Luther P, Baldwin D. Pioglitazone in the management of diabetes mellitus after transplantation. Am J Transplant 2004;4:2135–8.

[55] Willis SM, Kennedy A, Brant BP, et al. Effective use of thiazolidinediones for the treatment of glucocorticoid-induced diabetes. Diabetes Res Clin Pract 2002;58:87–96.

[56] Putz D, Kabadi UM. Insulin glargine in continuous enteric tube feeding. Diabetes Care 2002;25:1889–90.

[57] Park RH, Hansell DT, Davidson LE, et al. Management of diabetic patients requiring nutritional support. Nutrition 1992;8:316–20.

[58] Greci LS, Kailasam M, Malkani S, et al. Utility of HbA1c levels for diabetes case finding in hospitalized patients with hyperglycemia. Diabetes Care 2003;26:1064–8.

ELSEVIER
SAUNDERS

Med Clin N Am 92 (2008) 427–441

THE MEDICAL
CLINICS
OF NORTH AMERICA

Infectious Disease Emergencies

Nelson Nicolasora, MD[a], Daniel R. Kaul, MD[b],*

[a]Division of Infectious Disease, University of Michigan Medical School,
3120 Taubman Center 0378, Ann Arbor, MI 48109-0378, USA
[b]Transplant Infectious Disease Service, Division of Infectious Disease, University of Michigan
Medical Center, 3120 Taubman Center 0378, Ann Arbor, MI 48109-0378, USA

The severity of an infectious disease is largely determined by how the host responds to the virulence factors of the invading pathogen. Occasionally, this interaction (especially in immunocompromised patients) results in severe sepsis, septic shock, or its complications, which accounts for the majority of deaths attributable to infectious diseases in the developed world. Alternatively, local complications determine host survival (Table 1). The host–pathogen interaction and general principles of management of life-threatening infections are highlighted in Fig. 1.

In certain clinical situations (eg, severe sepsis, meningitis), rapid initiation of appropriate antibiotic therapy is a critical determinant of survival. In other diseases, "source control" (eg, debridement of infected tissue in necrotizing fasciitis) is urgently required. This article reviews principles of recognition and management of a selection of commonly encountered infectious disease emergencies, including sepsis, necrotizing soft tissue infections, acute meningitis, and the emerging issue of severe *Clostridium difficile* colitis. Less common but potentially deadly environmentally acquired or zoonotic pathogens are discussed, as are special patient populations, including the febrile returning traveler and the asplenic patient.

Sepsis

Sepsis, severe sepsis, and septic shock as defined by the consensus panel of the American College of Chest Physicians and the Society of Critical Care Medicine are outlined in Table 2 [1]. Classification of the spectrum of sepsis in a patient can be done with initial focused evaluation using the patient's vital signs and a minimal set of laboratory examinations with attention

* Corresponding author.
E-mail address: kauld@umich.edu (D.R. Kaul).

0025-7125/08/$ - see front matter © 2008 Elsevier Inc. All rights reserved.
doi:10.1016/j.mcna.2007.10.006   *medical.theclinics.com*

Table 1
Potential terminal events of an infectious process

Infectious process	Terminal event
Systemic disease with (eg, gram-negative bacteremia) or without bacteremia (eg, toxic shock syndrome, severe *C difficile* colitis)	Severe sepsis, septic shock, and its complications: acute respiratory distress syndrome, disseminated intravascular coagulation, multisystem organ dysfunction syndrome
Local effects	
Severe encephalitis or brain abscess	Brain herniation
Endocarditis	Severe congestive heart failure from valvular dysfunction or arrhythmia from conduction system involvement
Local toxin effects	Myocarditis and cardiogenic shock from diphtheria or respiratory failure from tetanus
TB cavitary disease or pulmonary aspergilloma	Asphyxiation from severe pulmonary hemorrhage
Severe epiglottis or diphtheritic membranes	Asphyxiation and upper airway obstruction
Typhoid ileitis	Peritonitis, shock, and hemorrhage from perforation

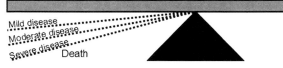

(A) INFECTIOUS AGENT(S):
toxins & other virulence factors

(B) HOST DEFENSES:
Natural barriers, humoral & cell-mediated immunity

+

+

(C) UNFAVORABLE HOST FACTORS
Increasing age
Breakdown of barriers
Acquired immunodeficiency syndrome
Diabetes mellitus
Cancer
Asplenia
End-organ disease
Neutropenia, lymphopenia
Chemotherapy, steroids & other immunosuppressive agents.

(D) MANAGEMENT
Resuscitative and supportive measures
Appropriate and timely antibiotics
Targeted diagnostics
Closer montioring (triaging)
Source control or anatomic repair: surgery, interventional radiology, etc.
Reduction of immunosuppression
Adjunctive medical therapy (e.g IVIG, activated protein C, etc.)

Mild disease
Moderate disease
Severe disease
Death

Health

Fig. 1. Diagramatic scheme showing interaction between (*A*) infectious agent (*B*) host defenses. In some instances, the virulence of the infecting agent coupled with (*C*) unfavorable host factors can overwhelm host defenses leading to severe disease. (*D*) General principles of disease management of infectious disease should be applied to restore health. IVIG, intravenous immunoglobulin.

Table 2
A summary of information needed during initial evaluation to classify severity of infection

	Clinical findings	
Vital signs	Temperature: > 38.4°C (100.4°F) or < 36°C (96.8°F)	Systolic blood pressure < 90 mm Hg or MAP < 70 mm Hg for at least 1 h despite adequate volume resuscitation, or the use of vasopressors to achieve the same goals
	Heart rate: > 90 beats/min	
	Respiratory rate: > 20 breaths/ min or Pa_{CO2} of < 32 mm Hg	
Abnormal labs	WBC: > 12,000/mm^3 or < 4000/mm^3 or > 10% immature neutrophils	

Sepsis: documented or suspected infection with two or more vital signs or laboratory criteria. Severe sepsis: sepsis with evidence of organ dysfunction. Septic shock: sepsis with persistent hypotension despite one hour of fluid resuscitation or use of vasopressors.

for signs of end-organ dysfunction (eg, mental status changes, and decreased urine output). As patients progress from sepsis to severe sepsis and septic shock, their prognosis worsens, and the need for urgent intervention and a higher level of care (eg, transfer to intensive care unit) increases. Patients who meet these criteria are a major challenge; a great variety of infectious agents may be responsible, and noninfectious etiologies (eg, pulmonary embolism, acute myocardial infarction, thrombotic thrombocytopenic purpura, and high-grade lymphoma) may mimic sepsis. In cases in which the cause is not immediately obvious, the clinical history needs to include comorbidities, travel and exposure history, previous microbial colonization or infection, immunosuppression, and recent hospitalization. Standard tests include a complete blood count, metabolic profile, chest radiography, electrocardiography, blood cultures (before antibiotics if possible), and an arterial blood gas in critical patients. Additional testing (eg, lumbar puncture, CT of the abdomen, and serologies for various infectious agents) is often necessary as directed by the clinical history and examination.

Adjunctive measures are a crucial aspect in the management of patients who have severe sepsis. Aggressive fluid resuscitation and vasopressors (eg, dopamine or norepinephrine) are generally indicated if the patient has refractory hypotension. Drotrecogen alpha (activated) has been demonstrated to reduce the risk of death of patients in who have severe sepsis [2]. This drug should be avoided in patients who have single-organ dysfunction or who are at high risk for catastrophic bleeding (eg, recent neurosurgery, thrombocytopenia). Achieving euglycemia with blood glucose levels less than 150 mg/dL (8.3 mmol/L) also improves outcome. Source control (ie, removal of the focus of infection) with the aid of surgery, interventional radiology, and other subspecialties should be an early priority.

A rational approach to empiric antimicrobial therapy forms a cornerstone in the management of these life-threatening infections. It is well established that delayed or microbiologically inadequate antibiotic therapy (ie, treatment with antibiotics to which the pathogen was later shown to be resistant) is associated with a worse outcome [3,4]. The choice of empiric antibiotics is complex, and a variety of factors, including drug allergy, drug–drug interactions, potential side effects, and ability to penetrate a particular site of infection, need to be considered. For community-acquired infections, resistant gram-negative rods (eg, *Pseudomonas aeruginosa*) generally do not have to be covered. Because of the increasing prevalence of community-acquired methicillin-resistant *Staphylococcus aureus* (MRSA) infections extending beyond obvious skin and soft tissue infections, vancomycin is reasonable pending further culture information [5]. If an intra-abdominal source is suspected, anaerobic coverage is required. For severe health care–associated or hospital-acquired infections, antimicrobial resistance is common, and empiric treatment has to be tailored according to institutional antibiotic resistance patterns, colonization history, likely site of infection, and previously used antimicrobials. Fig. 2 provides an overview of antibacterial spectrum of activity of commonly used drugs for critically ill patients who have hospital-acquired infections. In general, empiric treatment should cover

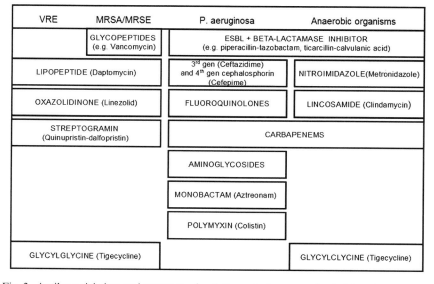

Fig. 2. Antibacterial class and spectrum of activity against common bacterial pathogens causing health care–associated infections. In general, empiric treatment of critically ill patients who have health care–associated infections requires treatment covering MRSA and *Pseudomonas aeruginosa*. Local institutional antibiotic resistant patterns, suspected site of infection, and patient history alter empiric antibiotic selection. Daptomycin is ineffective for pneumonia because it is inactivated by pulmonary surfactants. Aminoglycosides are rarely used alone except for urinary tract infections. The carbapenem ertapenem does not have reliable activity against *P aeruginosa*. Tigecycline has activity against most gram-negative organisms except *P aeruginosa*. ESBL, extended-spectrum beta lactams; VRE, vancomycin-resistant enterococcus; MRSA, methicillin-resistant *S aureus*; MRSE, methicillin-resistant *S epidermidis*.

MRSA and include a drug with activity against *P aeruginosa*. Coverage for vancomycin-resistant enterococcus may be warranted in patients who have a history of infection or colonization with this organism and severe sepsis.

The use of combination therapy for gram-negative infections is controversial; recent meta-analyses have not demonstrated a benefit, and no high-quality prospective study has been conducted using current antimicrobials in the population encountered in the modern hospital [6]. In addition, in patients who have fever and neutropenia, monotherapy with an extended spectrum beta lactam (eg, a carbapenem, antipseudomonal penicillin/beta-lactamase inhibitor, or third- or fourth-generation cephalosporin) is equivalent to or superior (ie, less toxicity) than combination therapy with two gram-negative agents (ie, addition of fluoroquinolone or aminoglycoside to beta-lactam) [7]. By increasing the "density" of antimicrobial use, gram-negative combination therapy promotes the development of antibiotic-resistant organisms and superinfection. In addition, increased risk of nephrotoxicity has been a consistent finding when aminoglycosides are used as one agent in combination therapy [8]. The most important issue is to determine that the spectrum of empiric coverage includes the gram-negative rods most commonly isolated in similar patients in the treating hospital; this relies on knowledge of local antimicrobial sensitivities. In some hospitals, this can generally be accomplished with one gram-negative agent. Once a pathogen has been identified, therapy should be narrowed. If combination therapy for gram-negative infection was initiated, one agent can usually be stopped when the patient improves.

Candida spp. are the fourth most common hospital blood stream isolate, and delay in initiation of appropriate therapy has been associated with increased mortality [9]. Thus, in patients who have severe sepsis and who are at high risk for candidemia (eg, a patient who has had recent abdominal surgery or who has a central venous catheter who becomes septic on broad-spectrum antibiotics), empiric treatment for *Candida spp.* with an azole (eg, fluconazole) or echinocandin (eg, anidulafungin, caspofungin, or micafungin) is appropriate. Patients who have extensive prior treatment with an azole (eg, fluconazole) should be empirically treated with echinocandins because of the risk of fluconazole-resistant candida species. Because of their toxicity, polyenes (ie, amphotericin products) are generally not used in this situation.

Special patient population—the asplenic patient

In the patient who does not have a spleen, certain organisms (eg, *Streptococcus pneumonia, Hemophilus influena, Neisseria meningitides,* or *Babesia microti*) may cause rapidly overwhelming infection with high mortality rates. In addition to patients who have congenital asplenia or who have had surgical removal of the spleen, so-called "functional asplenia" with similar risk may result from diseases such as sickle cell anemia or thalassemia. At the first sign of infection, prompt clinical evaluation, including blood cultures

and initiation of antibiotics with activity against encapsulated organisms
(eg, ceftriaxone), is indicated pending culture results. Asplenic patients
who are bitten by a dog or cat should also receive amoxicillin/clavulinic
acid or another antibiotic (eg, ceftriaxone) with activity against *Capnocyto-
phaga canimorsus*, which may cause purpura fulminans in this patient
population. Vaccination against *S pneumonia* and *H influenza* type B and
N meningitides (with the meningococcal vaccine, diphtheria conjugate) is indicated in patients who have asplenia or expected asplenia [10].

Skin and soft tissue infections

Skin and soft tissue infections are common indications for hospital admission. Cellulitis, which is infection of the superficial and subcutaneous layers of
the skin, may require close observation and intravenous antibiotics, but in
many patients can be treated as outpatients. Infections involving deeper
structures (ie, fascia or muscle) may be immediately life threatening. From
the point of view of the treating physician, the most important decision is
differentiating deeper necrotizing infections requiring urgent surgical intervention from more superficial cellulitis [11]. Clinical risk factors for deeper
or necrotizing soft tissue infections include trauma or abdominal surgery,
diabetes mellitus, alcoholism, and renal disease. The presence of purple or
red bullous lesions, pain on palpation over contiguous but superficially unaf-
fected areas, indistinct margins, crepitus, loss of sensation distal to the
affected area, and rapid progression suggest a deeper infection. Systemic toxicity (eg, renal failure, hypotension, and acidosis) can also be considered
a "warning sign" for a deeper or necrotizing infection, but it is often a late
finding. Other laboratory parameters that may help discriminate between
superficial and necrotizing soft tissue infections include C-reactive protein
greater than 150 mg/dL, white blood cell count greater than 15,000 cells/μl,
hemoglobin less than 13.5 g/dL, and sodium less than 135 mmol/L [12]. Plain
films may demonstrate gas in the soft tissues, and MRI or CT may reveal
abscess or evidence of enhancement, edema, or thickening in the fascia.
The lack of gas in the soft tissue does not exclude a diagnosis of a necrotizing
infection. The absence of abnormal findings in the fascia on MRI makes
necrotizing fasciitis less likely; its presence, however, may occur with simple
cellulitis. Rapid progression of the extent of the involved area or clinical
deterioration in uncertain cases suggests the need for surgical exploration.
Another option in ambiguous cases is biopsy or surgical exploration to determine if the fascia is involved because observation of the deeper soft tissue is
the only definitive method to make the diagnosis.

Management of deeper necrotizing infections of the skin and soft tissue
requires a combined medical and surgical approach, and repeated and sometimes extensive surgical debridement is often necessary. These infections
may be monomicrobial or polymicrobial, and this usually cannot be determined when the decision for initial antibiotic therapy is made. Thus, initial

therapy should include coverage of the most common pathogens (eg, beta hemolytic *streptococci*, *S aureus*, *E coli*, and *Clostridium perfringens*). Combination therapy with a beta-lactam/beta-lactamase inhibitor (eg, ampicillin-sulbactam or piperacillin-tazobactam) combined with clindamycin (to decrease toxin production) is recommended. Clindamycin may be stopped if toxin-producing bacteria (eg, beta hemolytic *streptococci* or *S aureus*) are not isolated. Patients who are allergic to penicillin may be treated with an aminoglycoside or fluoroquinolone in combination with clindamycin [13]. Community-associated MRSA has been described as a causative agent in necrotizing fasciitis (typically with more purulence and a more indolent course), and, given the increasing frequency of this pathogen in skin and soft tissue infections in general, many experts recommend the addition of vancomycin for unstable patients until culture data are available [14,15]. Intravenous immune globulin has been used in patients who have severe group A strep infections, but the efficacy of this treatment is unproven.

Special patient populations/pathogens

Although immunosuppressed patients are at increased risk of necrotizing soft tissue infections, the principles of diagnosis and management of skin and soft tissue infection outlined previously are not significantly different in most immunosuppressed patients. Some heavily immunosuppressed patients (eg, neutropenic patients) may develop cutaneous manifestations of systemic infections (eg, ecthyma gangrenosum), and empiric treatment should include coverage of *P aeruginosa*.

Skin and soft tissue infections in immunocompromised individuals warrant consideration of *Vibrio vulnificus*. *V vulnificus*, like other vibrios, is commonly found in warm estuarial and marine environments. Mortality as high as 50% in immunocompromised patients (including patients who have cirrhosis or hemochromatosis or patients who abuse alcohol) has been reported [16]. *V vulnificus* infection should be suspected in patients who give a history of ingestion of raw seafood or wound infection after exposure to seawater who later develop sepsis with associated hemorrhagic bullous skin lesions progressing to necrosis. *V vulnificus* grows without difficulty in standard blood culture media or on nonselective media (such as blood agar) routinely used for wound cultures. Preferred treatments include ceftazidime 2 g IV every 8 hours, ceftriaxone 1 g IV every 24 hours, or cefotaxime 2 g IV every 8 hours. Many experts combine any of these agents with doxycycline 100 mg IV or orally twice a day. Fluroquinolones are alternatives to cephalosphorins in cases of allergy [17].

Acute meningitis

Acute meningitis is a potentially life-threatening infection in which symptoms develop over hours to a few days. Rapid diagnosis, determination of etiology, and institution of therapy is essential to decrease mortality and morbidity. Typical signs and symptoms of acute bacterial meningitis may include severe headache, photophobia, fever, and stiff neck and may progress to delirium and seizure. Skin, conjunctiva, and mucous membranes should be examined closely for the petechial or ecchymotic lesions associated with *N menigitidis*. Pneumococcus may cause purpura fulminans, disseminated intravascular coagulation, widespread purpura, and gangrene of the extremities. In patients who have suggestive symptoms, lumbar puncture is required to make the diagnosis and identify the infectious cause.

Patients who have immunocompromised state, papilledema, change in mental status, focal neurological deficit, or a history of central nervous system disease are at greater risk for mass lesion, which may increase the risk of herniation at the time of lumbar puncture. Patients who do not have such risk factors should undergo urgent lumbar puncture followed by institution of antimicrobial therapy. Patients who have such risk factors should have a head CT before lumbar puncture is performed, but antimicrobial therapy should not be delayed [18].

Virtually all patients who have bacterial meningitis have cerebrospinal fluid (CSF) leukocytosis (ie, 100–10,000 cells/mm^3) with an elevated protein concentration and reduced glucose. If the patient has not recently received antibiotic therapy, cultures will be positive in about 75% of patients, and Gram stain of CSF will be positive in 60% to 90% of patients [18]. For patients who have negative Gram stains who have received previous antimicrobial therapy, latex agglutination tests for *S pneumonia*, *N meningitides*, and *H influenza* may be helpful in determining etiology. In patients who have suspected *N meningitides*, droplet precautions should be instituted until treatment has been administered for 48 hours. Close household or school contacts of a proven case of *N meningitides* should receive chemoprophylaxis with rifampin 600 mg twice a day for 2 days or a single 500-mg dose of ciprofloxacin. Most health care workers, unless they had close contact with the respiratory secretions of the source patient, do not require chemoprophylaxis.

Various laboratory or clinical parameters (eg, procalcitonin levels, c-reactive protein, and CSF formula findings) have been studied to differentiate aseptic meningitis due to "routine" viral pathogens from bacterial meningitis with negative Gram stains [19,20]. Although these methods require further validation and greater clinical availability, some institutions have ready availability of polymerase chain reaction (PCR) for enterovirus from the CSF. If results can be obtained rapidly, patients may be discharged and avoid unnecessary antibiotic therapy. Clinicians admit and observe many patients who have negative Gram stain pending the availability of culture results. In uncertain cases (particularly if antibiotic therapy was given before lumbar puncture or if the CSF formula or clinical picture is highly suggestive of bacterial meningitis), a full course of 10 to 14 days of therapy is administered.

In patients who have a negative Gram stain or who cannot immediately undergo lumbar puncture, empiric therapy should cover *S pneumonia*,

N meningitides, and *H influenza*; a third-generation cephalosporin (eg, ceftriaxone 2 g IV every 12 hours) is combined with vancomycin (15–20 mg/kg IV every 12 hours). The need for vancomycin is based on the increasing incidence of penicillin-resistant pneumococcus. Alternative agents for allergic patients include carbapenems and fluroquinolones. For patients at risk for *Listeria monocytogenes* (eg, immunosuppressed patients, patients > 50 years old, and patients who have malignancy), ampicillin (2 g IV every 4 hours) should be added. Patients who have had recent neurosurgical or other medical procedures involving structures contiguous to the central nervous system should be treated with a meropenem or cefepime in addition to vancomycin to treat hospital-acquired gram-negative organisms. Patients who have negative Gram stain and mental status changes or focal neurologic signs should be treated with acyclovir (10 mg/kg IV every 8 hours) for possible Herpes Simplex virus (HSV) meningoencephalitis. Temporal lobe hemorrhage, lymphocytic pleocytosis, and normal glucose are suggestive of HSV meningoencephalitis. A PCR for HSV DNA on the CSF is the diagnostic test of choice, and if negative, acyclovir can be usually be discontinued. After a pathogen has been identified, therapy can be narrowed. Aqueous penicillin G 24 million units daily is sufficient to treat penicillin-sensitive *S pneumonia*. The use of adjunctive corticosteroids to decrease morbidity and mortality has long been controversial; however, a recent randomized trial indicated a reduction in morbidity and mortality in adults who had pneumococcal meningitis treated with dexamethasone 10 mg IV every 6 hours for 4 days. The first dose must be given before or concurrent with the first dose of antimicrobials, and if *S pneumonia* is not isolated, the dexamethasone should be stopped [21].

Special patient populations/pathogens

Immunosuppression alters the differential diagnosis and presentation of meningitis or meningoencephalitis. In addition to the routine community-aquired pathogens discussed previously, additional viruses (eg, *Cytomegalovirus*, human Herpes virus 6), fungi (eg, *Cryptococcus neoformans*, endemic fungi), and bacteria (eg, *Nocardia spp.*) need to be considered. Immunosuppressed patients are much more likely to develop central nervous system disease if infected with West Nile virus. If no etiology is readily apparent on Gram stain of CSF, a cryptococcal antigen should be sent on CSF, and empiric treatment for *Listeria monocytogenes* is indicated. Infectious disease consultation is strongly recommended for immunosuppressed patients who have meningitis or menigoencephalitis.

Two neurologic illnesses worth discussing are rabies and botulism. Major animal reservoirs of the rabies virus are bats, raccoons, skunks, and foxes, with bats being the most common source in the United States [22]. After an average incubation period of 1 to 3 months, prodromal flu-like symptoms progress rapidly to hallucinations and delirium or ascending flaccid paralysis. The virus may be detected from the saliva, CSF, serum, or central nervous system tissue using reverse transcriptase PCR. Nuchal skin samples including at least 10 hair follicles/6 mm size can be sent to the CDC for direct fluorescent antibody testing. Once patients exhibit hydrophobia, paralysis, or signs of encephalitis, treatment is mostly supportive. A single case survived after drug-induced coma and treatment with ribavirin and amantidine [23]. This investigational protocol is available by contacting Dr. Rodney Willoughby at Children's Hospital of Wisconsin (414-266-2000).

Botulism results from neurotoxin produced by *Clostridium botulinum* and may be acquired from food (typically home canned) or an infected wound. Clinical symptoms generally include symmetric cranial neuropathies and descending paralysis without fever or significant sensory abnormalities [24]. Toxin assays may be conducted on food and clinical specimens by the CDC. Treatment consists of supportive measures and early (<24 hours after symptoms if possible) administration of specific antitoxin available from the CDC (404 639-2206). Wounds should be debrided. Although no evidence exists of its efficacy, some clinicians treat with aqueous penicillin G 20 million units daily.

C difficile enteritis

For many years, *C difficile* was generally considered a "nuisance pathogen" with relatively low morbidity and mortality [25]. In the past decade, hospitals throughout North America have reported severe outbreaks of *C difficile* colitis with increased numbers of cases, poor reponse to therapy, and severe disease with much higher rates of colectomy and death [25–27]. These outbreaks are due to a hypertoxin-producing strain that has acquired resistance to fluoroquinolones; this class of antibiotics has been implicated as a risk factor for acquiring *C difficile* colitis in the hospital setting [28]. Proton pump inhibitor use seems to be a risk factor in the inpatient and outpatient settings [29,30]. Severe cases, including deaths, have been reported in patients who have not had significant recent antibiotic use or health care environment exposure [31].

For the hospitalist, a high index of suspicion and awareness of local institutional *C difficile* rates are essential. Clinical clues suggestive of *C difficile* colitis as a cause of diarrhea in the antibiotic-treated patient include rapid increase in white blood cell count, recent episode of *C difficile* colitis, and thickened colon observed on CT of the abdomen. Although no randomized trial has been conducted, some studies have suggested poor response to metronidazole [25], and patients who have evidence of severe disease (eg, white blood cell count > 20,000 cell/μL, sepsis) should be treated with oral vancomycin (125–500 mg qid). Patients who have ileus may require gentle enemas with vancomycin, and the addition of intravenous metronidazole (500 mg every 6–8 hours), which has enterohepatic circulation, may be helpful. In severely ill patients, early surgical consultation is recommended.

Fever in the returning traveler

Fever in the returning traveler may be caused by "routine pathogens" (eg, community-acquired respiratory viruses, bacterial pneumonia, and Epstein-Barr virus) or more "exotic" pathogens that are less familiar to most clinicians in the developed world. An exhaustive review of this topic is beyond the scope of this article, and the differential diagnosis in an individual traveler depends on region of travel, specific exposures, and adherence to prescribed prophylactic regimens and pretravel vaccination. Physicians should concentrate initial diagnostic efforts on ruling out the most common potentially deadly infections: malaria, typhoid fever, and dengue. In one series of 6957 febrile travelers seeking care, malaria was found in 21%, dengue in 6%, and typhoid fever in 2% [32]. Because clinical syndromes associated with these three infections overlap, evaluation of febrile travelers (assuming exposure to areas where these diseases are endemic) should include blood smears for malaria, blood cultures for typhoid fever, and serologies for dengue. Treatment for malaria depends on the identified species and risk for resistance in the geographic area in which it is acquired. Possible regimens for *Plasmodium falciparum* (the most dangerous species) include quinine sulfate 10 mg/kg of the salt every 8 hours for 3 to 7 days combined with doxycycline 100 mg twice daily for 7 days. Typhoid fever is usually treated with 500 to 750 mg ciprofloxacin orally twice a day for 7 to 14 days; strains acquired in Asia may be resistant, and ceftriaxone 2 g IV daily or azithromycin 1 g orally followed by 500 mg daily are alternative treatments pending culture and sensitivity results. No specific treatment for dengue fever is available.

Zoonotic/tickborn pathogens with sepsis-like presentations

Some less common environmentally acquired or zoonotic pathogens may cause fulminant septic-like clinical syndromes with a significant morbidity and mortality if appropriate treatment is not instituted early. Although certain clinical findings (eg, rash, cytopenias, and conjunctival suffusion) may be helpful, any patient who has an undifferentiated septic presentation without a clear etiology should be queried on animal and environmental exposures. Exposures to question include ticks (eg, rocky mountain spotted fever, ehrlichiosis), lakes/ponds (eg, leptospirosis), rodents (eg, plague, rat bite fever), and farm or wild animals (eg, Q fever, tularemia). If the exposure and clinical picture are suggestive, empiric treatment based on likely pathogens (often with doxycycline) may be indicated. Season is relevant because most rickettsial diseases are much more common in the warmer months.

Leptospirosis

Leptospirosis may be acquired in most parts of the United States, with the highest rates observed in Hawaii. Animals excrete leptospires into standing water, and humans are infected though contact with this water [33]. Most cases are mild and resolve without treatment; severe leptospirosis is a multisystem disease with renal and hepatic dysfunction (ie, Weil's syndrome) being most prominent. Striking features may include a highly elevated bilirubin with only mild transaminitis and conjunctival suffusion [34]. Diagnosis relies on serology, but seroconversion may occur late, requiring repeat serologies. Thus, in suspected cases, empiric treatment with penicillin or doxycycline is indicated.

Q fever

Coxiella burnetti is a small, gram-negative rod acquired from exposure to farm animals and rarely household pets or ticks. The organism is present in highest numbers in the placenta, so attending the birth of infected animals is a major risk factor [35]. Most patients develop a self-limited influenza-like illness, but multisystem organ failure or endocarditis may occur [36]. The organism cannot be grown with routine media, and diagnosis relies on serologic testing. Doxycycline is first-line therapy; fluoroquinolones or macrolides are alternative treatments.

Plague

Plague remains endemic in the western United States, and most cases occur in the Southwest. *Yersinia pestis* is transmitted by fleas to rodent populations, and humans in contact with fleas or infected rodent carcasses may become infected. After a brief incubation period (up to a week), symptoms most commonly include bubos (tender swollen lymph nodes), but 10% to 25% of patients develop undifferentiated sepsis without bubos [37]. Diagnosis is most commonly made by culture of blood, sputum, or aspiration of a bubo; serologic tests are available. Streptomycin has long been the mainstay of therapy; alternatives include gentamicin and doxycycline. Respiratory isolation should be continued until at least 48 hours of antimicrobials have been administered and sputum cultures are shown to be negative.

Tularemia

Francisella tularensis is a zoonoses that is prevalent throughout the Northern hemisphere. Humans may be infected by an insect vector or by direct contact with an infected animal. After an up to 21-day (but generally shorter) incubation period, the most common clinical manifestation is ulceroglandular tularemia, which is a discrete ulcer with regional lymphadenopathy. Undifferentiated septic presentations (typhoidal or respiratory tularemia) may occur, with the exposure history being the only clue to diagnosis [38]. The organism is difficult to grow, and diagnosis generally relies on serology. Treatment has generally been with streptomycin 10 mg/kg IM twice a day for 10 days; doxycycline or gentamicin are alternatives.

Other rickettsial diseases and erhlichiosis

The diseases in this category of greatest concern in North America include Rocky Mountain spotted fever (RMSF), murine typhus, human monocytic ehrlichiosis (HME), and human granulocytic erhlichiosis (HGE). The combination of fever, headache, and rash should prompt questioning for exposure to these diseases. With the exception of murine typhus, which is transmitted by fleas, all of the previously mentioned diseases are transmitted by ticks. RMSF, HGE, and HME are most common in a band stretching from Virginia to Oklahoma. Murine typhus is most commonly seen in Texas. The spectrum of clinical manifestations ranges from a nonspecific febrile illness to multisystem organ failure; the latter is more common with RMSF. The absence of rash does not exclude the diagnosis, and transaminitis or thrombocytopenia is common. Diagnosis and decision to treat is generally based on clinical suspicion and exposure history, although circulating morulae are frequent in the blood smears of patients who have HGE. Diagnosis is generally confirmed with serology. Treatment, generally effective if instituted early, is with doxycycline.

Hantavirus

Hantavirus species were first described to cause disease in North America in the early 1990s. Human infection occurs by contact with infected rodents. Hantavirus pulmonary syndrome, the clinical syndrome observed in North America, is characterized by a flu-like illness followed by noncardiogenic pulmonary edema and shock. Hantavirus pulmonary syndrome has a mortality rate of 50%. Diagnosis is by means of serology, and ribavirin has been used as therapy with mixed results [39].

References

[1] Bone RC, Sibbald WJ, Sprung CL. The ACCP-SCCM consensus conference on sepsis and organ failure. Chest 1992;101:1481–3.
[2] Bernard GR, Vincent JL, Laterre PF, et al. Efficacy and safety of recombinant human activated protein C for severe sepsis. N Engl J Med 2001;344:699–709.
[3] Harbarth S, Nobre V, Pittet D. Does antibiotic selection impact patient outcome? Clin Infect Dis 2007;44:87–93.
[4] Kumar A, Roberts D, Wood KE, et al. Duration of hypotension before initiation of effective antimicrobial therapy is the critical determinant of survival in human septic shock. Crit Care Med 2006;34:1589–96.
[5] Fridkin SK, Hageman JC, Morrison M, et al. Methicillin-resistant *Staphylococcus aureus* disease in three communities. N Engl J Med 2005;352:1436–44.
[6] Paul M, Benuri-Silbiger I, Soares-Weiser K, et al. Beta lactam monotherapy versus beta lactam-aminoglycoside combination therapy for sepsis in immunocompetent patients: systematic review and meta-analysis of randomised trials. BMJ 2004;328:668–82.
[7] Paul M, Soares-Weiser K, Leibovici L. Beta lactam monotherapy versus beta lactam-aminoglycoside combination therapy for fever with neutropenia: systematic review and meta-analysis. BMJ 2003;326:1111–20.

[8] Furno P, Bucaneve G, Del Favero A. Monotherapy or aminoglycoside-containing combinations for empirical antibiotic treatment of febrile neutropenic patients: a meta-analysis. Lancet Infect Dis 2002;2:231–42.

[9] Garey KW, Rege M, Pai MP, et al. Time to initiation of fluconazole therapy impacts mortality in patients with candidemia: a multi-institutional study. Clin Infect Dis 2006;43:25–31.

[10] Melles DC, de Marie S. Prevention of infections in hyposplenic and asplenic patients: an update. Neth J Med 2004;62:45–52.

[11] Anaya DA, Dellinger EP. Necrotizing soft-tissue infection: diagnosis and management. Clin Infect Dis 2007;44:705–10.

[12] Wong CH, Wang YS. The diagnosis of necrotizing fasciitis. Curr Opin Infect Dis 2005;18: 101–6.

[13] Stevens DL, Bisno AL, Chambers HF, et al. Practice guidelines for the diagnosis and management of skin and soft-tissue infections. Clin Infect Dis 2005;41:1373–406.

[14] Miller LG, Perdreau-Remington F, Rieg G, et al. Necrotizing fasciitis caused by community-associated methicillin-resistant *Staphylococcus aureus* in Los Angeles. N Engl J Med 2005; 352:1445–53.

[15] Moran GJ, Krishnadasan A, Gorwitz RJ, et al. Methicillin-resistant *S. aureus* infections among patients in the emergency department. N Engl J Med 2006;355:666–74.

[16] Mead PS, Slutsker L, Dietz V, et al. Food-related illness and death in the United States. Emerg Infect Dis 1999;5:607–25.

[17] Liu JW, Lee IK, Tang HJ, et al. Prognostic factors and antibiotics in *Vibrio vulnificus* septicemia. Arch Intern Med 2006;166:2117–23.

[18] Tunkel AR, Hartman BJ, Kaplan SL, et al. Practice guidelines for the management of bacterial meningitis. Clin Infect Dis 2004;39:1267–84.

[19] Gerdes LU, Jorgensen PE, Nexo E, et al. C-reactive protein and bacterial meningitis: a meta-analysis. Scand J Clin Lab Invest 1998;58:383–93.

[20] Viallon A, Zeni F, Lambert C, et al. High sensitivity and specificity of serum procalcitonin levels in adults with bacterial meningitis. Clin Infect Dis 1999;28:1313–6.

[21] de Gans J, van de Beek D. Dexamethasone in adults with bacterial meningitis. N Engl J Med 2002;347:1549–56.

[22] Krebs JW, Mandel EJ, Swerdlow DL, et al. Rabies surveillance in the United States during 2004. J Am Vet Med Assoc 2005;227:1912–25.

[23] Willoughby RE Jr, Tieves KS, Hoffman GM, et al. Survival after treatment of rabies with induction of coma. N Engl J Med 2005;352:2508–14.

[24] Sobel J. Botulism. Clin Infect Dis 2005;41:1167–73.

[25] Bartlett JG. New drugs for Clostridium difficile infection. Clin Infect Dis 2006;43:428–31.

[26] Pepin J, Valiquette L, Alary ME, et al. Clostridium difficile-associated diarrhea in a region of Quebec from 1991 to 2003: a changing pattern of disease severity. CMAJ 2004;171:466–72.

[27] Pepin J, Valiquette L, Cossette B. Mortality attributable to nosocomial Clostridium difficile-associated disease during an epidemic caused by a hypervirulent strain in Quebec. CMAJ 2005;173:1037–42.

[28] Pepin J, Saheb N, Coulombe MA, et al. Emergence of fluoroquinolones as the predominant risk factor for Clostridium difficile-associated diarrhea: a cohort study during an epidemic in Quebec. Clin Infect Dis 2005;41:1254–60.

[29] Dial S, Alrasadi K, Manoukian C, et al. Risk of Clostridium difficile diarrhea among hospital inpatients prescribed proton pump inhibitors: cohort and case-control studies. CMAJ 2004;171:33–8.

[30] Dial S, Delaney JA, Schneider V, et al. Proton pump inhibitor use and risk of community-acquired Clostridium difficile-associated disease defined by prescription for oral vancomycin therapy. CMAJ 2006;175:745–8.

[31] Centers for Disease Control and Prevention (CDC). Severe *Clostridium difficile* associated disease in populations previously at low risk four states, 2005. MMWR Morb Mortal Wkly Rep 2005;54:1201–5.

[32] Wilson ME, Weld LH, Boggild A, et al. Fever in returned travelers: results from the GeoSentinel Surveillance Network. Clin Infect Dis 2007;44:1560–8.

[33] Bharti AR, Nally JE, Ricaldi JN, et al. Leptospirosis: a zoonotic disease of global importance. Lancet Infect Dis 2003;3:757–71.

[34] Kaul DR, Flanders SA, Saint S. Clinical problem-solving. Clear as mud. N Engl J Med 2005; 352:1914–8.

[35] Maurin M, Raoult D. Q fever. Clin Microbiol Rev 1999;12:518–53.

[36] Bonilla MF, Kaul DR, Saint S, et al. Clinical problem-solving: ring around the diagnosis. N Engl J Med 2006;354:1937–42.

[37] Prentice MB, Rahalison L. Plague. Lancet 2007;369:1196–207.

[38] Tarnvik A, Berglund L. Tularaemia. Eur Respir J 2003;21:361–73.

[39] Muranyi W, Bahr U, Zeier M, et al. Hantavirus infection. J Am Soc Nephrol 2005;16: 3669–79.

ELSEVIER
SAUNDERS

THE MEDICAL
CLINICS
OF NORTH AMERICA

Med Clin N Am 92 (2008) 443–465

Diagnosis and Management of Venous Thromboembolism

Tracy Minichiello, MD[a],*, Patrick F. Fogarty, MD[b]

[a]Division of Hospital Medicine, Department of Medicine, University of California,
505 Parnassus Avenue, Box 0131, San Francisco, CA 94143, USA
[b]Division of Hematology/Oncology, Department of Medicine, University of California,
505 Parnassus Avenue, Room M-1286, San Francisco, CA 94143–1270, USA

Venous thromboembolic disease (VTE), which includes lower-extremity deep vein thrombosis (DVT) and pulmonary embolism (PE), is a major public health concern. In the general population, the annual incidence of VTE has been estimated at approximately 100 per 100,000 persons [1–3], and PE causes up to 200,000 deaths annually in the United States [4].

In hospitalized patients, the prevalence of VTE is approximately 100 times higher than in the general population [1], and varies with indication for admission. Among inpatients not given thromboprophylaxis, the frequency of VTE ranges from 10% to 20% in medical patients up to 80% in high-risk surgical and critical care patients [4]. The frequency of the most devastating consequence of VTE, fatal PE, has been reported to range from 0.01% among low-risk surgical patients to 5% among hospitalized patients who have multiple risk factors [5]. Early, accurate diagnosis and prompt, appropriate treatment of VTE is essential to reducing morbidity and mortality from this disorder.

Diagnosis of venous thromboembolism

In recent years, strategies for assessing pretest probability of VTE have been developed. The original Wells Prediction Rule for DVT [6] comprised a scoring system based on nine clinical characteristics; a score of greater than or equal to 3 (highest pretest probability) was associated with a prevalence of DVT of 17% to 85%, compared with a prevalence of 0% to 13% in

* Corresponding author.
E-mail address: tminichiello@medicine.ucsf.edu (T. Minichiello).

0025-7125/08/$ - see front matter © 2008 Elsevier Inc. All rights reserved.
doi:10.1016/j.mcna.2007.12.001   medical.theclinics.com

those patients with the lowest pretest probability (Wells score of ≤ 0) [7]. The Rule has since been updated to provide for a "likely" or "unlikely" pretest probability of DVT (Table 1). In the Wells Prediction Rule for PE (Table 2) a score of greater than or equal to 7 (highest pretest probability) correlates with a prevalence of PE of 38% to 78%, compared with a 1% to 3% prevalence among patients with the lowest pretest probability (Wells score of 0–1) [7]. Although the evidence in support of clinical prediction models is strong [7], the value of these methodologies may be highest when combined with D-dimer assessment [8].

D-dimers are generated through degradation of fibrin that has been cross-linked, and indicate recent activity of the coagulation system. The test is sensitive but not very specific for VTE, and a negative D-dimer result (typically reported as <500 ng/mL) can exclude the diagnosis, particularly in patients with a low pretest probability, averting the need for diagnostic imaging [9]. The highest sensitivity (approximately 95%) exists with ELISA. Agglutination-based assays are less sensitive; indeed, the negative predictive value of non–ELISA-based D-dimer testing may be particularly poor among patient groups with an increased prevalence of VTE, such as elderly or hospitalized individuals [10]. The negative predictive value of D-dimer testing is strengthened when combined with a low pretest probability result from a clinical prediction rule. In this scenario, the incidence of VTE may be as low as 0.5% at 3-months follow-up, whereas patients with a moderate or high pretest probability despite negative D-dimer show a higher frequency of DVT (3.5% and 21.4%, respectively) [8].

Table 1
Pretest probability of DVT: the Wells Prediction Rule

Clinical characteristic	Score
Active cancer (patient receiving treatment for cancer within the previous 6 mo or currently receiving palliative treatment)	1
Paralysis, paresis, or recent plaster immobilization of the lower extremities	1
Recently bedridden for 3 d or more, or major surgery within the previous 12 wk requiring general or regional anesthesia	1
Localized tenderness along the distribution of the deep venous system	1
Entire leg swollen	1
Calf swelling at least 3 cm larger than that on the asymptomatic side (measured 10 cm below tibial tuberosity)	1
Pitting edema confined to the symptomatic leg	1
Collateral superficial veins (nonvaricose)	1
Previously documented DVT	1
Alternative diagnosis at least as likely as DVT	−2
Interpretation:	
DVT likely	≥ 2
DVT unlikely	<2

Abbreviation: DVT, deep vein thrombosis.

Adapted from Wells PS, Anderson DR, Rodger M, et al. Evaluation of d-Dimer in the diagnosis of suspected deep vein thrombosis. N Engl J Med 2003;349:1227–35; with permission. Copyright © 2003, Massachusetts Medical Society.

Table 2
Pretest probability of PE: the Wells Prediction Rule

Clinical characteristic	Score
Previous PE or deep vein thrombosis	+1.5
Heart rate > 100 beats per minute	+1.5
Recent surgery or immobilization	+1.5
Clinical signs of deep vein thrombosis	+3
Alternative diagnosis less likely than PE	+3
Hemoptysis	+1
Cancer	+1
Interpretation:	
High probability of PE	≥7
Moderate probability of PE	2–6
Low probability of PE	0–1

Abbreviation: PE, pulmonary embolism.

Data from Wells PS, Anderson DR, Rodger M, et al. Derivation of a simple clinical model to categorize patients probability of pulmonary embolism: increasing the models utility with the SimpliRED d-dimer. Thromb Haemost 2000;83:416–20.

Elevated D-dimer levels are characteristic of recent trauma or bleeding and are also frequently detected in the setting of hospitalization, advanced age, and malignancy, further reducing the positive predictive value of the D-dimer assay in those patient groups [11].

Diagnosis of deep vein thrombosis

Investigation for DVT usually is initiated when a patient is observed to have any of the following: calf or lower-extremity swelling (present in 88% of individuals ultimately diagnosed with DVT); pain or tenderness in the affected extremity (56%); or increased warmth or erythema (30%–40%) [12]. The Homans' sign (posterior calf tenderness on passive dorsiflexion of the foot) is present in fewer than 15% of cases of DVT, and a palpable cord is detectable in only 6% [12]. Alternatively, DVT may be discovered in an asymptomatic patient by radiographic imaging performed for other reasons, or in a patient who has been diagnosed with PE.

Doppler ultrasonography is recommended as the initial test for the radiographic diagnosis of lower-extremity DVT, because of its wide availability; noninvasive nature; low cost; and high sensitivity (89%–100%) and specificity (86%–100%) for symptomatic DVT [13,14]. Sensitivity is highest for proximal DVT, and decreases for distal lesions. Typical findings on Doppler ultrasonography include direct observation of an occlusive intraluminal thrombus, noncompressibility of a vein, or reduced or absent blood flow by color Doppler. Comparison with prior ultrasound studies (if available) may be helpful when assessing for DVT recurrence, because symptoms of the postthrombotic syndrome (PTS) or other conditions in the previously affected extremity may be similar to those of acute thrombosis.

Despite its extensive use in clinical trails and status as the gold standard diagnostic method for identification of DVT, contrast venography is not recommended for routine evaluation of DVT, because of patient discomfort, interobserver variability in interpretation, and high cost, among other factors [15]. Impedance plethysmography [16] and MRI [17] are generally not as accessible as Doppler ultrasonography in most institutions, but may have a role for evaluation of recurrent DVT.

Thrombi that are detected in the veins of the calf are generally accepted to have a lower potential for proximal propagation, leading to a reduced clinical concern for evolution to PE [18]. Although withholding anticoagulation may be acceptable in asymptomatic patients with distal lower-extremity DVT, serial imaging over a period of 1 to 2 weeks is recommended to ensure absence of clot extension [19]. In contrast, if a patient has symptoms (eg, pain, swelling) in the affected extremity, treatment should be administered as for proximal DVT (see later).

Diagnosis of pulmonary embolism

Typically, evaluation for PE is pursued when a patient complains of sudden shortness of breath; chest pain; hemoptysis; or when clinical findings, such as tachypnea (70% of patients with PE), tachycardia (43%), hypoxia (18%), or hypotension (10%), are present [12]. Alternatively, PE may be incidentally detected when performing imaging of the thorax for other reasons. Three main categories of overall clinical presentation exist: (1) massive PE marked by persistent hemodynamic instability; (2) submassive PE marked by evidence of right ventricular (RV) strain on echo, ECG, or right heart catheterization, without hemodynamic compromise; and (3) nonmassive PE marked by lack of RV compromise and normal hemodynamics.

The gold standard for diagnosis of PE is the pulmonary angiogram. This procedure is associated with a mortality rate of less than 0.5% and a slightly higher rate of other complications, including contrast nephropathy, cardiac arrhythmias, and cardiac perforation [20]. Ventilation perfusion scanning is noninvasive, but results are frequently nondiagnostic. Helical CT scanning is noninvasive, typically readily available, and has sensitivity for PE of up to 90% and a specificity of 95% [21]. Although sensitivity declines for detection of distal thrombi, negative CT results are associated with a low frequency (approximately 1%) of subsequent detection of clinically significant VTE, especially in the setting of a low clinical probability of VTE [22,23]. A diagnostic algorithm involving a low-probability clinical prediction rule, negative D-dimer assessment, and negative CT has been evaluated, showing a low frequency (<1.5%) of subsequent fatal and nonfatal VTE [24]. MRA has better sensitivity for lobar thromboses than for segmental or subsegmental lesions [25]; high cost and limited availability, among other issues, have hindered widespread use of this diagnostic modality.

Abnormalities of the transthoracic echocardiogram in patients with PE include RV hypokinesis, RV hypertrophy, and tricuspid regurgitation, and may be prognostic. For instance, RV dysfunction is associated with a doubling of PE-related mortality, although the effect may be most pronounced in hypotensive patients [26]. In one retrospective analysis of normotensive patients who presented with PE, however, RV hypokinesis remained an independent predictor of early death (hazard ratio, 1.94) [27]. Further data are required to clarify the role of echocardiogram in the initial assessment of patients with PE. Two tests, brain natriuretic peptide and serum troponin level, lack sufficient specificity to be useful in the diagnosis of PE, but may be helpful in determining prognosis. Elevated brain natriuretic peptide levels (>90 pg/mL) in patients who present with acute PE are associated with adverse clinical outcomes, including need for thrombolysis, requirement for cardiopulmonary resuscitation, and death [28]. Elevations in troponin levels indicate cardiac injury and are associated with an increased incidence of 30-day mortality [29]. In one study, a concomitant troponin level of greater than 0.07 μg/L and brain natriuretic peptide level of 600 ng/L were associated with a 33% mortality at 40 days, compared with no deaths among patients with normal levels [30]. Insufficient data exist, however, to lead to a recommendation that these adjunctive laboratory tests be performed at presentation in all patients.

Treatment of venous thromboembolism

The mainstay of treatment for VTE is anticoagulation. Anticoagulants do not dismantle thrombi directly; rather, they prevent propagation of the thrombus while the endogenous fibrinolytic system works to decrease the clot burden. In most cases, treatment of VTE should be based on confirmatory diagnostic studies, but if the pretest probability is high enough, anticoagulation may be started empirically pending definitive testing. Before initiation of anticoagulation, baseline laboratory studies should be obtained including urinalysis, Hemoccult, hemoglobin, hematocrit, platelet count, prothrombin time, International Normalized Ratio (INR), activated partial thromboplastin time (aPTT), blood urea nitrogen, and creatinine. Suggested anticoagulation regimens according to presentation are listed in Table 3.

Parenteral agents for the acute treatment of VTE include weight-based unfractionated heparin (either intravenously [31,32] or subcutaneously dosed [33]); weight-based low-molecular-weight heparin (LMWH) [34,35]; and the synthetic anti-Xa agent, fondaparinux (see Table 3) [36,37].

Intravenous unfractionated heparin typically is administered by an initial bolus (loading) dose followed by a continuous infusion; ensuing dose adjustments should be made using a standard nomogram [38,39]. Weight-based, subcutaneous unfractionated heparin also may be used with aPTT monitoring and dose adjustment to maintain the aPTT in therapeutic range

Table 3
Suggested anticoagulation regimens for the initial treatment of VTE

Event	Treatment (choose one)
DVT, lower extremity	**LMWH**
	Enoxaparin, 1 mg/kg subcutaneously twice daily
	Enoxaparin, 1.5 mg/kg subcutaneously daily
	Tinzaparin, 175 units/kg subcutaneously daily
	Dalteparin, 200 units/kg subcutaneously daily
	Subcutaneous UFH: aPTT monitoring
	15,000 units or 17,500 units every 12 h (initial dose for patients weighing 50–70 kg and >70 kg, respectively) with aPTT monitoring
	Subcutaneous UFH: no aPTT monitoring
	330 units/kg × 1 then 250 units/kg every 12 h
	Fondiparinux
	7.5–10 mg subcutaneously daily, depending on weight
	IV UFH
	80 units/kg bolus (minimum, 5000 units; maximum, 10,000 units) followed by a continuous infusion of 18 units/kg/h.
	Note: begin warfarin concurrent with initial dose of parenteral anticoagulant as selected above
DVT, upper extremity	**See DVT, lower extremity**
	Consider thrombolysis in appropriate candidates
Nonmassive PE	**See DVT, lower extremity**
	Risk stratification suggested to guide additional therapy and triage
Submassive PE	**See DVT, lower extremity**
	Risk stratification suggested to guide additional therapy
	Thrombolysis in selected patients
Massive PE	**IV UFH**
	Thrombolytic therapy (choose one)
	Alteplase, 100-mg infusion over 2 h, followed by IV UFH
	Alteplase, 100-mg bolus (if cardiac arrest)
	Urokinase, 4400 IU/kg loading dose over 10 min followed 4400 IU/kg/h for 12 h
	Note: for urokinase, heparin infusion should be administered concurrently
VTE and CrCl <30 mL/min	**UFH** (see DVT, lower extremity)
VTE and cancer	**Dalteparin** (see DVT, lower extremity)
	Tinzaparin (see DVT, lower extremity)
	Use LMWH as initial treatment and for at least 3–6 mo

Abbreviations: aPTT, activated partial thromboplastin time; CrCl, creatinine clearance; DVT, deep vein thrombosis; LMWH, low-molecular-weight heparin; PE, pulmonary embolism; UFH, unfractionated heparin; VTE, venous thromboembolism.

[40,41]. More recently, it has been shown that weight-based, subcutaneous unfractionated heparin without aPTT-based dose adjustment was as safe and effective as LMWH in the acute treatment of VTE. Interestingly, no association between a low aPTT and recurrent VTE or between a high aPTT and bleeding complications was observed [42].

LMWH and unfractionated heparin are equally efficacious for the acute treatment of DVT and nonmassive PE, both reducing the risk of early recurrence to approximately 3% [43,44]. Given the ease of dosing, lack of need for laboratory monitoring, trend toward superiority in prevention of recurrence and lower bleeding rates in systematic reviews, and ease of transition to the outpatient arena, LMWH is the recommended agent [40]. Some LMWHs can be dosed once or twice daily, without a significant difference in major bleeding or VTE recurrence [45,46]. Once-daily dosing with some LMWH preparations, however, may not be appropriate for patients with renal insufficiency, obesity, pregnancy, or active malignancy.

Fondaparinux, administered subcutaneously once daily, has been compared with LMWH for acute treatment of DVT [35] and unfractionated heparin for acute treatment of PE [37]. A weight-based regimen has been shown to be equally effective as LMWH or unfractionated heparin in preventing recurrent VTE with no difference in bleeding or mortality. Fondaparinux has a very long half-life (17 hours) and currently there is no antidote for easy reversal of the anticoagulant effect.

Warfarin is generally started at daily doses ranging from 2.5 to 10 mg and can be initiated along with a parenteral anticoagulant for the acute treatment of VTE. Selection of the starting dose of warfarin should include consideration of ethnicity, weight, age, nutritional status, and thyroid function (Box 1); concomitant medications should also be considered (Box 2). In

---

Box 1. Initiation of warfarin therapy in the hospitalized patient

- Usual initiation dose = 5 mg
- Consider higher initial dose (eg, 7.5 mg) in the following populations
  1. Weight >85 kg
  2. African American patients
  3. Clinical hypothyroidism
  4. Concomitant medications that decrease warfarin effect[a]
- Consider lower initial dose (eg, 2.5 mg) in the following populations
  1. Frail or advanced age (>75 years)
  2. Asian patients
  3. Hepatic insufficiency
  4. Malnutrition or poor oral intake
  5. Clinical hyperthyroidism
  6. High bleeding risk
  7. Concomitant medications that increase warfarin effect[a]

---

[a] See Box 2.

Box 2. Effect of selected agents on the INR in warfarin-anticoagulated patients

↑ *INR*
Erythromycin
Metronidazole
Fluconazole
Itraconazol
Ketoconazole
SMX-TMP
Amiodarone
Cimetidine
Phenytoin
Statins
Alcohol

↓ *INR*
Phenobarbital
Rifampin, rifabutin
Carbamazepine
Vitamin K
Phenytoin (chronic use)
Sucralfate
Ginseng
Alcohol

---

hospitalized patients, a starting daily dose of 5 mg usually results in timely achievement of a therapeutic INR without excessive bleeding [47,48]. Various polymorphisms for the CYP2C9 gene in the cytochrome P-450 system correlate with impaired warfarin metabolism [49,50], whereas polymorphisms in the VKORC1 gene in the vitamin K eposide reductase complex correlate with warfarin sensitivity or resistance [51,52]. Recently, algorithms have been developed to predict the starting dose of warfarin based on genetic variables, clinical data, and initial INR values [53]. Outcomes studies evaluating the clinical impact of genetic testing to guide warfarin therapy have not been completed and recommendations to test patients before initiation are premature.

In hospitalized patients, the INR should be monitored daily during warfarin initiation. As a vitamin K antagonist, warfarin depletes vitamin K–dependent coagulation factors with the shortest half-life first. Activities of factor VII (accounting for the initial rise in INR), and protein C (a natural anticoagulant, resulting in a transient hypercoagulable state) are reduced initially, followed by factor IX, factor X, and prothrombin. The half-lives of these factors are 12 hours, 45 hours, and 60 hours, respectively; an average of 5 days is required to achieve a steady-state reduction. For this reason, the parenteral anticoagulant should be continued for a minimum of 5 days, and at least and until the INR is greater than 2.0 on 2 consecutive days.

Both LMWH and fondaparinux are cleared by the kidneys, leading to accumulation in patients with renal insufficiency, and fondaparinux is contraindicated in patients with a creatinine clearance less than 30 mL/min. Treatment with unfractionated heparin is preferred. If the creatinine clearance is between 30 and 50 mL/min, LMWH may be used, but anti-Xa levels (drawn after ≥ 24 hours on therapy, 4–6 hours after a given dose) should be monitored. LMWH also has less predictable pharmacokinetics in this group of patients, and should be used with caution in patients weighing less than 50 kg. Anti-Xa monitoring is advised in these patients.

Thrombolysis

Thrombolytic agents activate the fibrinolytic system, resulting in more rapid resolution of a thrombus than with use of anticoagulation alone. Because the risk of bleeding is increased with use of these agents, patients who may benefit from thrombolysis should be selected carefully.

The pharmacologic approach to therapy in patients with nonmassive PE and most DVT involves only anticoagulation. Although there are no prospective randomized studies evaluating the efficacy of thrombolysis in patients with massive PE, the extremely high in-hospital mortality rate (approaching 30%) and potentially improved outcomes on subgroup analysis [44] have led to recommendations for use of thrombolysis in this setting [40]. In contrast, administration of thrombolytic agents for submassive PE remains controversial. Mortality from submassive PE, despite initial hemodynamic stability, is significant and ranges from 4% to 13% [54]. A single randomized, controlled trial of systemic thrombolysis for submassive PE compared with usual care with anticoagulation alone [55] showed a significant difference in the primary outcome (combined end point of treatment escalation and mortality) between the treatment groups, favoring thrombolysis. The difference, however, was related entirely to escalation of treatment, and the groups were similar in terms of mortality and recurrent VTE. A large European trial is underway to define better the risks and benefits of thrombolysis in patients with submassive PE.

Large proximal iliofemoral DVT has been associated with an increased risk of PTS. Manifestations of PTS can range from mild swelling of the affected leg on exertion or assumption of dependent positioning to constant pain, swelling, and inability to bear weight for any length of time. Because PTS is thought to be related to valvular incompetence, which is related to rates of recanalization, it has been postulated that more rapid and complete clearing of a significant intraluminal thrombus may lead to reduced risk for

PTS. Indeed, registry data show that patients with acute thrombosis (symptoms <10 days) who are treated with catheter-directed thrombolysis and achieve complete resolution of the thrombus have higher 1-year patency rates than those who do not achieve complete lysis [56]. A single, small randomized trial evaluating thrombolytic therapy versus conventional anticoagulation for acute proximal DVT [57] showed a 6-month patency rate of 72% in patients who received catheter-directed thrombolysis, compared with 12% in patients treated with anticoagulation alone. Given the increased bleeding risk associated with thrombolysis, the decision to pursue this therapy must be considered carefully. Ideally, only patients with significant proximal disease who are at low risk of bleeding, and find themselves in a center experienced with this approach, should be regarded as eligible. Although there are currently no randomized controlled trails of the use of thrombolytic agents in the management of upper-extremity DVT, reports of improved outcomes in selected cases has led the 7th ACCP Conference on Antithrombotic and Thrombolytic Therapy to propose that thrombolytics be considered in patients who have a low risk of bleeding and recent onset of symptoms [40]. Otherwise, the initial therapy in patients with acute upper-extremity DVT should mirror that of DVT of the lower extremity.

Cancer-related venous thromboembolism

None of the components of Virchow's triad (underlined in the bulleted points next) can be underestimated in their potential to promote and maintain a prothrombotic state in the cancer patient:

- Chemotherapy, cytokines induced by tumor cells, and malignant cells themselves can all lead to endothelial damage.
- Tumors may produce a circulating procoagulant or stimulate disseminated intravascular anticoagulation resulting in a hypercoagulability.
- Venous compression by metastatic disease or bulky lymphadenopathy can result in stasis.

Patients with cancer-related thrombosis have a threefold higher rate of recurrence while on oral anticoagulation compared with patients with non–cancer-related thrombosis. There may also be an increased risk of bleeding associated with warfarin therapy in cancer patients [58].

Some LMWHs seem to be more effective than warfarin in preventing recurrent thrombosis in patients with cancer and VTE, as evidenced in a recent trial that evaluated the efficacy of extended-duration treatment (6 months) with the LMWH dalteparin versus standard long-term treatment with warfarin. In this study, the frequency of VTE recurrence was 17% in the warfarin group, compared with 9% in the dalteparin group. There was no significant difference in bleeding events between the two groups. American College of Chest Physicians in their 2004 recommendations suggest at least

3 to 6 months of LMWH, with once-daily tinzaparin or once-daily dalte-parin, for acute treatment of cancer-related VTE because of this significant reduction in symptomatic recurrences [40].

Outpatient management of venous thromboembolism

Most DVT is now treated in the outpatient arena, a practice that is strongly supported by the evidence [59]. One recent study highlighted a num-ber of factors that may be associated with higher risk of earlier complica-tions, and identify patients who might benefit from inpatient treatment. Cancer, bilateral DVT, renal insufficiency, congestive heart failure, weight less than 70 kg, and immobility predicted a higher risk of recurrence or bleeding complications [60].

Scant evidence is available regarding outpatient treatment of PE. The FIDO trial, based in Canada, compared unmonitored weight-based subcu-taneously dosed unfractionated heparin with LMWH for the acute treat-ment of DVT or PE; over one third of patients with symptomatic PE were able to be treated entirely as outpatients [42]. One small prospective cohort study found outpatient treatment of PE to be safe and effective for selected patients, but required admission for those patients with hemody-namic instability, hypoxia requiring oxygen therapy, severe pain, high risk of major bleeding, or a concomitant condition requiring hospitalization [61]. In the United States, however, most patients with suspected acute PE are treated in the hospital, at least initially.

Adjunctive therapy for venous thromboembolism

All patients diagnosed with DVT should be prescribed a graduated com-pression stocking for the affected lower extremity; ideally, these should exert 30 to 40 mm Hg pressure at the ankle. The stocking should be worn for 1 to 2 years on the affected leg. When combined with long-term anticoagulation, graduated compression stocking may reduce the incidence and severity of PTS, in some cases by up to 50% [62,63].

Although historically it was thought that bed rest was safest for prevent-ing PE in patients with acute proximal DVT, this has not been supported in the literature [64]. Early ambulation with compression may decrease both propagation of the thrombus and development of PTS [65,66].

Inferior vena cava filters

The use of inferior vena cava (IVC) filters is becoming increasingly com-mon. The only generally agreed on indication for placement of an IVC filter is prevention of PE in a patient with an acute DVT in the setting of absolute contraindication to anticoagulation. The following additional uses of caval filters have also been described: to prevent PE in patients with free-floating ileofemoral thrombus, in chronic thromboembolic pulmonary hypertension, in acute PE and significant underlying cardiopulmonary disease, in cases of recurrent PE despite adequate anticoagulant therapy, and in patients undergoing thrombolysis. In other settings, placement of IVC filters should be avoided if at all possible. Complications associated with filter placement include migration, insertion site infections, and vessel penetration. IVC thrombosis following placement of IVC filters occurs commonly; rates are reported to be between 2% and 10%, although one study that provided long-term follow-up found rates to be as high as 20% to 30% [67].

The only randomized trial evaluating the use of IVC filters to prevent PE in patients with proximal ileofemoral DVT showed that, compared with patients who received anticoagulation alone, those who received IVC filter placement in addition to anticoagulant therapy had lower rates of symptomatic PE at 14 days (1.1% versus 4.8%; 95% confidence interval [CI], 0.05–1.05) and 2 years (3.4% versus 6.3%; 95% CI, 0.21–1.41) but higher rates of DVT at 2 years (20.8% versus 11.6%; 95% CI, 1.09–2.94) [68]. An 8-year follow-up study of this trial was recently published, which again found decreased rates of symptomatic PE in patients with IVC filter but increased rates of DVT [69]. There was no difference in the rates of PTS. No randomized controlled data on the performance of these devices in patients in the acute phase who are not concurrently anticoagulated are available.

If an IVC filter must be placed in a patient with a temporary contraindication to anticoagulation, it is recommended to start a full course of anticoagulation as soon as deemed safe. Guidelines created by the Thrombosis Interest Group of Canada are available on-line and have been recently reviewed (www.tigc.org).

Within the past several years, certain types of IVC filters have been approved for temporary use and retrieval; these are most useful for individuals with venous thrombosis who have a time-limited barrier to use of anticoagulants (eg, impending surgery). A retrospective review found retrievals, performed between days 1 and 139 postplacement, successful in 85% of patients [70]; anticoagulation was not interrupted for filter retrieval. Retrieval failures were attributed to thrombus within the filter (50%) and technical difficulties, including tilting of the filter, and embedding in the vessel wall (50%) [70]. The rate of success of retrieval probably declines as time progresses, so to avoid inadvertent conversion of a temporary filter to a permanent one, it is critical to arrange close follow-up for patients postplacement so that removal actually occurs.

Etiology of venous thromboembolism

Understanding the risk factors for thrombosis helps providers estimate the risk of recurrence and make appropriate recommendations regarding duration of treatment. The most important predictor of recurrence is the presence or absence of removable (eg, transient) risk factors at the time of the event (Table 4) [71]. Assessment for a transient risk factor is best

Table 4
Risk of recurrent VTE after stopping anticoagulant therapy

Variable	Relative risk of recurrence
Transient risk factor	0.5
Persistent risk factor	≥ 2
Cancer	< 3
Discontinuation of estrogen	< 1
Unprovoked VTE	≥ 2
Distal DVT versus proximal DVT or PE	0.5
Venal caval filter	< 1.8
Protein C, S, antithrombin deficiencies	1–3
Heterozygous factor V Leiden	1–2
Homozygous factor V Leiden	4.1
Heterozygous prothrombin gene mutation G20210A	1–2
Heterozygous for both factor V Leiden and G20210A prothrombin gene	2–5
Factor VIII level > 200 IU/dL	< 6
Antiphospholipid antibodies	2–4
Hyperhomocysteinemia	2.7
Second versus first episode of VTE	< 1.5

Abbreviations: DVT, deep vein thrombosis; PE, pulmonary embolism; VTE, venous thromboembolism.

Adapted from Kearon C. Long-term management of patients after venous thromboembolism. Circulation 2004;110(Suppl I):I-10–I-18; with permission.

performed at the time of presentation, when patient recall is highest for such factors as trauma; medications (oral contraceptives, hormone-replacement therapy, exposure to heparin); prolonged air travel; immobilization; or recent surgery. Additionally, VTE is associated with a number of systemic diseases (Table 5). It is the duty of the treating clinician to search for associated diseases that may change management and uncover a previously undiagnosed disorder.

Cancer

Approximately 10% of patients who present with unprovoked events are diagnosed with cancer within a few years of presentation with VTE [72]. This risk is highest in the first 1 to 6 months after presentation and declines over the subsequent 2 years.

In addition to a thorough history and physical examination, current practice for cancer screening includes performing a complete blood count, liver function tests, calcium level, urinalysis, chest radiograph, and age-appropriate malignancy screening. A recent trial of screening for occult malignancy in patients with idiopathic VTE randomized patients to the current practice versus extensive screening, including abdominal ultrasound, CT scan, barium swallow, sigmoidoscopy and colonoscopy, Hemoccult assessment, sputum cytology and tumor markers, mammography, Pap smear, and prostate-specific antigen. The authors found malignancy in 13% of the

Table 5
Systemic diseases associated with thrombosis

Systemic disease	Clinical features	Diagnostic data
Inflammatory bowel disease	Bloody diarrhea, aphthous ulcers, arthritis, rash	Histologic analysis of intestinal biopsy specimens
Nephrotic syndrome	Periorbital edema, peripheral edema	Urine protein analysis
Behçet's disease	Oral ulcers, genital ulcers, ophthalmologic issues	—
Myeloproliferative disorders (P. Vera, essential thrombocytosis)	Pruritis, plethora	CBC, JAK-2 mutation
Sickle cell disease	Anemia, sickle crises	Evaluation of the blood smear, hemoglobin electrophoresis
Antiphospholipid antibody syndrome	Livedo, arthritis, rash	Lupus anticoagulant, ELISA for anticardiolipin antibody IgG and IgM (assess ≥ 3 mo after acute event)
Cancer	Weight loss, night sweats	CBC, LFTS, PSA, pap smear, routine cancer screening
Paroxysmal nocturnal hemoglobinuria	Hemolytic anemia	CBC, flow cytometry for CD55, CD59
Pregnancy	Amenorrhea	Urine pregnancy test (all women of childbearing age)

Abbreviations: CBC, complete blood count; LFTs, liver function tests; PSA, prostate-specific antigen.

intervention group with only a single case of malignancy subsequently identified, whereas 10% of the control group was found to have a malignancy at 2-year follow-up. Those malignancies identified by extensive screening were earlier stage; however, there was no difference in cancer-related mortality at 2 years [73]. Given the lack of a survival advantage and the significant cost, extensive cancer screening currently cannot be recommended; a cost-effectiveness analysis is underway.

Thrombophilia

About 50% of patients presenting with unprovoked VTE have laboratory evidence of an inherited thrombophilic disorder. Deficiencies in protein C, S, and antithrombin tend to present a higher risk for first and recurrent VTE and present at a younger age, whereas heterozygosity for the factor V Leiden or prothrombin gene mutations are weaker risk factors (see Table 4). Sending a thrombophilia work-up at the time of acute thrombosis is associated with high rate of false positivity, because acute thrombosis may result in decreased levels of protein C, protein S, and antithrombin, and increased anticardiolipin antibodies, appearance of lupus anticoagulants, and elevated factor VIII levels. Moreover, heparin can decrease antithrombin levels, warfarin decreases proteins C and S, and both warfarin and heparin can interfere with lupus anticoagulant assessment. For these reasons, it is best to delay testing in most patients until 3 months after the event. If a clear transient risk factor for thrombosis is present and there is no family history, however, testing is not likely to change management and should be deferred.

Duration of anticoagulation

Decisions regarding the duration of anticoagulation beyond the usual treatment of VTE must take into consideration both the risk of clinically significant recurrent thrombosis were anticoagulation to be discontinued [71] and the risk of bleeding caused by anticoagulation. This assessment must be performed on a case-by-case basis and should be repeated annually in patients who are being managed with indefinite anticoagulation. Patient preferences must also be considered.

The major determinant of risk of recurrence is the clinical scenario surrounding the initial event. The risk of recurrence after anticoagulation is stopped is much lower if the event was provoked by a removable risk factor [74,75]: the more significant the removable risk factor, the lower the risk of recurrence. The following may also influence decisions regarding duration of anticoagulation or extension of anticoagulation beyond the usual treatment period:

- Location of the thrombosis: For instance, patients who present with isolated calf vein thrombosis have a lower risk of recurrence (RR, 0.5) compared with those with proximal vein thrombosis. Concern over recurrence may be enhanced, however, if the initial event occurred in a particularly problematic site, such as dural sinus, mesenteric vessel, and so forth.
- Type of thrombosis: In patients who initially present with PE, the risk that a recurrent event also will be PE is higher than in patients who initially present with DVT [76].
- Cancer: Patients with active malignancy and VTE have a recurrence risk that is two to three times that of patients with non–cancer-related thrombosis.

Importantly, results from the laboratory work-up of thrombophilia typically have little impact on decisions regarding duration of anticoagulation, with the exception of detection of the antiphospholipid antibody syndrome (which usually mandates indefinite anticoagulation) and perhaps discovery of (rarer) serious, familial disorders (eg, antithrombin deficiency).

Duration of anticoagulation: current clinical practice

Studies have shown that anticoagulation with a vitamin K antagonist for less than 3 months after detection of VTE is associated with higher risk of recurrence, whereas extended duration therapy is associated with the lowest risk of recurrence [59]. Current recommendations for duration of therapy according to presentation and other clinical risk factors are outlined in Table 6 [40].

The goal INR for initial treatment of VTE with warfarin is 2.5 (range INR, 2.0–3.0); patients whose thrombosis occurred in the setting of a transient, reversible risk factor may receive 3 months of treatment, whereas patients with an idiopathic event usually receive a minimum of 6 to 12 months of treatment, although recurrent rates rise once anticoagulation is discontinued regardless of the duration.

Intensity of anticoagulation

After a minimum of 3 months of full-intensity warfarin, treatment with lower-intensity warfarin (goal INR, 1.5–2.0) was tested in the extended treatment of unprovoked VTE in the PREVENT trial [77]. At 1-year follow-up, low-intensity warfarin was associated with an incidence of recurrence of 2.6% per patient-year versus 7.2% per patient-year in the placebo arm. In the ELATE trial, however, full-intensity therapy was superior to

Table 6
Recommendations for duration of therapy from the 7th ACCP Conference on Antithrombotic and Thrombolytic Therapy: evidence-based guidelines

Scenario	Duration of therapy	Additional comments
Transient risk factor[a]	3 mo	Give VTE prophylaxis in any subsequent high-risk setting
Isolated calf vein thrombosis	3 mo	—
Unprovoked thrombosis	6–12 mo	Consider indefinite anticoagulation
Cancer-related VTE	Continue while cancer active, metastatic, or undergoing therapy	Treatment with LMWH (dalteparin or tinzaparin) recommended for first 3–6 mo
Recurrent VTE	Indefinite	—
Significant underlying thrombophilia[b]	12 mo	Consider indefinite anticoagulation

Abbreviations: LMWH, low-molecular-weight heparin; VTE, venous thromboembolism.

[a] Major transient risk factors include major surgery, major trauma, major hospitalization, plaster cast immobilization. Minor transient risk factors include pregnancy; hormonal therapy; prolonged airline travel (>8 h).

[b] Significant thrombophilia includes documented antiphospholipid antibody syndrome; two or more thrombophilic conditions (combined factor V Leiden and prothrombin 20210 gene mutation); antithrombin deficiency; protein C deficiency; protein S deficiency; hyperhomocysteinemia; persistently elevated factor VIII levels.

Data from Buller HR, et al. Antithrombotic therapy for venous thromboembolic disease: the Seventh ACCP Conference on Antithrombotic and Thrombolytic Therapy. Chest 2004; 126(3 Suppl):401S–428S.

low-intensity therapy (0.6% recurrent VTE per patient-year versus 1.9% recurrence per patient year, respectively); there was no difference in major bleeding between the groups [78]. Full-intensity warfarin is preferred for extended-duration treatment, because it is more effective than low-intensity treatment, and is not associated with an increase in major bleeding rates over a low-intensity program. Patients may prefer the convenience of low-intensity anticoagulation, however, because INR monitoring may be performed less frequently.

Further risk stratification

Committing a patient to lifelong anticoagulation is clearly not without risk. Because up to 70% of patients with unprovoked thrombosis do not experience recurrence, reserving indefinite therapy for only those who are at highest risk seems to be the best approach. There are increasing data available to help individualize this assessment of risk.

Prandoni and colleagues [79] examined patients with unprovoked thrombosis for evidence of residual vein obstruction by ultrasound at 3 months postdiagnosis (and serially thereafter, if residual vein obstruction was present). Evidence of residual vein obstruction was associated with a higher risk of VTE recurrence once anticoagulation was stopped, compared with those without residual vein obstruction (23% versus 4%, respectively, over 2 years).

A number of cohort studies have now shown that patients with elevation in D-dimers measured approximately 30 days after cessation of an adequate course of anticoagulation are at increased risk of recurrence compared with those patients with normal or low D-dimers [80–82]. Palareti and colleagues [83] performed D-dimer testing (measured by qualitative assay 1 month after cessation of anticoagulation) in patients with a first occurrence of unprovoked VTE who had received a minimum of 3 months of anticoagulation. Patients with a negative D-dimer remained off anticoagulation, whereas patients with positive D-dimer were randomized to either restart anticoagulation or remain off therapy. At an average follow-up time of 18 months, patients with an elevated D-dimer level who did not receive anticoagulation had a recurrence rate of 15%, compared with 3% among patients in whom anticoagulation had been resumed because of an elevated D-dimer and 6% among patients who remained off anticoagulation in response to a normal D-dimer. Given concerns about the persistent risk of VTE recurrence rate after discontinuation of anticoagulation despite a negative D-dimer and uncertainties regarding interpretation of clinical trials results that are based on qualitative versus quantitative D-dimer assays, the role of routine D-dimer testing to determine duration of anticoagulation for idiopathic VTE is still debated. Another large management trial is underway that may help to clarify these issues.

In patients with PE, RV dilation on presentation is a predictor of short-term adverse outcome. Further, more recent data suggest that persistent RV dilation at the time of discharge also predicts for a higher risk of recurrent VTE over the subsequent 2 to 3 years (30%, compared with 3% and 11%, respectively, in those with regression of RV dilation or no RV dilation on admission) [84].

Improving safety of anticoagulation

Anticoagulants are among the most common drugs associated with medication errors [85]. The Institute for Healthcare Improvement has included the prevention of harm from anticoagulants in its recently launched 5 Million Lives Campaign (http://www.ihi.org/IHI/Programs/Campaign/). Additionally, as a 2008 National Patient Safety Goal, the Joint Commission has proposed the addition of a requirement to "reduce the likelihood of patient harm associated with the use of anticoagulation therapy."

Inpatient anticoagulation services, staffed and managed by pharmacists, can be indispensable in advancing safe in-hospital practices surrounding the use of anticoagulation. Such services have been associated with a reduction in supratherapeutic INRs, fewer bleeding incidents, decreased length of stay, and decreased readmission for bleeding complications [86,87].

One specific focus of the proposed patient safety provisions concerns the discharge process for patients who have received therapeutic-dose anticoagulation during the hospital admission and who have been directed to continue anticoagulation as an outpatient. Communication between inpatient and outpatient providers at the time of discharge is critical. Inpatient providers should furnish those who will see the patient in follow-up for management of their anticoagulation with detailed information including discharge medications, recent INR trend, recent warfarin daily doses, and the recommended timing of the initial postdischarge INR measurement. Before discharge, patients and family members should also receive intensive education about anticoagulation therapy, highlighting (for patients discharged on warfarin) the importance of diet issues (including alcohol use), prescription and over-the-counter medications, and herbal preparations. Patients should be familiar with the signs and symptoms of bleeding or recurrent thrombosis and should be explicitly instructed to seek medical attention if they are concerned about either of these complications. Providers must emphasize the potential risks of anticoagulant therapy, the narrow therapeutic window, and the need for meticulous follow-up.

References

[1] Heit JA, Melton LJ 3rd, Lohse CM, et al. Incidence of venous thromboembolism in hospitalized patients vs community residents. Mayo Clin Proc 2001;76(11):1102–10.
[2] White RH. The epidemiology of venous thromboembolism. Circulation 2003;107(23 Suppl 1): I4–8.

[3] Silverstein MD, Heit JA, Mohr DN, et al. Trends in the incidence of deep vein thrombosis and pulmonary embolism: a 25-year population-based study. Arch Intern Med 1998;158(6): 585–93.

[4] Horlander KT, Mannino DM, Leeper KV. Pulmonary embolism mortality in the United States, 1979–1998: an analysis using multiple-cause mortality data. Arch Intern Med 2003; 163(14):1711–7.

[5] Geerts WH, Pineo GF, Heit JA, et al. Prevention of venous thromboembolism: the Seventh ACCP conference on antithrombotic and thrombolytic therapy. Chest 2004;126(3 Suppl): 338S–400S.

[6] Wells PS, Hirsh J, Anderson DR, et al. Accuracy of clinical assessment of deep-vein thrombosis. Lancet 1995;345(8961):1326–30.

[7] Segal JB, Eng J, Tamariz LJ, et al. Review of the evidence on diagnosis of deep venous thrombosis and pulmonary embolism. Ann Fam Med 2007;5(1):63–73.

[8] Fancher TL, White RH, Kravitz RL. Combined use of rapid D-dimer testing and estimation of clinical probability in the diagnosis of deep vein thrombosis: systematic review. BMJ 2004; 329(7470):821.

[9] Stein PD, Hull RD, Patel KC, et al. D-dimer for the exclusion of acute venous thrombosis and pulmonary embolism: a systematic review. Ann Intern Med 2004;140(8):589–602.

[10] Brotman DJ, Segal JB, Jani JT, et al. Limitations of D-dimer testing in unselected inpatients with suspected venous thromboembolism. Am J Med 2003;114(4):276–82.

[11] Goldhaber SZ, Simons GR, Elliott CG, et al. Quantitative plasma D-dimer levels among patients undergoing pulmonary angiography for suspected pulmonary embolism. JAMA 1993; 270(23):2819–22.

[12] Anderson FA Jr, Wheeler HB, Goldberg RJ, et al. A population-based perspective of the hospital incidence and case-fatality rates of deep vein thrombosis and pulmonary embolism. The Worcester DVT Study. Arch Intern Med 1991;151(5):933–8.

[13] Kearon C, Julian JA, Newman TE, et al. Noninvasive diagnosis of deep venous thrombosis. Mcmaster Diagnostic Imaging Practice Guidelines Initiative. Ann Intern Med 1998;128(8): 663–77.

[14] Tapson VF, Carroll BA, Davidson BL, et al. The diagnostic approach to acute venous thromboembolism. Clinical practice guideline. American thoracic society. Am J Respir Crit Care Med 1999;160(3):1043–66.

[15] Leizorovicz A, Kassai B, Becker F, et al. The assessment of deep vein thromboses for therapeutic trials. Angiology 2003;54(1):19–24.

[16] Huisman MV, Buller HR, ten Cate JW. Utility of impedance plethysmography in the diagnosis of recurrent deep-vein thrombosis. Arch Intern Med 1988;148(3):681–3.

[17] Moody AR, Pollock JG, O'Connor AR, et al. Lower-limb deep venous thrombosis: direct MR imaging of the thrombus. Radiology 1998;209(2):349–55.

[18] Moser KM, LeMoine JR. Is embolic risk conditioned by location of deep venous thrombosis? Ann Intern Med 1981;94(4 pt 1):439–44.

[19] Huisman MV, Buller HR, ten Cate JW, et al. Serial impedance plethysmography for suspected deep venous thrombosis in outpatients. The Amsterdam General Practitioner Study. N Engl J Med 1986;314(13):823–8.

[20] Stein PD, Athanasoulis C, Alavi A, et al. Complications and validity of pulmonary angiography in acute pulmonary embolism. Circulation 1992;85:462–8.

[21] Mullins MD, Becker DM, Hagspiel KD, et al. The role of spiral volumetric computed tomography in the diagnosis of pulmonary embolism. Arch Intern Med 2000;160(3): 293–8.

[22] Quiroz R, Kucher N, Zou KH, et al. Clinical validity of a negative computed tomography scan in patients with suspected pulmonary embolism: a systematic review. JAMA 2005; 293(16):2012–7.

[23] Musset D, Parent F, Meyer G, et al. Diagnostic strategy for patients with suspected pulmonary embolism: a prospective multicentre outcome study. Lancet 2002;360(9349):1914–20.

[24] van Belle A, Buller HR, Huisman MV, et al. Effectiveness of managing suspected pulmonary embolism using an algorithm combining clinical probability, D-dimer testing, and computed tomography. JAMA 2006;295(2):172–9.

[25] Oudkerk M, van Beek EJ, Wielopolski P, et al. Comparison of contrast-enhanced magnetic resonance angiography and conventional pulmonary angiography for the diagnosis of pulmonary embolism: a prospective study. Lancet 2002;359(9318):1643–7.

[26] ten Wolde M, Sohne M, Quak E, et al. Prognostic value of echocardiographically assessed right ventricular dysfunction in patients with pulmonary embolism. Arch Intern Med 2004;164(15):1685–9.

[27] Kucher N, Rossi E, De Rosa M, et al. Prognostic role of echocardiography among patients with acute pulmonary embolism and a systolic arterial pressure of 90 mm Hg or higher. Arch Intern Med 2005;165(15):1777–81.

[28] Kucher N, Printzen G, Goldhaber SZ. Prognostic role of brain natriuretic peptide in acute pulmonary embolism. Circulation 2003;107(20):2545–7.

[29] Giannitsis E, Muller-Bardorff M, Kurowski V, et al. Independent prognostic value of cardiac troponin T in patients with confirmed pulmonary embolism. Circulation 2000;102(2):211–7.

[30] Kostrubiec M, Pruszczyk P, Bochowicz A, et al. Biomarker-based risk assessment model in acute pulmonary embolism. Eur Heart J 2005;26(20):2166–72.

[31] Hull RD, Raskob GE, Brant RF, et al. Relation between the time to achieve the lower limit of the APTT therapeutic range and recurrent venous thromboembolism during heparin treatment for deep vein thrombosis. Arch Intern Med 1997;157(22):2562–8.

[32] Hull RD, Raskob GE, Brant RF, et al. The importance of initial heparin treatment on long-term clinical outcomes of antithrombotic therapy: the emerging theme of delayed recurrence. Arch Intern Med 1997;157(20):2317–21.

[33] Hommes DW, Bura A, Mazzolai L, et al. Subcutaneous heparin compared with continuous intravenous heparin administration in the initial treatment of deep vein thrombosis: a meta-analysis. Ann Intern Med 1992;116(4):279–84.

[34] Dolovich LR, Ginsberg JS, Douketis JD, et al. A meta-analysis comparing low-molecular-weight heparins with unfractionated heparin in the treatment of venous thromboembolism: examining some unanswered questions regarding location of treatment, product type, and dosing frequency. Arch Intern Med 2000;160(2):181–8.

[35] Gould MK, Dembitzer AD, Doyle RL, et al. Low-molecular-weight heparins compared with unfractionated heparin for treatment of acute deep venous thrombosis: a meta-analysis of randomized, controlled trials. Ann Intern Med 1999;130(10):800–9.

[36] Buller HR, Davidson BL, Decousus H, et al. Fondaparinux or enoxaparin for the initial treatment of symptomatic deep venous thrombosis: a randomized trial. Ann Intern Med 2004;140(11):867–73.

[37] Buller HR, Davidson BL, Decousus H, et al. Subcutaneous fondaparinux versus intravenous unfractionated heparin in the initial treatment of pulmonary embolism. N Engl J Med 2003; 349(18):1695–702.

[38] Raschke RA, Reilly BM, Guidry JR, et al. The weight-based heparin dosing nomogram compared with a "standard care" nomogram: a randomized controlled trial. Ann Intern Med 1993;119(9):874–81.

[39] Cruickshank MK, Levine MN, Hirsh J, et al. A standard heparin nomogram for the management of heparin therapy. Arch Intern Med 1991;151(2):333–7.

[40] Buller HR, Agnelli G, Hull RD, et al. Antithrombotic therapy for venous thromboembolic disease: the seventh ACCP conference on antithrombotic and thrombolytic therapy. Chest 2004;126(Suppl 3):401S–28S.

[41] Prandoni P, Carnovali M, Marchiori A. Subcutaneous adjusted-dose unfractionated heparin vs fixed-dose low-molecular-weight heparin in the initial treatment of venous thromboembolism. Arch Intern Med 2004;164(10):1077–83.

[42] Kearon C, Ginsberg JS, Julian JA, et al. Comparison of fixed-dose weight-adjusted unfrac-tionated heparin and low-molecular-weight heparin for acute treatment of venous thrombo-embolism. JAMA 2006;296(8):935–42.

[43] van Dongen CJ, van den Belt AG, Prins MH, et al. Fixed dose subcutaneous low molecular weight heparins versus adjusted dose unfractionated heparin for venous thromboembolism. Cochrane Database Syst Rev 2004;4:CD001100.

[44] Wan S, Quinlan DJ, Agnelli G, et al. Thrombolysis compared with heparin for the initial treatment of pulmonary embolism: a meta-analysis of the randomized controlled trials. Cir-culation 2004;110(6):744–9.

[45] Merli G, Spiro TE, Olsson CG, et al. Subcutaneous enoxaparin once or twice daily compared with intravenous unfractionated heparin for treatment of venous thromboembolic disease. Ann Intern Med 2001;134(3):191–202.

[46] Chong BH, Brighton TA, Baker RI, et al. Once-daily enoxaparin in the outpatient setting versus unfractionated heparin in hospital for the treatment of symptomatic deep-vein throm-bosis. J Thromb Thrombolysis 2005;19(3):173–81.

[47] Harrison L, Johnston M, Massicotte MP, et al. Comparison of 5-mg and 10-mg loading doses in initiation of warfarin therapy. Ann Intern Med 1997;126(2):133–6.

[48] Crowther MA, Ginsberg JB, Kearon C, et al. A randomized trial comparing 5-mg and 10-mg warfarin loading doses. Arch Intern Med 1999;159(1):46–8.

[49] Voora D, Eby C, Linder MW, et al. Prospective dosing of warfarin based on cytochrome P-450 2C9 genotype. Thromb Haemost 2005;93(4):700–5.

[50] Higashi MK, Veenstra DL, Kondo LM, et al. Association between CYP2C9 genetic variants and anticoagulation-related outcomes during warfarin therapy. JAMA 2002;287(13): 1690–8.

[51] Rieder MJ, Reiner AP, Gage BF, et al. Effect of VKORC1 haplotypes on transcriptional reg-ulation and warfarin dose. N Engl J Med 2005;352(22):2285–93.

[52] Wadelius M, Chen LY, Downes K, et al. Common VKORC1 and GGCX polymorphisms associated with warfarin dose. Pharmacogenomics J 2005;5(4):262–70.

[53] Millican E, Jacobsen-Lenzini PA, Milligan PE, et al. Genetic-based dosing in orthopaedic patients beginning warfarin therapy. Blood 2007;110(5):1511–5.

[54] Kreit JW. The impact of right ventricular dysfunction on the prognosis and therapy of normotensive patients with pulmonary embolism. Chest 2004;125(4):1539–45.

[55] Konstantinides S, Geibel A, Heusel G, et al. Heparin plus alteplase compared with heparin alone in patients with submassive pulmonary embolism. N Engl J Med 2002;347(15): 1143–50.

[56] Mewissen MW, Seabrook GR, Meissner MH, et al. Catheter-directed thrombolysis for lower extremity deep venous thrombosis: report of a national multicenter registry. Radiol-ogy 1999;211(1):39–49.

[57] Elsharawy M, Elzayat E. Early results of thrombolysis vs anticoagulation in iliofemoral venous thrombosis: a randomised clinical trial. Eur J Vasc Endovasc Surg 2002;24(3): 209–14.

[58] Prandoni P, Lensing AW, Piccioli A, et al. Recurrent venous thromboembolism and bleeding complications during anticoagulant treatment in patients with cancer and venous thrombo-sis. Blood 2002;100(10):3484–8.

[59] Segal JB, Streiff MB, Hoffman LV, et al. Management of venous thromboembolism: a sys-tematic review for a practice guideline. Ann Intern Med 2007;146(3):211–22.

[60] Trujillo-Santos J, Herrera S, Page MA, et al. Predicting adverse outcome in outpatients with acute deep vein thrombosis. findings from the RIETE registry. J Vasc Surg 2006;44(4): 789–93.

[61] Kovacs MJ, Anderson D, Morrow B, et al. Outpatient treatment of pulmonary embolism with dalteparin. Thromb Haemost 2000;83(2):209–11.

[62] Prandoni P, Lensing AW, Prins MH, et al. Below-knee elastic compression stockings to pre-
     vent the post-thrombotic syndrome: a randomized, controlled trial. Ann Intern Med 2004;
     141(4):249–56.
[63] Kolbach DN, Sandbrink MW, Hamulyak K, et al. Non-pharmaceutical measures for pre-
     vention of post-thrombotic syndrome. Cochrane Database Syst Rev 2004;1:CD004174.
[64] Junger M, Diehm C, Storiko H, et al. Mobilization versus immobilization in the treatment of
     acute proximal deep venous thrombosis: a prospective, randomized, open, multicentre trial.
     Curr Med Res Opin 2006;22(3):593–602.
[65] Partsch H, Kaulich M, Mayer W. Immediate mobilisation in acute vein thrombosis reduces
     post-thrombotic syndrome. Int Angiol 2004;23(3):206–12.
[66] Partsch H, Blattler W. Compression and walking versus bed rest in the treatment of prox-
     imal deep venous thrombosis with low molecular weight heparin. J Vasc Surg 2000;32(5):
     861–9.
[67] Hann CL, Streiff MB. The role of vena caval filters in the management of venous thrombo-
     embolism. Blood Rev 2005;19(4):179–202.
[68] Decousus H, Leizorovicz A, Parent F, et al. A clinical trial of vena caval filters in the preven-
     tion of pulmonary embolism in patients with proximal deep-vein thrombosis. Prevention du
     Risque d'Embolie Pulmonaire par Interruption Cave Study Group. N Engl J Med 1998;
     338(7):409–15.
[69] PREPIC Study Group. Eight-year follow-up of patients with permanent vena cava filters in
     the prevention of pulmonary embolism: the PREPIC (Prevention du Risque d'Embolie
     Pulmonaire par Interruption Cave) randomized study. Circulation 2005;112(3):416–22.
[70] Ray CE Jr, Mitchell E, Zipser S, et al. Outcomes with retrievable inferior vena cava filters:
     a multicenter study. J Vasc Interv Radiol 2006;17(10):1595–604.
[71] Lopez JA, Kearon C, Lee AY. Deep venous thrombosis. Hematology Am Soc Hematol
     Educ Program 2004;439–56.
[72] Murchison JT, Wylie L, Stockton DL. Excess risk of cancer in patients with primary venous
     thromboembolism: a national, population-based cohort study. Br J Cancer 2004;91(1):92–5.
[73] Piccioli A, Lensing AW, Prins MH, et al. Extensive screening for occult malignant disease in
     idiopathic venous thromboembolism: a prospective randomized clinical trial. J Thromb
     Haemost 2004;2(6):884–9.
[74] Levine MN, Hirsh J, Gent M, et al. Optimal duration of oral anticoagulant therapy: a ran-
     domized trial comparing four weeks with three months of warfarin in patients with proximal
     deep vein thrombosis. Thromb Haemost 1995;74(2):606–11.
[75] Schulman S, Rhedin AS, Lindmarker P, et al. A comparison of six weeks with six months of
     oral anticoagulant therapy after a first episode of venous thromboembolism. Duration of
     Anticoagulation Trial Study Group. N Engl J Med 1995;332(25):1661–5.
[76] Eichinger S, Weltermann A, Minar E, et al. Symptomatic pulmonary embolism and the risk
     of recurrent venous thromboembolism. Arch Intern Med 2004;164(1):92–6.
[77] Kearon C, Ginsberg JS, Kovacs MJ, et al. Comparison of low-intensity warfarin therapy
     with conventional-intensity warfarin therapy for long-term prevention of recurrent venous
     thromboembolism. N Engl J Med 2003;349(7):631–9.
[78] Ridker PM, Goldhaber SZ, Glynn RJ. Low-intensity versus conventional-intensity warfarin
     for prevention of recurrent venous thromboembolism. N Engl J Med 2003;349(22):2164–7,
     author reply 2164-7.
[79] Prandoni P, Lensing AW, Prins MH, et al. Residual venous thrombosis as a predictive factor
     of recurrent venous thromboembolism. Ann Intern Med 2002;137(12):955–60.
[80] Palareti G, Legnani C, Cosmi B, et al. Risk of venous thromboembolism recurrence: high
     negative predictive value of D-dimer performed after oral anticoagulation is stopped.
     Thromb Haemost 2002;87(1):7–12.
[81] Palareti G, Legnani C, Cosmi B, et al. Predictive value of D-dimer test for recurrent venous
     thromboembolism after anticoagulation withdrawal in subjects with a previous idiopathic
     event and in carriers of congenital thrombophilia. Circulation 2003;108(3):313–8.

[82] Eichinger S, Minar E, Bialonczyk C, et al. D-dimer levels and risk of recurrent venous thromboembolism. JAMA 2003;290(8):1071–4.

[83] Palareti G, Cosmi B, Legnani C, et al. D-dimer testing to determine the duration of anticoagulation therapy. N Engl J Med 2006;355(17):1780–9.

[84] Grifoni S, Vanni S, Magazzini S, et al. Association of persistent right ventricular dysfunction at hospital discharge after acute pulmonary embolism with recurrent thromboembolic events. Arch Intern Med 2006;166(19):2151–6.

[85] Fanikos J, Stapinski C, Koo S, et al. Medication errors associated with anticoagulant therapy in the hospital. Am J Cardiol 2004;94(4):532–5.

[86] Bond CA, Raehl CL. Pharmacist-provided anticoagulation management in United States hospitals: death rates, length of stay, Medicare charges, bleeding complications, and transfusions. Pharmacotherapy 2004;24(8):953–63.

[87] Dager WE, Branch JM, King JH, et al. Optimization of inpatient warfarin therapy: impact of daily consultation by a pharmacist-managed anticoagulation service. Ann Pharmacother 2000;34(5):567–72.

ELSEVIER
SAUNDERS

Med Clin N Am 92 (2008) 467–479

THE MEDICAL
CLINICS
OF NORTH AMERICA

Critical Care Medicine for the Hospitalist

Derek J. Linderman, MD[a], William J. Janssen, MD[a,b],*

[a]*Division of Pulmonary Sciences and Critical Care Medicine, University of Colorado Health Science Center, 4200 E 9th Ave., C272, Denver, CO 80262, USA*
[b]*Department of Medicine, National Jewish Medical and Research Center, K729B, 1400 Jackson St., Denver, CO 80206, USA*

More than 85% of hospitalists take care of patients in the intensive care unit (ICU) [1]. Those who do not almost certainly will be asked to participate in the care of these individuals at other points during hospitalization. It is important for hospitalists to be familiar with current practice guidelines and management principles for common ICU diagnoses. Two of the most common reasons for admission to the ICU include sepsis and respiratory failure. Sepsis is the tenth leading cause of death in the United States and the primary cause of death in the ICU [2]. Respiratory failure caries an equally high mortality; more than one third of patients with acute respiratory failure do not survive to discharge [3]. Another frequent diagnosis in the ICU is anemia, which can be potentially life threatening. The management of these common diagnoses has evolved in recent years as new data have emerged that impact morbidity and mortality. The aim of this article is to review some of these important topics in critical care medicine, including the latest management recommendations for sepsis, the use of noninvasive ventilation in respiratory failure, and practice guidelines for transfusion in critically ill patients.

Sepsis and septic shock

There are more than 750,000 cases of sepsis in the United States each year, which result in 210,000 deaths [2]. The incidence has doubled in the last two decades and the trend is expected to continue, with estimates that by 2020 the United States will experience 1 million additional cases

---

* Corresponding author. Department of Medicine, National Jewish Medical and Research Center, K729B, 1400 Jackson St., Denver, CO 80206.
E-mail address: janssenw@njc.org (W.J. Janssen).

0025-7125/08/$ - see front matter © 2008 Elsevier Inc. All rights reserved.
doi:10.1016/j.mcna.2007.10.005 *medical.theclinics.com*

annually. The primary reasons for this dramatic increase are aging of the population, increased frequency of invasive procedures, and the development of antibiotic-resistant organisms. In addition to the clinical burden of sepsis, the financial impact is significant. Sepsis accounts for 40% of total ICU expenditures and costs more than $16 billion each year [2].

Until recently, no single agent or treatment strategy has demonstrated sufficient efficacy to warrant routine use. Several new therapies have emerged that seem to impact morbidity and survival, however, including early goal-directed therapy, activated protein C, and the use of low-dose corticosteroids. This article discusses these new interventions and the early management of sepsis.

Sepsis is a clinical syndrome that begins with a localized infection followed by systemic inflammation and widespread tissue injury. If left untreated, tissue hypoperfusion, hypotension, and organ damage ensue. The severity of sepsis is best classified using criteria established by the American College of Chest Physicians and Society of Critical Care Medicine (Table 1) [4]. It is important to note that the systemic inflammatory response syndrome is a widespread inflammatory response that results from any insult (eg, trauma, pancreatitis, transfusion reaction). Systemic inflammatory response syndrome caused by infection is termed "sepsis."

Table 1
Classification of sepsis by stage

Stage of sepsis	Features
Systemic inflammatory response syndrome	Must have at least two of the following: 1. Temperature $> 38°C$ or $< 36°C$ 2. Heart rate > 90 beats/min 3. Respiratory rate > 20 breaths/min or $Paco_2$ < 32 mm Hg 4. White blood cell count $> 12,000$ cells/mm^3 or < 4000 cells/mm^3, or $> 10\%$ immature (band) forms
Sepsis	Systemic inflammatory response syndrome plus presumed infection[a]
Severe sepsis	Sepsis with one of the following: 1. organ dysfunction 2. hypoperfusion 3. hypotension
Septic shock	Sepsis with 1. hypotension despite adequate fluid resuscitation[b] 2. hypoperfusion

[a] The diagnosis of infection does not require positive cultures. Infection can be presumed from clinical findings, such as infiltrates on a chest radiograph, bacteria in the urine, or the presence of white blood cells in an otherwise sterile space.

[b] Patients who require vasopressors or inotropic therapy despite adequate fluid resuscitation are in septic shock.

Sepsis results from complex interactions between the infecting micro-organism and the host inflammatory, coagulation, and immune responses. Early sepsis is characterized by a proinflammatory state in which neutro-phils are activated and high levels of inflammatory cytokines are present. Proteases, prostaglandins, and leukotrienes released from inflammatory cells damage the vascular endothelium, which results in leakage of pro-tein-rich fluid from the capillaries and release of nitric oxide, a potent vaso-dilator. Vasodilatation of the arterial capillary networks and venous capacitance beds results in low peripheral vascular resistance with reflexive tachycardia and hypotension. In most patients, the cardiac output is initially high. As sepsis progresses, however, myocardial suppression may occur, leading to inadequate cardiac output.

The aforementioned physiologic derangements are often compounded by hypovolemia. Patients who have sepsis often have poor oral fluid intake and large insensible water losses through the skin and respiratory tract. The end result is a state of regional and systemic hypoperfusion. Perfusion is also im-paired on a microscopic level. Injury to the vascular endothelium coupled with a procoagulant state leads to platelet aggregation and microvascular thrombosis. Microvascular defects are further exacerbated by changes in erythrocyte biochemistry that cause the red cells to become rigid and lose their ability to deform in an already compromised microcirculation. Treat-ment of sepsis requires prompt correction of these abnormalities to correct microvascular and systemic hypoperfusion. Prolonged impairment of oxy-gen delivery leads to tissue hypoxia, multiple organ failure, and death.

The first step in the management of patients who have sepsis is to assess airway stability, respiration, and perfusion. Mechanical ventilation should be considered in patients with unstable blood pressure, encephalopathy, se-vere sepsis, or septic shock. Etomidate is an ultrashort-acting sedative agent commonly used for endotracheal intubation. It should be avoided in pa-tients who have sepsis because it can cause adrenal insufficiency and may worsen survival [5].

Tissue perfusion can be improved through correction of hypovolemia, im-provement of blood pressure, and augmentation of cardiovascular oxygen de-livery. Early goal-directed therapy with targeted achievement of physiologic endpoints improves survival [6]. Goals for the first 6 hours of care include reaching (1) central venous pressure between 8 and 12 mm Hg, (2) mean arte-rial pressure more than 65 mm Hg, and (3) central venous oxygen saturation (S_cvO_2) more than 70%. These endpoints are best achieved by sequential use of intravenous fluids, vasopressors, inotropic agents, and blood transfusion.

Intravenous fluids should be administered immediately after the sepsis syndrome is recognized. Fluid resuscitation can proceed through any avail-able intravenous access; however, in patients who have severe sepsis or septic shock, a central venous catheter should be placed to facilitate fluid adminis-tration and monitoring of venous filling pressures and S_cvO_2 [6]. The central venous pressure and S_cvO_2 can be obtained from a well-positioned internal jugular or subclavian central venous catheter (femoral venous catheters do not accurately reflect central venous measurements). Pulmonary artery catheters can provide similar information and information about left-sided filling pressures. Use of pulmonary artery catheters does not improve outcomes, however, and tends to have higher complication rates [7]. Most patients who have severe sepsis can be managed appropriately with a central venous catheter.

Intravenous fluids should be administered rapidly as boluses. No evidence suggests superiority of crystalloids over colloids, although the volume of distribution is greater for crystalloids, which mandates larger infusion volumes. Crystalloids (eg, normal saline or Ringer's lactate) should be administered at a rate of 500 to 1000 mL over 30 minutes. Colloids should be given at a rate of 300 to 500 mL every 30 minutes. The central venous pressure and mean arterial blood pressure should be assessed immediately after each fluid bolus. Intravenous fluid boluses should be repeated until the central venous pressure reaches 8 to 12 mm Hg, pulmonary edema develops, or the pulmonary capillary wedge pressure exceeds 18 mm Hg. Most patients require 6 to 10 L of crystalloid for initial resuscitation [8].

Vasopressors are required for patients who remain hypotensive despite fluid resuscitation. Norepinephrine and dopamine are potent vasoconstrictors and should be used as first-line agents. They should be administered as continuous infusions and titrated to maintain a mean arterial blood pressure more than 65 mm Hg. Vasopressin is an antidiuretic hormone analog with weak vasoconstrictive effects. It is not recommended as a first-line agent for septic shock but may have a role in refractory cases. Two small studies have suggested that a fixed infusion dose of 0.04 U/min lowers norepinephrine requirements and improves creatinine clearance [9,10].

Once hypovolemia and hypotension have been corrected, the clinician must reassess the patient for evidence of continued hypoperfusion. Two clinically useful markers of perfusion are serum lactate and the central venous oxygen saturation. The S_cvO_2 can be measured by drawing a blood gas from the distal port of a central venous catheter or by using one of several commercially available central venous catheters capable of continuous S_cvO_2 measurement. A rising serum lactate or an S_cvO_2 less than 70% suggests tissue hypoxia and inadequate systemic oxygen delivery. Oxygen delivery can be augmented by improving cardiac output or increasing the oxygen-carrying capacity of blood. The latter is achieved by transfusion of packed red blood cells and should be considered when the hematocrit is less than 30% [6]. Cardiac output can be improved by use of inotropic agents. Dobutamine is the drug of choice in patients with shock. Doses between 3 and 12 $\mu g/kg/min$ can improve the cardiac index by 20% to 40% [11,12]. Peripheral vasodilatation and tachycardia can result; dobutamine is often used with a vasoconstrictor, such as norepinephrine.

Antibiotics should be administered at the same time that physiologic derangements are being corrected. The time from diagnosis to initiation of antibiotic therapy is the strongest predictor of mortality in sepsis [13]. Inappropriate initial antibiotic selection is unfortunately common and occurs in up to one third of cases [14]. Prompt identification and control of the infection site are essential. A careful history and physical examination often provide clues to the source of infection. Blood cultures, a chest radiograph, and urinalysis with culture are recommended for all patients. Additional diagnostic studies (eg, abdominal CT or lumbar puncture) should be driven by clinical clues.

In some instances an infectious cause is not readily apparent. Empiric broad-spectrum antibiotics should be administered to cover gram-positive and -negative bacteria. Antifungal agents should be considered in patients who have prolonged neutropenia or hematologic malignancies. The rates of methicillin-resistant *Staphylococcus aureus* infection are increasing in hospitalized patients and in the community [15,16]. Intravenous vancomycin should be considered in all patients until methicillin-resistant *S aureus* has been excluded. Once a microbial pathogen has been isolated, antibiotic therapy should be tailored to provide more narrow and appropriate coverage.

The use of corticosteroids in severe sepsis and septic shock has gained recent favor. Evidence suggests that a large proportion of critically ill patients suffer from relative adrenal insufficiency [17]. Hypothalamic, pituitary, and adrenal gland function are impaired by proinflammatory cytokines. The adrenal glands also can be damaged directly by infection, hemorrhage, and ischemic infarction or inhibited by drugs such as etomidate and ketoconazole. Adrenal function is commonly assessed by measuring a baseline serum cortisol level and examining the adrenal gland response to adrenocorticotropin-releasing hormone (ACTH). A baseline cortisol level of less than 15 μg/dL is generally considered insufficient in critically ill patients [18]. Conversely, baseline cortisol levels more than 34 μg/dL generally indicate adequate adrenal reserve. When the baseline cortisol level is between 15 and 34 μg/dL, the response to ACTH should be used as a guide.

One multicenter, randomized, controlled trial of patients who had septic shock showed reduced mortality in patients who had relative adrenal insufficiency (defined by a post-ACTH cortisol level increase $\leq$ 9 μg/dL) who were treated with a combination of 50 mg intravenous hydrocortisone four times daily and once-daily fludrocortisone (50 μg orally) for 7 days [19]. Corticosteroid administration did not improve mortality in patients who responded to ACTH (change in cortisol > 9 μg/dL). Other randomized, controlled trials have demonstrated significant effects on shock reversal with hydrocortisone [20]. A second multicenter, randomized, double-blind, placebo control trial is currently underway in Europe to verify these findings.

Patients in septic shock with a baseline cortisol level of more than 34 μg/dL are at high risk for death [17]. Because their adrenal glands are capable of producing cortisol, it is unlikely that they will benefit from steroid replacement. Until the results of ongoing studies are released, we recommend that all patients in septic shock have serum cortisol levels measured at baseline and then 60 minutes after a 250-μg dose of intravenous ACTH. Corticosteroids should be administered until test results have returned. Table 2 serves as a guide for determining when to continue corticosteroid treatment.

Activated protein C is an endogenous protein that inhibits thrombin formation, enhances fibrinolysis, and modulates inflammation. Reduced levels are found in most patients who have sepsis, which has been hypothesized to contribute to microvascular thrombosis and dysregulation of the coagulation cascade. The only commercially available source of recombinant human activated protein C is drotrecogin alpha. Several large clinical trials have explored the use of this agent in patients with severe sepsis or septic shock and have demonstrated a significant survival benefit in selected patients who are treated within the first 48 hours of diagnosis [21,22]. The benefit is most pronounced when therapy is started within 24 hours and in patients with multiorgan failure [23].

The APACHE II scoring system predicts mortality in critically ill patients based on physiologic parameters, laboratory data, age, and the presence of chronic disease [24]. Patients with higher scores are sicker and more likely to die. Patients with an APACHE II score of less than 25 do not benefit from drotrecogin alpha and are not candidates for therapy [25]. Drotrecogin alpha is administered as a constant infusion for 96 hours at a rate of 24 μg/kg/h. The major risk is bleeding, which is seen in up to 2.4% of patients [23]. The infusion should be stopped 2 hours before surgery or invasive procedures. It can be restarted 12 hours after surgery or 2 hours after less invasive procedures. The bleeding risk is greatest in patients with a platelet count less than 30,000/μL. If platelet levels drop below this threshold during the course of infusion, platelets should be transfused. Because of the significant risk of bleeding and the complexity of patient selection, consultation with a critical care specialist or infectious disease expert should be considered before using drotrecogin alpha.

Transfusion in the intensive care unit

Anemia is a common condition in critically ill patients. Forty percent to 50% of patients admitted to the ICU receive at least one transfusion during hospitalization, and 85% of patients with an ICU stay of 1 week or more receive a transfusion [26,27]. Despite an average admission hemoglobin level

Table 2
Recommendations for Corticosteroid Treatment in Septic Shock.

Baseline cortisol	< 15 μg/dL	15–34 μg/dL		> 34 μg/dL
Change in cortisol following ACTH		≤ 9 μg/dL	> 9 μg/dL	
Corticosteroids indicated?	Yes	Yes	No	No

of 11.3 g/dL, the median time to first transfusion is only 2 days [28]. Patients who remain in the ICU for more than 7 days have a constant transfusion requirement of one to two units of red blood cells per week [26,27]. Given such high resource use and the potential risk of adverse events, there has been significant interest in understanding why critically ill patients require frequent transfusions and when the balance of risks and benefits tips in favor of transfusion.

Multiple factors lead to anemia in the ICU. One of the most obvious causes is acute blood loss related to either invasive procedures or gastrointestinal bleeding. A second cause is phlebotomy, which can account for more than 40 mL of blood loss per day [28]. Intravascular hemolysis also can contribute to anemia, particularly in patients with disseminated intravascular coagulation. In addition to suffering red cell loss, critically ill patients have an underproduction anemia characterized by abnormal use of iron stores and diminished production of erythropoietin [29].

Although there are benefits to giving blood, several risks are associated with transfusion. Transmission of infection, although low because of modern screening methods, is one such risk. Other risks include volume overload, hemolytic reactions, and immunomodulatory effects. Immune system modulation can manifest in one of two ways: activation or down-regulation. Immune system down-regulation can increase the risk of infection and cancer recurrence in patients who have received allogenic blood transfusion. Typical transfusion reactions, transfusion-related acute lung injury, and the rare but serious transfusion-associated graft-versus-host disease are caused by donor or recipient leukocyte activation to foreign antigens [29].

Red blood cell transfusion has become an important component of the initial management of patients who have septic shock [6]. The mechanism by which red cell transfusion improves tissue perfusion remains unclear, however. Studies in septic euvolemic patients have shown that erythrocyte transfusion increases oxygen delivery but tissue oxygen extraction actually decreases and myocardial minute work increases [30]. Red blood cell storage techniques may provide a partial explanation. Depletion of 2,3-diphosphoglycerate in stored blood causes a left shift in the oxygen-dissociation curve. This shift enhances the ability of red cells to bind oxygen but prevents oxygen release at the tissue level. Storage also may result in loss of cellular antioxidants, which leads to cellular rigidity and sludging in the microcirculation. Depletion of antioxidants also can lead to conversion of hemoglobin to methemoglobin, which further impairs unloading of oxygen [29].

Given the potential risks of red blood cell transfusion and the possibility that transfusion of blood may not yield significant benefits, there has been great interest in determining when a patient ideally should receive transfusion. One of the first studies to shed light on transfusion practices in the ICU showed that 85% of patients who stayed in the ICU for 1 week or more received transfusion on average of 9.5 units of red blood cells [27].

Patients who required more than 5 units of blood had more ventilator days, more days in the ICU, and higher mortality rates compared with patients who received fewer (or no) transfusions. Most transfusions for nonacute blood loss either had no indication noted or were given solely for a low hematocrit [26]. A randomized trial was performed to see if outcomes differed between a restrictive transfusion group (target hemoglobin 7–9 g/dL) and a liberal transfusion group (target hemoglobin 10–12 g/dL). There was a lower mortality rate during hospitalization in the restrictive group, but 30- and 60-day mortality rates were not significantly different between the two. Patients in the restrictive transfusion group who were less ill (APACHE II score ≤ 20) and younger (age ≤ 55) had a significantly lower 30-day mortality then their counterparts in the liberal group. There was no mortality difference between the two transfusion strategies in patients with known cardiac disease. More cardiac events were seen in the liberal transfusion group [31].

Patients with cardiovascular disease traditionally have been considered a group that benefits from a higher hematocrit. Recent data suggested that patients with acute coronary syndromes who undergo erythrocyte transfusion actually may have a higher mortality, however [32]. Randomized trials support this notion and indicate that a restrictive transfusion strategy is safe in critically ill patients who have coronary artery disease [31,33]. The exact level at which blood should be transfused is unknown. For example, one study demonstrated that elderly patients who were admitted to the ICU with acute coronary syndromes and a hematocrit less than 24% benefited from transfusion [34]. Their counterparts who had hematocrit levels of more than 24% did not benefit from transfusion, and patients with hematocrit levels more than 36% were harmed. In contrast, younger patients with coronary disease may be able to tolerate hemoglobin transfusion thresholds as low as 7 g/dL (or hematocrit of 21%) [33].

The following approach is recommended for patients who do not have active bleeding. Patients who have severe sepsis or septic shock should receive red blood cells as part of an acute resuscitation algorithm if the hematocrit is less than 30% and there is evidence of tissue hypoperfusion despite adequate volume resuscitation and correction of hypotension. Once tissue hypoperfusion has been corrected, a restrictive transfusion strategy should be adopted to maintain a hematocrit more than 21%. This hematocrit level is appropriate for most patients in ICU, including those with stable coronary disease. Patients with acute coronary syndromes may benefit from a higher hematocrit level, although the absolute level remains controversial. We suggest that a hematocrit of 24% is reasonable for many patients with acute coronary syndromes but advocate an approach in which the treating physician takes all clinical variables into account rather than just a laboratory value.

Because transfusion of packed red blood cells carries potential harm, there has been significant interest in other methods to safely increase hemoglobin levels, namely administration of exogenous recombinant human erythropoietin. Results have been disappointing. Taken together, the results of several large trials demonstrate no improvement in survival, hospital length of stay, or days free of mechanical ventilation in patients treated with erythropoietin compared with placebo [35–38]. Erythropoietin may increase hemoglobin levels in patients managed with a restrictive transfusion strategy [36] and may reduce the number of transfusions required per patient [37], but the magnitude of these changes is small and unlikely to provide significant clinical benefit. Trauma patients may be an exception to this rule. Subgroup analysis of a recent large trial showed a survival benefit in trauma victims treated with erythropoietin compared with placebo [38]. This trial also documented an increased incidence of thrombotic events in patients treated with erythropoietin. In our opinion, the current data do not support the routine use of erythropoietin in the medical or surgical ICU. A possible exception is trauma patients, although further studies are needed in this group.

Respiratory failure and noninvasive ventilation

Respiratory failure is a frequent cause of admission to the ICU. There are nearly 330,000 episodes of acute respiratory failure in the United States each year [3]. Of these episodes, almost 20% are treated with endotracheal intubation and mechanical ventilation [3]. Although mechanical ventilation remains the definitive therapy, noninvasive positive pressure ventilation (NPPV) is increasingly used for hypercapnic and hypoxic respiratory failure. The benefit of this modality is that patients can avoid potential risks and complications of invasive ventilation, such as ventilator-associated pneumonia, sinusitis, prolonged use of sedation, and tracheal stenosis.

NPPV is a pressure support mode of ventilation in which the patient receives ventilatory support through the use of a tight-fitting mask. Ventilatory support can be provided through continuous administration of positive airway pressure (CPAP) or through biphasic administration of pressure (bilevel). With CPAP, the patient receives a constant level of pressure support that is maintained throughout the respiratory cycle. Bilevel ventilation provides a high level of pressure support during inspiration known as inspiratory positive airway pressure and a lower level of pressure during exhalation, which is termed expiratory positive airway pressure. Additional parameters that can be adjusted for NPPV include the fraction of inspired oxygen, a backup respiratory rate to help reduce apneas, and a rise time that determines how long the inspiratory pressure is delivered.

Typically the inspiratory pressure is titrated upward to increase a patient's tidal volume and is the first parameter to adjust in hypercapnic respiratory failure. Expiratory pressure works much like positive end expiratory pressure during conventional ventilation. It helps recruit atelectatic or partially consolidated alveolar units, thereby improving oxygenation. It also helps to stent open the easily collapsible airways seen in patients with obstructive sleep apnea, tracheomalacia, and chronic obstructive pulmonary disease. Expiratory positive airway pressure is most beneficial for patients with hypoxemic respiratory failure but is also being used in patients with obstructive lung disease and hypercapnea. In addition to improving gas exchange, NPPV can ease the work of breathing and prevent respiratory muscle fatigue.

There are various interfaces for noninvasive ventilation. Typical devices are either a nasal mask that covers just the nose or a full-face mask that fits over the nose and mouth. Additional interfaces include nasal pillows that fit in the nostrils and helmets that may cover the entire face or head. All interfaces require a good seal so that the set pressure is delivered and not allowed to leak out. Patient comfort and good fit of the mask are important determinants of whether NPPV succeeds or fails.

Chronic obstructive pulmonary disease is one of the most common conditions in which NPPV is used. During severe disease exacerbations, the use of NPPV reduces intubation rates and improves mortality [39–42]. NPPV also reduces hospital length of stay by an average of 5.6 days [41,42]. NPPV also has been well studied in respiratory failure associated with acute cardiogenic pulmonary edema. The application of positive pressure to the thorax works to improve respiratory mechanics and reduces transudation of fluid across the alveolar membrane. Cardiac preload and afterload are reduced, which improves cardiac output. There is a significant reduction in the rate of intubation and mortality in patients with pulmonary edema receiving NPPV compared with standard therapy [43,44].

There is debate as to whether CPAP is superior to bilevel NPPV in treatment of acute pulmonary edema. Although CPAP is clearly superior to standard therapy alone, the use of bilevel NPPV did not meet statistical significance for mortality when compared with standard therapy in two meta-analyses [43,44]. This difference is most easily attributable to a smaller number of patients and fewer studies using bilevel. There is also concern that bilevel may increase the risk of myocardial infarction. In a randomized trial that compared bilevel ventilation with CPAP, the rates of myocardial infarction were higher in the bilevel group [45]. Importantly, this risk was not borne out when bilevel was compared with standard therapy [44,45]. Although the benefits of NPPV in patients with respiratory failure caused by cardiogenic pulmonary edema are clear, further investigation is needed to clarify whether CPAP is safer and more efficacious than bilevel.

Hypoxemic respiratory failure can result from various causes, including pneumonia, acute pulmonary edema, acute lung injury, acute respiratory distress syndrome, and atelectasis. The benefits of NPPV in this group as a whole are unclear. Some studies suggest an overall reduction in ICU length of stay and mortality, whereas others do not [46]. Heterogeneity in the cause and underlying physiology most likely accounts for the discrepancies. Two groups of patients with hypoxemic respiratory failure that do seem to benefit from NPPV are immunosuppressed patients with acute pneumonia and postoperative patients who have undergone lung resection [47]. Even in these groups the failure rate of NPPV remains high. NPPV should be instituted with caution in patients with hypoxemic respiratory failure. Close patient monitoring is essential, and mechanical ventilation should be considered quickly if there is any evidence of treatment failure.

It should be noted that the positive pressures used in the aforementioned clinical trials were relatively high and may be greater than many physicians are accustomed to using. The average inspiratory positive airway pressure setting was 15 to 20 cm H_2O, and the typical expiratory positive airway pressure used was 5 cm H_2O [39,40,43]. These higher pressures may be necessary to achieve the reported reductions in intubation rates and mortality. Initiation and titration of noninvasive ventilation requires well-trained respiratory therapists and may require consultation with a pulmonary specialist. Patients with hemodynamic instability are not candidates for NPPV. Other exclusion criteria include gastrointestinal bleeding and emesis, which place patients at high risk for aspiration, encephalopathy, or patient agitation that compromise the patient's ability to interact with the NPPV system, and facial deformities or trauma, which prohibits use of a tight-fitting mask.

NPPV has clear benefits for patients with hypercapnic respiratory failure from chronic obstructive pulmonary disease and hypoxemic respiratory failure from acute cardiogenic pulmonary edema. NPPV is the standard initial therapy in these conditions provided that a contraindication does not exist. Widespread use of NPPV in other scenarios, such as hypoxemic respiratory failure, is not recommended, although select groups tend to do better than others. Intubation and mechanical ventilation should be instituted promptly if a patient is not improving in a timely manner.

Summary

Sepsis, anemia, and respiratory failure are common entities in the ICU and result in significant morbidity and mortality. Recent advances with documented improvement in clinical outcomes include the use of early goal-directed therapy, low-dose corticosteroids, and activated protein C in septic shock, practices that minimize red blood cell transfusion in the ICU, and the use of NPPV in patients with acute respiratory failure from pulmonary edema and chronic obstructive pulmonary disease.

References

[1] Lindenauer PK, Pantilat SZ, Katz PP, et al. Hospitalists and the practice of inpatient medicine: results of a survey of the National Association of Inpatient Physicians. Ann Intern Med 1999;130:343–9.

[2] Angus DC, Linde-Zwirble WT, Lidicker J, et al. Epidemiology of severe sepsis in the United States: analysis of incidence, outcome, and associated costs of care. Crit Care Med 2001; 29(7):1303–10.

[3] Behrendt CE. Acute respiratory failure in the United States: incidence and 31-day survival. Chest 2000;118(4):1100–5.

[4] Levy MM, Fink MP, Marshall JC, et al. 2001 SCCM/ESICM/ACCP/ATS/SIS International Sepsis Definitions Conference. Crit Care Med 2003;31(4):1250–6.

[5] Absalom A, Pledger D, Kong A. Adrenocortical function in critically ill patients 24 h after a single dose of etomidate. Anaesthesia 1999;54(9):861–7.

[6] Rivers E, Nguyen B, Havstad S, et al. Early goal-directed therapy in the treatment of severe sepsis and septic shock. N Engl J Med 2001;345(19):1368–77.

[7] ARDS Clinical Trials Network. Pulmonary-artery versus central venous catheter to guide treatment of acute lung injury. N Engl J Med 2006;354(21):2213–24.

[8] Rackow EC, Falk JL, Fein IA, et al. Fluid resuscitation in circulatory shock: a comparison of the cardiorespiratory effects of albumin, hetastarch, and saline solutions in patients with hypovolemic and septic shock. Crit Care Med 1983;11(11):839–50.

[9] Dunser MW, Mayr AJ, Ulmer H, et al. Arginine vasopressin in advanced vasodilatory shock: a prospective, randomized, controlled study. Circulation 2003;107(18):2313–9.

[10] Patel BM, Chittock DR, Russell JA, et al. Beneficial effects of short-term vasopressin infusion during severe septic shock. Anesthesiology 2002;96(3):576–82.

[11] De Backer D, Berre J, Zhang H, et al. Relationship between oxygen uptake and oxygen delivery in septic patients: effects of prostacyclin versus dobutamine. Crit Care Med 1993; 21(11):1658–64.

[12] Jardin F, Sportiche M, Bazin M, et al. Dobutamine: a hemodynamic evaluation in human septic shock. Crit Care Med 1981;9(4):329–32.

[13] Kumar A, Roberts D, Wood KE, et al. Duration of hypotension before initiation of effective antimicrobial therapy is the critical determinant of survival in human septic shock. Crit Care Med 2006;34(6):1589–96.

[14] Leibovici L, Paul M, Poznanski O, et al. Monotherapy versus beta-lactam-aminoglycoside combination treatment for gram-negative bacteremia: a prospective, observational study. Antimicrob Agents Chemother 1997;41(5):1127–33.

[15] Miller LG, Perdreau-Remington F, Rieg G, et al. Necrotizing fasciitis caused by community-associated methicillin-resistant *Staphylococcus aureus* in Los Angeles. N Engl J Med 2005; 352(14):1445–53.

[16] Fridkin SK, Hageman JC, Morrison M, et al. Methicillin-resistant *Staphylococcus aureus* disease in three communities. N Engl J Med 2005;352(14):1436–44.

[17] Annane D, Sebille V, Troche G, et al. A 3-level prognostic classification in septic shock based on cortisol levels and cortisol response to corticotropin. JAMA 2000;283(8):1038–45.

[18] Cooper MS, Stewart PM. Corticosteroid insufficiency in acutely ill patients. N Engl J Med 2003;348(8):727–34.

[19] Annane D, Sebille V, Charpentier C, et al. Effect of treatment with low doses of hydrocortisone and fludrocortisone on mortality in patients with septic shock. JAMA 2002;288(7): 862–71.

[20] Minneci PC, Deans KJ, Banks SM, et al. Meta-analysis: the effect of steroids on survival and shock during sepsis depends on the dose. Ann Intern Med 2004;141(1):47–56.

[21] Bernard GR, Vincent JL, Laterre PF, et al. Efficacy and safety of recombinant human activated protein C for severe sepsis. N Engl J Med 2001;344(10):699–709.

[22] Vincent JL, Bernard GR, Beale R, et al. Drotrecogin alfa (activated) treatment in severe sepsis from the global open-label trial ENHANCE: further evidence for survival and safety and implications for early treatment. Crit Care Med 2005;33(10):2266–77.

[23] Vincent JL, Angus DC, Artigas A, et al. Effects of drotrecogin alfa (activated) on organ dysfunction in the PROWESS trial. Crit Care Med 2003;31(3):834–40.

[24] Knaus WA, Draper EA, Wagner DP, et al. APACHE II: a severity of disease classification system. Crit Care Med 1985;13(10):818–29.

[25] Abraham E, Laterre PF, Garg R, et al. Drotrecogin alfa (activated) for adults with severe sepsis and a low risk of death. N Engl J Med 2005;353(13):1332–41.

[26] Corwin HL, Parsonnet KC, Gettinger A. RBC transfusion in the ICU: is there a reason? Chest 1995;108(3):767–71.

[27] Corwin HL, Gettinger A, Pearl RG, et al. The CRIT study: anemia and blood transfusion in the critically ill: current clinical practice in the United States. Crit Care Med 2004;32:39–52.

[28] Vincent JL, Baron JF, Reinhart K, et al. Anemia and blood transfusion in critically ill patients. JAMA 2002;288(12):1499–507.

[29] Raghavan M, Marik PE. Anemia, allogenic blood transfusion, and immunomodulation in the critically ill. Chest 2005;127(1):295–307.

[30] Dietrich KA, Conrad SA, Hebert CA, et al. Cardiovascular and metabolic response to red blood cell transfusion in critically ill volume-resuscitated nonsurgical patients. Crit Care Med 1990;18(9):940–4.

[31] Hébert PC, Wells G, Blajchman MA, et al. A multicenter, randomized, controlled clinical trial of transfusion requirements in critical care. N Engl J Med 1999;340(6):409–17.

[32] Rao SV, Jollis JG, Harrington RA, et al. Relationship of blood transfusion and clinical outcomes in patients with acute coronary syndromes. JAMA 2004;292(13):1555–62.

[33] Hébert PC, Yetisir E, Martin C, et al. Is a low transfusion threshold safe in critically ill patients with cardiovascular diseases? Crit Care Med 2001;29(2):227–33.

[34] Wu WC, Rathore SS, Wang Y, et al. Blood transfusion in elderly patients with acute myocardial infarction. N Engl J Med 2001;345(17):1230–6.

[35] Corwin HL, Gettinger A, Rodriguez RM, et al. Efficacy of recombinant human erythropoietin in the critically ill patient: a randomized double-blind placebo-controlled trial. Crit Care Med 1999;27(11):2346–50.

[36] Corwin HL, Gettinger A, Pearl RG, et al. Efficacy of recombinant human erythropoietin in the critically ill patient: a randomized controlled trial. JAMA 2002;288:2827–35.

[37] Zarychanski R, Turgeon AF, McIntyre L, et al. Erythropoietin-receptor agonists in critically ill patients: a meta-analysis of randomized controlled trials. CMAJ 2007;177(7):725–34.

[38] Corwin HL, Gettinger A, Fabian TC, et al. Efficacy and safety of epoetin alfa in critically ill patients. N Engl J Med 2007;357(10):965–76.

[39] Brochard L, Mancebo J, Wysocki M, et al. Noninvasive ventilation for acute exacerbations of chronic obstructive pulmonary disease. N Engl J Med 1995;333(13):817–22.

[40] Çelikel T, Sungur M, Cehan B, et al. Comparison of noninvasive positive pressure ventilation with standard medical therapy in hypercapneic acute respiratory failure. Chest 1998; 114(6):1636–42.

[41] Keenan SP, Sinuff T, Cook DJ, et al. Which patients with acute exacerbation of chronic obstructive pulmonary disease benefit from noninvasive positive-pressure ventilation? A systematic review of the literature. Ann Intern Med 2003;138(11):861–70.

[42] Peter JV, Moran JL, Phillips-Hughes J, et al. Noninvasive ventilation in acute respiratory failure: a meta-analysis update. Crit Care Med 2002;30(3):555–62.

[43] Masip J, Roque M, Sánchez B, et al. Noninvasive ventilation in acute cardiogenic pulmonary edema: systematic review and meta-analysis. JAMA 2005;294(24):3124–30.

[44] Peter JV, Moran JL, Phillips-Hughes J, et al. Effect of non-invasive positive pressure ventilation (NIPPV) on mortality in patients with acute cardiogenic pulmonary oedema: a meta-analysis. Lancet 2006;367:1155–63.

[45] Mehta S, Jay GD, Woolard RH, et al. Randomized, prospective trial of bilevel versus continuous positive airway pressure in acute pulmonary edema. Crit Care Med 1997;25(4): 620–8.

[46] Keenan SP, Sinuff T, Cook DJ, et al. Does noninvasive positive pressure ventilation improve outcome in acute hypoxemic respiratory failure? A systematic review. Crit Care Med 2004; 32(12):2516–23.

[47] Lellouche F. Noninvasive ventilation in patients with hypoxemic acute respiratory failure. Curr Opin Crit Care 2007;13:12–9.

**ELSEVIER
SAUNDERS**

Med Clin N Am 92 (2008) 481–490

THE MEDICAL
CLINICS
OF NORTH AMERICA

Index

Note: Page numbers of article titles are in **boldface** type.